Body, Capital, and Screens

Body, Capital, and Screens

Visual Media and the Healthy Self in the 20th Century

Edited by
Christian Bonah
and Anja Laukötter

Routledge
Taylor & Francis Group
LONDON AND NEW YORK

This project has received funding from the European Research Council (ERC) under the European Union's Horizon 2020 research and innovation programme (grant agreement No. 694817).

First published in 2020 by Amsterdam University Press Ltd.

Published 2025 by Routledge
4 Park Square, Milton Park, Abingdon, Oxon OX14 4RN
605 Third Avenue, New York, NY 10158

Routledge is an imprint of the Taylor & Francis Group, an informa business

ISBN: 9789462988293 (hbk)
ISBN: 9781041176251 (pbk)
ISBN: 9781003691709 (ebk)
NUR 670

Cover illustration: Sascha Kürschner, 'FEELING REAL' from the series 'PURSUIT OF HAPPINESS'
Cover design: Coördesign, Leiden

DOI: 10.5117/9789462988293

Table of Contents

List of Figures

List of Tables

Acknowledgements

This book began life with the inaugural conference of the international research project 'The healthy self as body capital: Individuals, market-based societies, body politics and visual media in the twentieth century Europe', held in Strasbourg from 23 to 25 February 2017. The editors would like to thank all participants for their stimulating input during this outstanding event. The presentations and discussions influenced this book in many ways.

The research project and the book are funded by the European Research Council (ERC) under the European Union's Horizon 2020 research and innovation programme (grant agreement No. 694817) and receive significant support from the University of Strasbourg, the Research Unit SAGE (UMR 7363), and the Max Planck Institute for Human Development Berlin (Center for the History of Emotions). We owe gratitude to Tricia Close Koenig, Thérèse Vicente, Lionel Boutton, Fatima Gomis, and Assia Hammali for material support with our research and Elisabeth Fuchs for translation work and subtitling (all University of Strasbourg). We would also like to thank our editor at Amsterdam University Press, Maryse Elliott, for her support in the production of the book.

Moreover, we thank our contributors for their inspiring ideas and in-depth research. We would like to thank the artists VALIE EXPORT for her collaboration with one of the chapters and Sascha Kürschner for working with us on the book cover. We hope that his drawing 'FEELING REAL' from his series 'PURSUIT OF HAPPINESS' provides a fitting visual prelude to an interesting read.

Finally, the editors would like to thank Karola Rockmann (Max Planck Institute for Human Development, Center for the History of Emotions) for her tremendous editorial work on this book. We feel fortunate to have worked with such a capable, reliable, thorough, and ever-patient colleague!

Visual Media and the Healthy Self in the 20th Century: An Introduction

Christian Bonah and Anja Laukötter

Abstract

To introduce *Body, Capital, and Screens* as a series of in-depth case studies at the intersection of film and media studies and the social and cultural history of the body, we have chosen, as with all of the contributions, a film emblematic for the chapter's specific thematic focus: *Victoire de la vie/Victory of life* (FR, 1937) by Henri Cartier-Bresson. Through these images, we intend to detail our approach illustrating how the material and social aspects of moving images have served as a hyphen between body politics, on the one hand, and the market as the 20th century's primary form of social and economic organization, on the other. We lay out the framework for connecting bodies and capital with the significance of a century's worth of utility media culture.

Keywords: health, capital, Cartier-Bresson, *Victoire de la vie/Victory of life*, Spanish Civil War, children, documentary impulse, media, film

Body, Capital, and Screens: Visual Media and the Healthy Self in the 20th Century is about how the material and social aspects of moving images have served as a link between body politics, on the one hand, and the market as the 20th century's primary form of social and economic organization, on the other. The book is the product of work undertaken by the international research group 'The healthy self as body capital: Individuals, market-based societies, body politics and visual media in the twentieth century Europe'.[1]

1 This project has received funding from the European Research Council (ERC) under the European Union's Horizon 2020 research and innovation programme (grant agreement No. 694817), https://bodycapital.unistra.fr, accessed 19 September 2018.

Bonah, C. and A. Laukötter (eds.), *Body, Capital, and Screens: Visual Media and the Healthy Self in the 20th Century*. Taylor & Francis Group, 2020
DOI 10.5117/9789462988293_INTRO

The group's historiographical research, carried out with a cultural-studies bent, focusses on visual media (ranging from documentary and amateur film to television and the internet) and the body and their relation to a variety of health issues. In turn, the group seeks to connect this visual history of the body with economic history.[2]

We conceive visual media not merely as a mirror or expression of the things they depict, but as media and art endowed with their own distinct, interactive, performative power. Furthermore, we think that studying them is essential for a number of reasons: because their distribution has grown considerably over the past century; because they transcend spatial boundaries, whether they be those of nations, social groups, or professional associations; because their utilitarian character and their use as tools of promotion and communication links them to market-economic principles. Visual media are, for us, a vantage point. They have produced a form of knowledge and scientific objectivity with and without words,[3] transforming word-based health politics by channelling it into an increasing variety of visual communications media. This has ultimately proven essential for the enactment of beliefs about health and body practices in the communication societies of the 20th century.

Our approach is distinct from a history *of* bodies on screens (film history) and a body history *with* moving images (history of representations). Instead, our goal has been to write, through the cipher of visual sources, a history of the interaction between bodies and visual media, both on-screen and off-screen. By placing primacy on the 'through', our analysis positions moving images as our starting point. We treat moving images as a corpus of sources, analysing their language, context, and interdependencies with their contents. Finally, our approach takes visual media as a historical source that can complement—and sometimes serve as an alternative to—written sources. They can also serve as counter-archives to dominant state-organized visual sources,[4] recording what the Magnum Photo Agency characterized as the pulse of a time. In short, visual material might be seen as the 20th century's paramount archival source.[5]

The authors have chosen to work with the concept of 'body capital' in order to open space for a new perspective on economically grounded health practices that is founded in a rigorous, inductive analysis of visual

2 Berghoff and Vogel, *Wirtschaftsgeschichte als Kulturgeschichte*.

3 Daston and Galison, *Objectivity*.

4 Amad, *Counter-Archive*.

5 Mitman and Wilder, *Documenting the World*.

culture. Just as the engine was a key metaphor in depictions of the body in films and written sources from the first half of the 20th century,[6] the body conceived as capital became a leading visual and non-visual metaphor at its end. As a form of capital, the body has been treated as a means of production, a source of value to be protected, managed, and harvested, a source of value constantly at risk, a value that promises future returns. But our use of body capital is not metaphorical. It stems from the economic concept of capital and its use in sociological criticism. On the one hand, the concept confronts the reality of the prevalent use of 'human capital', defined as embedding resources in people.[7] On the other, it draws on Pierre Bourdieu's notions of cultural or social capital, which he developed to explain social inequalities and domination as consequences of economic capitalization.[8] As we will outline later, body capital provides a framework for studying the interdependencies between bodies, screens, and markets. This framework opens a new perspective on questions about the commodification of bodies and the marketization of health,[9] about the links between health and aesthetic appearance, and, most importantly, about the increasing imperative to measure and make measurable bodies and capital.[10]

As a heuristic concept, body capital should not be seen as another bead on the already long string of body-related capitals, such as health

6 Rabinbach, *Human Motor.*

7 Becker, 'Investment in Human Capital'.

8 Bourdieu and Passeron, *La reproduction*; Bourdieu, *Esquisse d'une théorie*; Bourdieu, 'Les trois états'; Bourdieu, 'Forms of Capital'.

9 Commodification is used here in a wide sense, beyond commodification of body parts in organ transplants; Scheper-Hughes and Wacquant, *Commodifying Bodies*. We are referring to processes of transforming health practices and behaviours into sanitary objects and goods. For example, for cleanliness, there is hypoallergenic soap; for tuberculosis prevention, there is proper nutrition, vitamin supplements, and Bacillus Calmette–Guérin (BCG) vaccines; for obesity, there are anti-obesity drugs, etc. Health products, of course, cover the most visible preventive and therapeutic agents/medicines—from vitamin D pills replacing exposure to sunlight, vitamin supplements complementing fresh fruit, or lifestyle drugs such as Viagra—but they also cover an increasingly diverse array of self-monitoring devices—from thermometers and scales to blood sugar or hypertension monitors, fitness watches, and sleep monitors—increasingly tracking and measuring our lives and quantifying ourselves. Greene et al., *Therapeutic Revolutions*.

10 Measurement and measurement devices are core values and tools in 20th-century economics and biomedicine, helping ensure that people make decisions in an allegedly rational manner. They deal with individuals as discrete units. They are localized and determined. They also have a temporal component where investments link the present to future outcomes. Capital is a bridge between now and the future. Grossman, 'On the Concept'.

capital,[11] emotional capital,[12] symbolic capital,[13] psychological capital,[14] mental capital,[15] or erotic capital.[16] The analytical concept of body capital, in contrast, combines the economic notion of a resource that enables the production of more resources with the sociological notion of symbolic capital that produces the social in terms of accumulation, objectivation, instrumentalization, and interiorization. Most important for our research is the analytical horizon opened by the concept of body capital, which enables us to trace the interconnections between visual media—long conceived of as indispensable tools for the 'invisible government'[17]—and the 'invisible hand' of the market. Many of the chapters in this book seek to detail this interconnection beyond the more self-evident relations between promotion, advertisement, and corporate public relations.[18]

Our work begins with images. Visual media provide not only the primary material of the book, but also give it its organizational principle. Each article begins with an analysis of a film, this introduction being no exception. Our choice for the introduction is photographer Henri Cartier-Bresson's film *Victoire de la vie* ('Victory of life', 1937).

The first images of the documentary sound film show children in the streets, a toddler, a woman walking by observing girls playing and jumping, and a group of older boys working, cleaning the street (Figure 0.1). The scene is Madrid: a long panning shot down a central street of the Spanish capital shows us crowded sidewalk markets and queues in front of shops. A voice from the off comments: 'Madrid continues to live under the spell of bombing.'[19] Cut. A soldier filmed from the back slowly patrolling the empty streets. A group of children on the ground in a circle. A passage between two defence walls with gun shafts. Off-voice: 'The war zone where no one lives.'[20] The camera then moves into a dark area beyond the walls, then a cut to scenes of destruction. Then there is a shot of a cameraman filming a soldier seated on a chair among the ruins. The streets are blocked off by barricades, with uneasy citizens moving haltingly through them.

11 Grossman, 'On the Concept'.
12 Thomson, *Emotional Capital.*
13 Brunnett, *Die Hegemonie symbolischer Gesundheit.*
14 Luthans et al., *Psychological Capital.*
15 Weehuizen, 'Mental Capital'.
16 Hakim, *Erotic Capital*; Neveu, 'Les sciences sociales'.
17 Bernays, *Propaganda*; Lippmann, *Public Opinion.*
18 Bonah, 'In the Service'.
19 'Madrid la martyre continue à vivre au son des canons'.
20 'La zone de guerre où personne ne vit'.

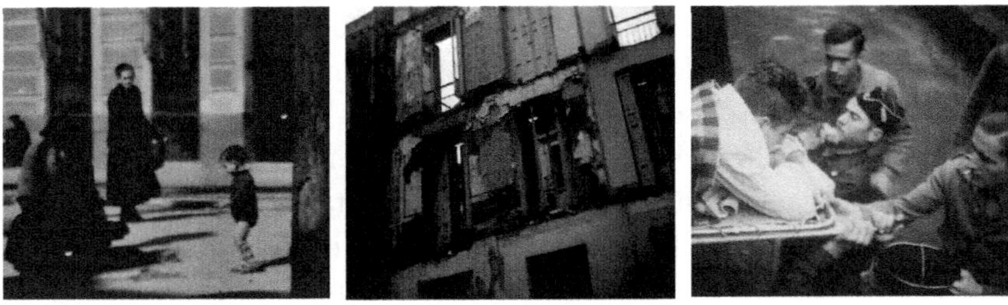

0.1. Three stills from *Victoire de la vie* ('Victory of life', 1937).

Wide-angle shots from below document the destruction of houses and churches, magnifying the devastation of living conditions. These images of a war zone are presented as the effects of military conflict. This thematic framework is not only established by images of children and the camera's focus on their bodies, but also by informative tables and animation that explain the situation. Images of sanatoria and dispensaries follow before we see factories manufacturing sanitary products. Cartier-Bresson then films the training of stretcher-bearers and shows the departure of soldiers and life on the front. The camera follows the movement of mobile hospitals. Images of care are underlined with shots of wounded, but nevertheless rescued soldiers. We see images of the hospitals like the Murcia, a military hospital in Barcelona, and images of the well-known Ritz Hotel, which was used as a hospital during the war. After showing their exterior, Cartier-Bresson then takes us inside to see how they care for their patients, the arrangement of the hospital, doctors performing surgery, and wounded people lying in wait. Various animations describe the Barcelona hospital's services before asking viewers for donations. This request is followed by images of amputees struggling to adapt to a life without legs. At the Spanish border Puigcerda, we see refugee children playing and dancing. At the convalescent centre in the city of Benicassim near Valencia, we see images of the wounded and their rehabilitation before we see how men leave for battle.

Victoire de la vie was created by the French photographer, artist, and director Henri Cartier-Bresson, who, in 1937, decided to travel with his camera team throughout Spain to shoot a documentary on the work being done by the American medical unit American Medical Bureau in the Spanish Civil War. He produced it for Frontier Films, an organization born out of Nykino, a militant cooperative of film-makers based in New York.[21] Debates within the 1930s

21 The film is credited to Henri Cartier. Cartier-Bresson's political communist engagement between 1936 and 1946 and his militant utility film-making with Ciné-Liberté after an experience as Renoir's assistant for the 1936 election communist campaigning film *La vie est à nous* was

French left on the 'new culture' provide context for Henri Cartier-Bresson's film, and can help us understand why militant organizations, political groups, and trade unions produced films like *Victoire de la vie* in the times of the Popular Front.[22] Jean-Richard Bloch, an influential representative of the 'new culture' movement, published several texts encouraging the left to integrate new media into their work in order to escape the constraints of traditional literary culture.[23] The awareness that radio, photography, and film were vital forms of expression and communication was quite widespread at that time. But, before 1935, leftist organizations did not have the means necessary to produce anything of real force. This situation changed in the spring of 1936, when a series of strikes triggered an influx of membership that brought new funds to parties and organizations. The union movement was so massive that, in the span of a month, the majority of film technicians had become union members, almost from zero. This allowed organizations sympathetic to the leftist cause to invest in production.[24] Many of the technologies and forms of moving images and the different types of screens analysed in this book correspond to Bloch's sense of novelty.[25] Mass communication, cutting-edge artistic forms, and technological novelty remained an enduring promise of moving images everywhere. In short, the moving images literally had, or were at least attributed with, the power to move things.

As a French Popular Front film, internationalist and pacifist in its message, *Victoire de la vie* was part of a broader movement of social documentation in film that included the Farm Administration films in the United States

concealed in order not to compromise his entry into the United States immediately after the Second World War. Assouline, *Henri Cartier-Bresson*.

22 Among the militant organizations, some of the most important include the films produced by the French Section of the Workers' International (SFIO), the General Confederation of Labour (CGT), and the French Communist Party (PCF) with Humanity. From May 1935 until early 1937, the SFIO was the most systematic producer of films under the impetus of Marceau Pivert, one of the few politicians really interested in cinema. The film service of the Socialist Federation of the Seine produced, in all, about fifteen pieces of 'proletarian counter-news'. Ory, *La Belle Illusion*.

23 Ory, *La Belle Illusion*.

24 The militant cinema of the Popular Front sought to associate films of a new spirit (social, union, popular) with a new style of producing. From this point of view, the Front's emblematic film remains Jean Renoir's *La Marseillaise*, an unfinished but remarkable 1937 attempt at a cooperative production financed by viewers.

25 Here, one can identify three kinds of modernity: 'modernism' as a supranational artistic filmic avant-garde; 'modernization', engaging bodily practices in connection with industrial production processes; and 'modernity' as a particular mode of historical life associated with patterns of consumption and advertising. The distinction is borrowed and adapted from: Elsaesser, 'Propagating Modernity', p. 236.

and the Empire Marketing Board films in the United Kingdom. These films mixed information and education with counterviews in order to unveil political manipulation and hegemonies, and, at the same time, to shape perceptions and orientate behaviours.

The film *Victoire de la vie* captures the book's thematic scope and form well. This volume focusses on visual media that informed and educated people about life and health and improving health practices, a strong example being Cartier-Bresson's documentary film. At the centre of our investigations are visual (mass) media, useful/utility film and *inédits* (amateur, family, and private visual media), and television. We are interested in forms of documentary depiction of bodily realities. Related visual materials, such as mainstream films or still images like posters or exhibitions, will only be considered insofar as they are immediately relevant to the production and reception of documentary film. Our central interest, in other words, is not the Hollywood/Pathé-style fictional portrayal of health, body, and illness.[26]

Carefully directed by Henri Cartier-Bresson, *Victoire de la vie* was produced to support Republican Spain and make known the activities of the Centrale Sanitaire Internationale in order to obtain moral and financial support. To this end, he shows the health efforts and mobilization of Republican Spain, on the front lines and behind the scenes, and the medical solidarity of foreign countries coordinated by the International Health Centre (CSI). Films like *Victoire de la vie* that document the world and at the same time try to change it were produced in abundance during the 20th century. Studying their visual characteristics lies at the heart of this book. The scope of the book, however, sweeps wider. The authors seek to demonstrate that visual media played a constitutive role in the cultural history of the body in the 20th century and to detail some of the ways in which mass media have helped shape and influence our bodily conditions and our self-awareness or understanding of them.

Body Capital

The core idea of the book is, to a great extent, inspired by Pierre Bourdieu's influential sociological work *Distinction: A Social Critique of the Judgement of Taste*.[27] Bourdieu identifies economic, social, and cultural capital as forces

26 Harper and Moor, *Signs of Life*; Reagan et al., *Medicine's Moving Pictures*; Friedman, *Cultural Sutures*.

27 Bourdieu, *La distinction*; Bourdieu, *Esquisse d'une théorie*; Bourdieu and Passeron, *La reproduction*; Bourdieu, 'Forms of Capital'.

in order to describe individuals' positions in (French) societies. Going one step further, we argue that understanding the increasingly marketized world of the 20th century demands supplementing this tripartite conception of capital with a fourth term. The concept of body capital introduced in this book is founded on the conviction that the (healthy) body has evolved into a new (fourth) currency. Succinctly put, it denotes an individual resource that can be nurtured and then mobilized, invested in and employed for future returns.

There are at least two compelling reasons for conceiving of the body as a new 'capital form'. One is that the concept of body capital allows us to stress the economic aspects of individual health in the 20th century. In the nineteenth and in beginning of the 20th century, state-run health programmes were primarily concerned with the useful and functioning body understood as a collective body. Over the run of the century, however, this focus shifted to place more emphasis on individual health and the promotion of practices of self-optimization. Supported by new health products in caring for themselves, individuals are able to bargain with their body capital in different social spheres. Perhaps more importantly, however, individuals have internalized health practices to such an extent that they create new subjectivities. An example of the significance of health in job markets in Western countries like Germany and France is that discrimination for being overweight can sometimes be just as strong as racial discrimination. The fit and slim body is recognized as an expression of self-discipline and high potential, while the overweight body is regarded as a marker of negatively connoted loss of control.[28] Thus, one could argue that it is not an option or a freedom to live a healthy life, but an imperative. The self-optimized individual, as Michel Foucault has described it, has become a key political tool of the liberal or capitalist system.[29] Over the last decade, the burgeoning field of the history of capital and capitalism has produced several path-breaking works on the processes, mechanisms, and effects of capitalism (including in health systems) on a micro and macro level in Western societies.[30] Yet, beyond a few select works, the role of visual media has largely been neglected in the extant literature.[31] It seems that visual media are primarily viewed as part of the cultural sphere, disconnected from issues of economics. This book

28 Jay Rowell, comment on the workshop *Capital and Capitalism* in Strasbourg 2017.

29 Foucault, *Le gouvernement de soi.*

30 See, for example, Illouz, *Cold Intimacies*; Budde, *Kapitalismus*; Kocka and Linden, *Capitalism*; Bänziger and Suter, *Histories of Productivity*; Donauer, 'Emotions at Work'; Ebbinghaus and Manow, *Comparing Welfare Capitalism*; Lengwiler and Madarász, *Das präventive Selbst.*

31 Berridge and Loughlin, *Medicine.*

cannot fill the gap with one fell stroke, but it might accomplish the more modest goal of encouraging further research in this direction. The concept of body capital was coined to bridge these spheres and to help analyse their interconnections and even interdependencies. Thus, the book aims to understand better the role that modern visual mass media have played in the shift in health paradigms over the span of two centuries. Dominant at the beginning of the 20th century was a national, biopolitical public-health paradigm characterized by collective bodies, workforce, and labour society. By the late 20th century, the paradigm shifted, as market forces and market fundamentalism increasingly came to determine the norms of what constitutes a better, healthier individual life. Visual media, as the book tries to show, not only reflect this historical process and development, but have, to a large extent, shaped it. In the 1990s, scholars like Lisa Cartwright undertook important theoretical reflections on film in the sciences, work that has recently been given a new life by scholars like Oliver Gaycken and Scott Curtis.[32] Still, theoretical work on the documentary depictions of body realities remains rare.[33] Our book addresses this research gap.

Second, the concept of body capital allows us to stress the high value attributed to the body in the 20th century. This is not to say that Pierre Bourdieu leaves out the body in his analysis of capital or in his overall theory. To the contrary, his key concepts all have a strong corporeal dimension, whether it be 'habitus' as a product and producer of practices, 'hexis' as a system of attitudes and movements, or, especially, the concept of 'incorporation' as the assimilation of structures and practices.[34] Without specifically focussing on the body, these theoretical frameworks clearly underline that the individual body is defined by economic, social, and cultural capital. These forms of capital motivate us to create knowledge on how to dress, move, and eat in different social settings. Perhaps more importantly, it is through them that our bodies are both defined and can redefine social structures and classes.

So, what does body capital do for us? As Christiane Reinecke has rightly argued, Bourdieu's theoretical framework and his empirical research for *Distinction* have to be understood in the context of French society in the 1960s. To a certain degree, Bourdieu misses the gradual dissolution of class structures, the processes of individualization and globalization, and the relevance of gender, race, sexuality, and age in the 20th century.[35] We would

32 Cartwright, *Screening the Body.*

33 Gaycken, *Devices of Curiosity*; Curtis, *Shape of Spectatorship.*

34 See Bourdieu, 'Zur Genese'; Bourdieu and Wacquant, *Réponses*; Fröhlich, 'Habitus und Hexis'.

35 Reinecke, 'Der (damalige) Geschmack'.

add the analytical category of the body to Reinecke's list. Even though Bourdieu had a clear notion of the relevance of the body, he generally placed it in the background. To bring the body out of the shadows and underline its increasing importance in the long run of the 20th century, we single it out and work with the concept of body capital.

The transformation of the body into a form of capital, at least on a conceptual level, has a strongly corporeal dimension.[36] It brings in and combines, as Andreas Reckwitz has put it, the 'cultural and the material, the symbolic and the objective'.[37] Moreover, the focus on the body makes it possible to consider affects and emotions, two phenomena largely neglected by Bourdieu.[38] As historian and anthropologist Monique Scheer—who draws on Bourdieu's concept of 'habitus'—has argued, the body has a strong historical dimension and is linked to embodied emotion practices.[39] Important for our work are the social and communicative aspects of emotions, which play a crucial role in the persuasiveness of media productions.[40] In this sense, the book aims to highlight theoretically and empirically the interactive force and performative power of films on subjects in the modern world: how these films worked to influence behaviours and attitudes towards one's own health and one's body, and how health became a form of investment for the future, one of the meanings of capital.

This is also the way we analyse *Victoire de la vie*. The film opens with a three- or four-year-old boy entering the frame from the right. The camera follows his movement in a panoramic shot, he looks briefly into the camera, and the boy then hesitantly turns to a sand pile in the grey street. At the same time, a woman enters the frame from the opposite side, observes him briefly, and passes by. A girl plays on the dirty sidewalk with a bucket. A group of children plays a jumping game on the sidewalk. In March 1937, Cartier-Bresson had shot a series of 31 photographs for the communist newspaper *Ce Soir*; this series was published on the front page. Produced in the context of a photo contest, the photo series 'The Lost Child' portrays children's misery. Henri Cartier-Bresson presents the children as in need: They are depicted playing simple games on the streets, chatting, dancing outside, and generally enjoying themselves as 'normal' children without paying attention to their desperate surroundings. These children are

36 Shilling, *Body and Social Theory*.

37 Reckwitz, 'Practices and their Affects', p. 115; Reckwitz, 'Habitus oder Subjektivierung?', p. 59.

38 Reckwitz, 'Practices and their Affects', p. 116.

39 Scheer, 'Are Emotions'. See also Eitler and Scheer, 'Emotionengeschichte als Körpergeschichte'.

40 Laukötter, 'Politik im Kino'.

representations of innocence. They are supported, helped, and educated by adults who clearly underline how happy they are to care for the children and enable them to live healthy lives. In that sense, these children are not only innocent but also the representation of the future of Spain. In reference to the film title, the children are the victory of life, icons and incarnations of what the bombs and the enemy has not—cannot—destroy. Against the backdrop of war and misery and severely wounded soldiers, these innocent children, with their healthy bodies, are the capital of a nearby and hopefully better and more secure future.

Both produced in and derived from visual media, body capital is a distinctive power and an economic currency. This provides the framework for the case studies in this volume. The case studies analyse the various interests, motivations, and practices of a range of various global, national, and local health institutions, different industries (media industries, pharmaceutical industries, health supplies industries, etc.), sciences (medicine, psychology, etc.), classes, specific interest groups (like self-help and activist groups), and, last but not least, visual media commissioned by both the state and private corporations.

Perspectives on Time and Spaces (and Their Hierarchies)

Much of what non-fiction television and other visual media produced in the 20th century was influenced by what Gregg Mitman has described as the century's 'documentary impulse', which was informed by the belief in the capacity of photographs and films to 'visually capture the world, order it, and render it useful for future generations'.[41] As we are concerned with the long-term efficacy of the production of images over the past century, our book explores utility and educational films,[42] television,[43] and amateur film/video.[44]

41 Mitman and Wilder, 'Introduction', p. 1.

42 Ostherr, *Medical Visions*; Acland and Wasson, *Useful Cinema*; Orgeron et al., *Learning*; Bonah et al., *Health Education Films*; Zimmermann, *Geschichte*; Hediger and Vonderau, *Films that Work*; Hediger et al., *Films That Work Harder*; Zimmermann, *Schaufenster Schweiz*.

43 Boon, 'Medical Films and Television'; Boon, *Films of Fact*; Bourdon, *Histoire de la télévision*; Delavaud and Maréchal, *Télévision*; Lafon, *Histoire de la télévision régionale*; Lévy, *Regards de la télévision française*; Poels, *Les trente glorieuses*; Sauvage and Veyrat-Masson, *Histoire de la télévision française*; Powell and Shandley, *German Television*; Gumbert, *Envisioning Socialism*; Soulages, *Les rhétoriques télévisuelles*.

44 Mattl et al., *Abenteuer Alltag*; Forster, 'Mitten hinein'; Odin, *Le film de famille*; Zimmermann, *Reel Families*.

Spanning three major media ages (film, TV, internet), we seek not to disregard their differences, but instead to focus on long-enduring structural elements. In this sense, our project might be seen as a *longue durée* contextualized media archaeology. Yet, while taking these differences and the historical development of each media into account, the book argues that there are also a variety of overlaps and mutual influences between these distinct media forms that pertain to their themes, formats, aesthetics, etc.[45]

Our comprehensive approach, which is anchored in our research on documentary films, is not an end in itself. On the contrary, including all different media seems necessary for developing an accurate understanding of how moving images displayed, impacted, transformed, produced, and represented bodies in the 20th century. Only by analysing and comparing various media formats is it possible to gain a well-rounded perspective on how the body became a medium and a site of embodied 'capital'. Studying issues of health in visual media over a longer time period, we intend to trace the above-mentioned shift in health policy and campaigns from the early 20th century to the present. While the former was dominated by a paternalistic state, with religious, political, or professional prescriptions mapping out 'ways to strength and beauty' (according to the UFA film, *Wege zu Kraft und Schönheit* 1924/1925), the latter moved towards a mode of governing bodies wholly justified on economic grounds, which, at least in theory, has, as its highest aim, the expansion of individual consumer choice. A *longue durée* approach on the visual material studied seems especially necessary if we take the massive changes in health systems and understandings of health and diseases throughout the 20th century into account.

The changes were immense: at the beginning of the century stood the invention of public health, the rapid emergence and diffusion of mechanically produced images and moving pictures, and a revolution in liberal economic theory and practice. By the end of the century, there was the reinvention of *new* public health, the internet revolution, and the economic crisis that gave birth to economic neoliberalism in the 1990s and 2000s. In the middle of this period, and central to our book, lie the industry-based therapeutic revolution and medicalization of society, the invention of television, the epidemiological transition (increased life expectancy and the emergence of chronic disease), and the golden age of the welfare state. All of this exerted a decisive and lasting influence on body practices and perceptions.

We start our book with the film *Victoire de la vie*. It is a militant film produced in the heyday of state propaganda before the Second World War

45 Hagener et al., *State of Post-Cinema*; Strauven, *Cinema of Attractions Reloaded*.

by a leading photojournalist and founder of the Magnum Photo cooperative picture agency. Thereby, and more generally throughout this book, we aim to dislocate and reframe classical boundaries of media studies—photography, film, TV, and internet—and of established historic periods—First World War, interwar period, Second World War, Cold War, etc. In doing so, we seek to uncover continuities in audiovisual and mass-media culture where classical historical accounts and disciplinary boundaries frequently suggest breaking points.

In this sense, Cartier-Bresson's *Victoire de la vie* exemplifies what is at stake. The first half of the century was dominated by the world wars. Accordingly, much of the political, economic, and social activity of this period was determined by military conflict, its causes, and its consequences. As *Victoire de la vie* shows, this can neither be restricted to the two world wars, nor to individual belligerent countries. What is evident from film archives is that military conflicts and preparation for them were forceful catalysts for audiovisual production and mobilization.

Visual media shaped the 20th century in significant ways. Interestingly, although many films—a point particularly pertinent as concerns their relationship to the body—were produced for specific spaces, they often ended up being received outside of these spaces. The term 'space' has a variety of meanings. One might think of professional spaces (as, for example, the laboratory, the clinic, industry, the pharmaceutical industries), social spaces (like schools, homes, activist groups, etc.), and even national and global spaces. Moreover, screening spaces vary, from large screens in cinemas, clubs, or civic spaces, whether they be indoors or outdoors; small screens in homes, schools, or public television sets; and other screens like computers, smartphones, and similar devices. The accessibility of these various types of screens is part of the production and reproduction of social hierarchies. Not all of these spaces and screens can be addressed in this book, but we have nevertheless sought to discuss a variety.

In her chapter on United Nations Educational, Scientific and Cultural Organization (UNESCO)-sponsored films in the 1940s and early 1950s, **Zoë Druick** elucidates how the spirit of transcending national boundaries has historically guided international approaches to film production. Envisioned to have a global reach, these films tried to educate people about peace, freedom, and cosmopolitan world citizenship. This chapter argues that these goals did, by no means, escape reinforcing hierarchies and making normative judgements: in combining reportage, documentary, and moral injunction, these films undermined not only the biopolitical orientation of the United Nations (UN), but also its supremacy in the Western world.

Moreover, she argues that, even though UNESCO's universalism aimed to debunk 'race' as a category in their official statements, it was perpetuated in their media text and production.

The decentring of the Western perspective is taken further in **Jean-Paul Gaudillière**'s contribution. Entering the debate on the production and reproduction of political and social hierarchies in visual media, his chapter analyses aspects of the north-south divide in film. It offers an account of discourses on body government, drawing on recent subaltern and world historiography of health outside Europe. Gaudillière's study begins by critiquing several films about the Global South that were produced by Western institutions and thus reproduce their viewpoints and biases. After pointing out these films' problematic aspects, Gaudillière proceeds to make a plea that scholars consider alternative visual records that originated in the Global South and argues for the need to provincialize Europe and North America. In this sense, the chapter poses a challenge both to Gaudillière's own selection of films as well as to the book as a whole, as the majority of films studied in this collection come from the West (Germany/GDR, Great Britain, France, United States).

But hierarchies with a highly normative dimension were propagated not only through transnational visual media productions, but also within national borders, as **Olaf Stieglitz** clearly shows. In his chapter on the expanding markets for participatory sports in the United States between the 1890s and the 1930s, he analyses how visual media like film and photography were integrated into the creation of normatively idealized bodies. The images of swimming helped introduce a scientific understanding of bodies and their motions to a broader audience. Moreover, these swimming bodies served as sites where the body as a modern, ubiquitous, and attractive, sexualized, marketable commodity was negotiated. Moreover, Stieglitz shows how these visual media addressed issues of gender, race, ethnicity, and age.

The next two chapters highlight voices of dissent. **Christian Bonah**'s chapter on sex education in French National Television around 1968 begins with an account of how mainstream television (after having become a mass media in France) and various prominent people believed that the 'invasion' of erotic depictions of the female body was a visual translation of the so-called sexual revolution.[46] Bonah shows that, while state-produced films and TV broadcasts can serve historians as a primary source, they should not be seen as the final statement on particular historical phenomena. Other

46 *L'invasion de la sexualité dans la vie quotidienne*, ORTF, 25 January 1971, 01:02:07, INA MediaPro database identification number CAF93024168.

audiovisual sources can be used as counter-archives to explore different framings of the same phenomena and the different aspects of history that they reveal.[47] From school television and pioneering experimental forms of participative television production to militant video productions, the counter-archives provide examples of marginal or subversive approaches, both in terms of the stakeholders involved and the content they showed. These subaltern sources reveal a series of attempts to put on film ordinary talk about sexuality, which were influenced by new developments in camera technology and the technique of direct cinema.

Sophie Delpeux's contribution analyses how Austrian artist VALIE EXPORT's video and body art of the late 1960s destabilized bourgeois understandings of the body and capitalist appropriations of art and media. This study on the artist's pastiches made of advertisements reveals a biting criticism of a male-engineered and male-dominated social reality. In this criticism, EXPORT makes clear that body capital is constructed by the male gaze. In contemporary art as a market, the value resides with what the artist embodies more so than what they produce or do. What EXPORT creates is a reverse form of body capital, where the artist's body as capital becomes a critique of economic capital and capitalization. Delpeux elucidates well Baudrillard's claim that the 'emancipation of woman and the emancipation of the body are logically and historically linked', at least in the Western traditions and hierarchies.[48]

Screens and Markets/Capital

Victoire de la vie is a typical non-fiction film, one of thousands produced in Europe and North America between the First and Second World Wars that straddle the line between documentary and propaganda and were produced to promote, educate, or agitate around a particular issue.[49] As engaged films with a message, these visual media intend to make the viewer realize or do things. They are performative in intent. This is one of our major concerns, hypotheses, and claims: Beyond their capacity to represent, films intervene, influence, co-produce, and may even condition the content that they document. We argue that moving images throughout the 20th century have participated in shaping the way we live and the world we live in. We

47 Amad, *Counter-Archive*.

48 Baudrillard, *Consumer Society*, p. 137.

49 Elsaesser, 'Propagating Modernity', p. 234.

consider them as an active force, not only as something that reveals or portrays. The question is then: What do these films do to make people do things (or fail to make them do)?

Cartier-Bresson's film is concerned with mobilizing international solidarity and funds for a cause. It demonstrates more generally that screens can serve as stages for public agendas, going beyond being mere surfaces of projection. Films that seek to promote a humanitarian mission or political solidarity, however, were not only a phenomenon of the social and political conflicts of the 1930s. They have a long history that includes the early volunteer society films of the 1920s and, after the Second World War, films produced by the American Cancer Society, the Association Française contre les Myopathies, and similar patient associations/charity organizations in the Western world.[50]

Beginning in the 1960s, television brought forth the telethon, a form of fundraising entertainment geared towards mobilizing audience compassion. One such example is addressed in more detail in the chapter by **Karen Lury** on the BBC's *Children in Need* telethon, a television broadcast that has been running for over 35 years. Lury's analysis connects how televisual grammar conceived as currency aligns with currency models within the economy of the National Health Service (NHS).

Viewed as a 'proletarian counter newsreel', *Victoire de la vie* needs to be read in connection with 1930s propaganda documentaries' practical aspects of informing, instructing, and indoctrinating. From the marching military music that introduces the first (dissonant) images of children playing, to the long sequences of the care of wounded soldiers reminiscent of post-First World War cripple films, Cartier-Bresson subverts these images to project his plea for international solidarity. In this sense, he aims at a 'visual (counter) construction of the social'.[51] But does this function in the way the director (or the group that commissioned the film) intended? And, if so, how? We have little information about where and how *Victoire de la vie* was screened and if it actually mobilized people as hoped. Questions about reception are essential and they surface early on in the history of utility films, as Anja Laukötter has shown elsewhere.[52] These questions are as important for producers as they are for historians, helping us not to misperceive the significance of a film or simply equate aesthetic quality with reception performance. Since early studies on the reception of health films conducted

50 Rabeharisoa and Callon, *Le pouvoir des malades*.

51 Mitchell, *What Do Pictures Want?*; Mitchell, 'What Do Pictures Really Want?'; Mitchell, *Picture Theory*.

52 Laukötter, 'Measuring Knowledge and Emotions'; Laukötter, 'Politik im Kino'.

in the 1920s, however, the issue of evaluating and measuring the performance and effectiveness of films has posed considerable difficulties.[53]

Luc Berlivet addresses this issue in his analysis of anti-alcohol health campaigns in France in the 1980s, which were part of new public-health strategies directly linked to booming advertisement agencies and practices. In the golden years of evidence-based medicine, health advertisements were informed by policy studies and field experiments in social psychology. In the same period, audience studies became an integral part of television programming, and, in telling fashion, telethons integrated a form of efficiency measure into their very format. At the centre of the set and programme was, and still is, the donation counter that tallies up the money raised, as Karen Lury's article on telethons analyses. Screen efficacy was simply translated into money. Measurement was immediate and integrated into the show, thus illustrating how the measurement directly influenced that which was being measured. At the same time, producers planned 'money shots', a term used to describe visual sequences they knew would trigger donations.

War is present throughout *Victoire de la vie*. It is not illustrated by explicit images of combat or bombardments, but rather through implicit images of destroyed churches and religious objects. War is mainly observed from latent scenes, not through war scenes, but in the documentation of destruction as a consequence of belligerence. Nevertheless, the film does take a political position. In order to remind the viewer of how the 'Army of Africa' and Nazi Germany supported Franco's troops, the director uses a simple shot filmed inside a fortified shelter taken over by the Republicans: One sees a swastika and the badge of the 'Army of Africa'. Moreover, Cartier-Bresson's depiction of Spanish men also has political implications: Shots show a soldier learning to read, wounded patients playing chess, a sequence taking place in the countryside where farmers give half of their harvest to the army (some of them even make a fist as a symbol supporting the army's efforts). Furthermore, in the film's last sequence, the militiamen leave for the front again by truck and on foot while this statement appears in superimposition: 'With such men Spain cannot die. The ideal for which they gave their blood is an ideal of peace. So the kids can grow up happy. For tomorrow's beautiful harvest. Spain with a big heart must live. Spain will live.'[54] This

53 See Laukötter, 'Measuring Knowledge and Emotions'. See also Laukötter, 'How Films Entered the Classroom'; Laukötter', 'Politik im Kino'.

54 'Avec de tels hommes. L'Espagne ne peut pas mourir. L'idéal pour lequel ils ont prodigué leur sang est un idéal de PAIX. Pour que leurs enfants grandissent dans la joie. Pour les belles moissons de demain. L'Espagne au grand coeur doit vivre. L'Espagne vivra.'

astonishing comment on Spain and its big heart anchors Cartier-Bresson's film in the territory of emotions. The narrator of *Victoire de la vie* aims to create solidarity in addressing the nation's 'big heart' and in linking it to the happiness of the children screened.

A similar linkage is addressed in **Anja Laukötter**'s chapter on the relevance of emotions in the creation of new subjectivities in films for East German youth from the 1960s. Analysing narrative strategies and film techniques, the chapter illustrates how these films encourage young people to navigate puberty by managing their emotions in the right way, all with the aim of defining individuals' position in a socialist society. In drawing on scientific knowledge, these films take on a performative role in mimicking the film's emotional suggestions to reach the ultimate aim of producing young socialist subjects.

In both cases, one might argue, using children as objects of concern functions to symbolize authenticity in these films and, at the same time, creates a perspective on a future with a new and better society. The use and sometimes abuse of child subjects in agitation and documentary films to appeal to the audience emotionally is widespread, from interwar social hygiene films,[55] to the series of six films the Nazis created to promote the sterilization of the mentally ill[56] in 1930s Germany, to British municipal films,[57] to regular appearances of children in telethons and similar broadcasts.

It is not necessarily the depicted child, but also the conveyed childhood experience that produces audience identification and emotionally captures the spectator. **David Cantor**'s chapter addresses this issue in its analysis of the nearsighted Mr. Magoo, one of the most popular animated figures in the American cinema of the 1950s. Cantor discusses Magoo's resurrection in advertisement in the early 1960s in order to show how Magoo's fading television career turned him into a market asset that enabled a new film producer to use him to a different end. When Magoo went commercial, health was coupled with other consumption goods that Magoo came to represent. In his health advertisement career, Magoo's 'inverse' body capital—namely, his visual handicap—was made into a comic resource intended to charm spectators into accepting difficult health information. The strategy of convincing people through laughter, light-heartedness, and comic slapstick is based on a protagonist behaving in a childlike manner.

55 Vignaux, *Jean Benoît-Lévy*; Bonah and Laukötter, 'Moving Pictures'; and Bonah and Laukötter, 'Introduction'.

56 Bonah and Lowy, 'La propagande sanitaire'.

57 Lebas, *Forgotten Futures*.

Playing with emotions to make people do things, trust in something, or overcome (childish) fear points to affinities between childhood and documentary film, where children not only symbolize innocence and hope in the future, but also lend the film authenticity. Cinematic realism depicted the sincere experience of childhood in order to spread messages about eminently political issues and ideas.

Techniques intended to suggest authenticity and reality are central to documentary visual media, which defines itself as something that informs, educates, and entertains; for example, the British Broadcasting Corporation (BBC) and the Office de radiodiffusion television française (ORTF). In his chapter, **Timothy M. Boon** discusses live, on-location television broadcasts from the 1950s, specifically in medical contexts. A new form of media that purported to give viewers a look at unmediated reality, Boon analyses how the camera and broadcast techniques used forced doctors and patients to 'play themselves', since, after all, cameras had to be set up and could not be hardwired into the doctors' eyes, cuts had to be made, etc. He details the grammars of authenticity that gave live, on-location TV the veneer of taking place in the here and now. Among the audiovisual techniques that sought to lend authenticity to film was the inclusion of children. After all, children do not play themselves, they simply play, whether they are in front of a camera or not. Boon analyses the live medical television show *Your Life in Their Hands* to reveal a different technique. The show purported to offer insight into issues concerning professional confidentiality and the sacredness of the doctor-patient relationship, all the while increasing its entertainment appeal by allowing people the illusion of watching something that was truly taking place combined with the thrill of peeping into events of a confidential, intimate nature. At the same time, live broadcasts outside ultimately constructed what was perceived as the individual's reality. 'Outside' meant filming at the real location; 'live' implied that television was broadcasting as things were happening. However, what was being *done* was *enacted*, since agents had to wait for the cameras and their teams to be ready. Thus, cameras did not just simply record what viewers ultimately came to perceive as live and on-site.

In comparing a World Health Organization (WHO) film on infectious diseases from 1948 with contemporary WHO videos and conspiracy videos on the Zika virus from social media, **Kirsten Ostherr** researches the challenges posed by the multiplication of different visual media, the rapid speed that has closed the gap between the moment of broadcast and the circulation of images, the practices of private archiving that elide established archival practices, and the issues involved when visual communication on social networks precedes state public-health intervention. While, in 1948, WHO films were produced in a top-down fashion, the analysis of social media from the early 2000s and their more horizontal structure indicates an erosion of the control and power of key national and international organizations. Taking a different approach to that of Zoë Druick and Jean-Paul Gaudillière, Ostherr deploys a global perspective and addresses new questions on new hierarchies and authority of knowledge, the social implications of access and use of information, and its datafication.

Organization of the Book

Body, Capital, and Screens: Visual Media and the Healthy Self in the 20th Century is a series of in-depth case studies at the intersection of film and media studies and the social and cultural history of the body. It investigates relationships between film, television, private and public actors of the health sector, and economic development. Our book brings together new research from Europe and North America. Our outlook is international, covering France, Britain, Germany and the German Democratic Republic (GDR), the United States, and global institutions. It discusses key actors and the moving images that depict them in the mass-media society of the 20th century and its neoliberal market features.

In order to underscore the central status of films, each chapter of this book starts and closes with a vignette from a film emblematic of the chapter's specific thematic focus. The chapters are not limited to one film, but instead use the selected film to develop an argument on the specific aspect of body capital explored in depth throughout the chapter using other visual material.

We sought to include chapters that interact with one another and have tried to indicate here some of their interconnections. We hope that the reader identifies more overlaps and communication between the articles while reading.

In a sense, our approach adheres to the most accepted in visual culture studies, analysing the social construction of the visible and the visible construction of the social. The new element in our work is the connection we establish with bodies and capital and the significance we attribute to visual media in this relationship, a significance that has held for a century's worth of utility media culture. Accordingly, we have arranged the chapters in line with three different aspects of body capital: grammars of film/television and body capital, which stresses structural elements and different approaches to analysing these media; interiorized body capital, which relates to different bodily dimensions of capital, embodiment, and their normative implications; and hegemonies of body capital, which analyses the social construction of bodies and hierarchies. The book desires to provoke further discussions and explorations with the reader about the role of body capital in our visual world.

Works Cited

Films, Television Programmes, and Recordings

Children in Need, BBC, 1980–.

La Marseillaise, directed by Jean Renoir, Popular Front, 1937 (unfinished).

Victoire de la vie, directed by Henri Cartier-Bresson, Frontier Films for the Centrale Sanitaire Internationale, 1937.

Wege zu Kraft und Schönheit, directed by Wilhelm Prager, UFA, 1924/1925.

Your Life in Their Hands, BBC, 1958–1964, 1980–1986.

Books and Articles

Acland, Charles R., and Haidee Wasson, eds., *Useful Cinema* (Durham, NC: Duke University Press, 2011).

Amad, Paula, *Counter-Archive: Film, the Everyday, and Albert Kahn's Archives de la Planète* (New York: Columbia University Press, 2010).

Assouline, Pierre, *Henri Cartier-Bresson: L'œil du siècle* (Paris: Gallimard, 2001).

Bänziger, Peter-Paul, and Mischa Suter, eds., *Histories of Productivity: Genealogical Perspectives on the Body and Modern Economy* (New York: Routledge, 2017).

Baudrillard, Jean, *The Consumer Society: Myths and Structures* (London: Sage, 1998).

Becker, Gary S., 'Investment in Human Capital: A Theoretical Analysis', *Journal of Political Economy*, 70, 5.2 (1962), pp. 9–49, https://www.jstor.org/stable/1829103.

Berghoff, Hartmut, and Jakob Vogel, eds., *Wirtschaftsgeschichte als Kulturgeschichte: Dimensionen eines Perspektivenwechsels* (Frankfurt am Main: Campus, 2004).

Bernays, Edward L., *Propaganda* (New York: Horace Liveright, 1928).

Berridge, Virgina, and Kelly Loughlin, *Medicine, the Market and the Mass Media: Producing Health in the Twentieth Century* (London: Routledge, 2005).

Bonah, Christian, 'In the Service of Industry and Human Health: The Bayer Corporation, Industrial Film, and Promotional Propaganda, 1934–42', in *Health Education Films in the Twentieth Century*, ed. by Christian Bonah, David Cantor, and Anja Laukötter (Rochester: University of Rochester Press, 2018), pp. 85–142.

Bonah, Christian, David Cantor, and Anja Laukötter, eds., *Health Education Films in the Twentieth Century* (Rochester: University of Rochester Press, 2018).

Bonah, Christian, and Anja Laukötter, 'Moving Pictures and Medicine in the First Half of the 20th Century: Some Notes on International Historical Developments and the Potential of Medical Film Research', *Gesnerus*, 66, 1 (2009), pp. 121–146.

Bonah, Christian, and Anja Laukötter, 'Introduction: Screening Diseases: Films on Sex Hygiene in Germany and France in the First Half of the 20th Century', *Gesnerus*, 72, 1 (2015), pp. 5–14.

Bonah, Christian, and Vincent Lowy, 'La propagande sanitaire par le film documentaire en France et en Allemagne: Réflexions à partir de deux exemples du milieu des années 1930: L'œuvre Grancher et Erbkrank', in *Nazisme, science et médecine*, ed. by Christian Bonah, Anne Danion-Grilliat, Josiane Olff-Nathan, and Norbert Schappacher (Paris: Glyphe, 2006), pp. 167–192.

Boon, Timothy, *Films of Fact: A History of Science in Documentary Films and Television* (London: Wallflower, 2008).

Boon, Timothy, 'Medical Films and Television: Alternative Paths to the Cultures of Biomedicine', in *The Oxford Handbook of the History of Medicine*, ed. by Mark Jackson (Oxford: Oxford University Press, 2011), pp. 617–633.

Bourdieu, Pierre, *Esquisse d'une théorie de la pratique: Précédé de trois études d'ethnologie kabyle* (Geneva: Droz, 1972) [English translation: *Outline of a Theory of Practice*, trans. by Richard Nice (Cambridge: Cambridge University Press, 1977)].

Bourdieu, Pierre, *La distinction: Critique sociale du jugement* (Paris: Éditions de Minuit, 1979) [English translation: *Distinction: A Social Critique of the Judgment of Taste*, trans. by Richard Nice (Cambridge, MA: Harvard University Press, 1984).

Bourdieu, Pierre, 'The Forms of Capital', in *Handbook of Theory and Research for the Sociology of Education*, ed. by John G. Richardson (New York: Greenwood, 1986), pp. 46–58.

Bourdieu, Pierre, 'Les trois états du capital culturel', *Actes de la recherche en sciences sociales*, 30 (November 1979), pp. 3–6, doi:10.3406/arss.1979.2654.

Bourdieu, Pierre, 'Zur Genese der Begriffe Habitus und Feld', in *Schriften zu Politik und Kultur, vol. 2: Der Tote packt den Lebenden*, ed. by Margareta Steinrücke, trans. by Jürgen Bolder (Hamburg: VSA-Verlag, 1997), pp. 59–78.

Bourdieu, Pierre, and Jean-Claude Passeron, *La reproduction: Éléments d'une théorie du système d'enseignement* (Paris: Éditions de Minuit, 1970) [English translation: *Reproduction in Education, Society and Culture*, trans. by Richard Nice (London: Sage, 1977)].

Bourdieu, Pierre, and Loïc J. D. Wacquant, *Réponses: Pour une anthropologie réflexive* (Paris: Seuil, 1992).

Bourdon, Jérôme, *Histoire de la télévision sous de Gaulle*, new ed. (Paris: Presses des MinesParistech, 2014).

Brunnett, Regina, *Die Hegemonie symbolischer Gesundheit: Eine Studie zum Mehrwert von Gesundheit im Postfordismus* (Bielefeld: transcript, 2009).

Budde, Gunilla, ed., *Kapitalismus: Historische Annäherungen* (Göttingen: Vandenhoeck & Ruprecht, 2011).

Cartwright, Lisa, *Screening the Body: Tracing Medicine's Visual Culture* (Minneapolis: University of Minnesota Press, 1995).

Curtis, Scott, *The Shape of Spectatorship: Art, Science, and Early Cinema in Germany* (New York: Columbia University Press, 2015).

Daston, Lorraine, and Peter Galison, *Objectivity* (New York: Zone Books, 2007).

Delavaud, Gilles, and Denis Maréchal, *Télévision: Le moment expérimental* (Rennes: Apogée, 2011).

Donauer, Sabine, 'Emotions at Work—Working on Emotions: The Production of Economic Selves in Twentieth-Century Germany' (PhD thesis, Freie Universität Berlin, 2013).

Ebbinghaus, Bernhard, and Philipp Manow, eds., *Comparing Welfare Capitalism: Social Policy and Political Economy in Europe, Japan and the USA* (London: Routledge, 2001).

Eitler, Pascal, and Monique Scheer, 'Emotionengeschichte als Körpergeschichte: Eine heuristische Perspektive auf religiöse Konversionen im 19. und 20 Jahrhundert', *Geschichte und Gesellschaft*, 35, 2 (2009), pp. 282–313, doi: 10.13109/gege.2009.35.2.282.

Elsaesser, Thomas, 'Propagating Modernity: German Documentaries from the 1930s: Information, Instruction and Indoctrination', in *The Oxford Handbook of Propaganda Studies*, ed. by Jonathan Auerbach and Russ Castronovo (Oxford: Oxford University Press, 2013), pp. 237–260, doi:10.1093/oxfordhb/9780199764419.013.013.

Forster, Ralf, 'Mitten hinein ins Jugendleben: Die Amateurfilme von Bernd Maywald (1955–1967)', *Filmblatt*, 21, 60 (2016), pp. 73–84.

Foucault, Michel, *Le gouvernement de soi et des autres*, 2 vols. (Paris: Seuil, 2008–2009).

Friedman Lester D., ed., *Cultural Sutures: Medicine and Media* (Durham, NC: Duke University Press, 2004).

Fröhlich, Gerhard, 'Habitus und Hexis: Die Einverleibung der Praxisstrukturen bei Pierre Bourdieu', in *Grenzenlose Gesellschaft?, vol. 2, part 2: Ad-hoc-Gruppen, Foren*, ed. by Claudia Honegger and Hermann Schwengel (Opladen: Leske + Budrich, 1999), pp. 100–102.

Gaycken, Oliver, *Devices of Curiosity: Early Cinema and Popular Science* (Oxford: Oxford University Press, 2015).

Greene, Jeremy A., Flurin Condrau, and Elizabeth Siegel Watkins, eds., *Therapeutic Revolutions: Pharmaceuticals and Social Change in the Twentieth Century* (Chicago: University of Chicago Press, 2016).

Grossman, Michael, 'On the Concept of Health Capital and the Demand for Health', *Journal of Political Economy*, 80, 2 (1972), pp. 223–255.

Gumbert, Heather L., *Envisioning Socialism: Television and the Cold War in the German Democratic Republic* (Ann Arbor: University of Michigan Press, 2014).

Hagener, Malte, Vinzenz Hediger, and Alena Strohmaier, eds., *The State of Post-Cinema: Tracing the Moving Image in the Age of Digital Dissemination* (London: Palgrave Macmillan, 2016).

Hakim, Catherine, *Erotic Capital: The Power of Attraction in the Boardroom and the Bedroom* (New York: Basic Books, 2011).

Harper, Graeme, and Andrew Moor, eds., *Signs of Life: Medicine and Cinema* (London: Wallflower Press, 2005).

Hediger, Vinzenz, Florian Hoof, and Yvonne Zimmermann, eds., *Films That Work Harder: The Circulations of Industrial Cinema* (Amsterdam: Amsterdam University Press, forthcoming).

Hediger, Vinzenz, and Patrick Vonderau, eds., *Films that Work: Industrial Film and the Productivity of Media* (Amsterdam: Amsterdam University Press, 2009).

Illouz, Eva, *Cold Intimacies: The Making of Emotional Capitalism* (Cambridge: Polity Press, 2007).

Kocka, Jürgen, and Marcel van der Linden, eds., *Capitalism: The Reemergence of a Historical Concept* (London: Bloomsbury, 2016).

Lafon, Benoît, *Histoire de la télévision régionale: De la RTF à la 3, 1950–2012* (Bry-sur-Marne: INA, 2012).

Laukötter, Anja, 'How Films Entered the Classroom: The Sciences and the Emotional Education of Youth through Health Education Films in the United States and Germany, 1910–30', *Osiris*, 31, 1 (2016), pp. 181–200.

Laukötter, Anja, 'Measuring Knowledge and Emotions: Audience Research in Educational Films at the Beginning of the Twentieth Century', in *Health Education Films in the Twentieth Century*, ed. by Christian Bonah, David Cantor, and Anja Laukötter (Rochester: University of Rochester Press, 2018), pp. 305–325.

Laukötter, Anja, 'Politik im Kino: Eine Emotions- und Wissenschaftsgeschichte des Sexualaufklärungsfilms im 20. Jahrhundert' (Habilitation thesis, Humboldt Universität zu Berlin, 2018).

Lebas, Elizabeth, *Forgotten Futures: British Municipal Cinema 1920–1980* (London: Black Dog, 2011).

Lengwiler, Martin, and Jeanette Madarász, eds., *Das präventive Selbst: Eine Kulturgeschichte moderner Gesundheitspolitik* (Bielefeld: Transcript, 2010).

Lévy, Marie-Françoise, *Regards de la télévision française sur la famille: 105 émissions sélectionnées à travers les archives 1956–1986* (Paris: IDEF, 1987).

Lippmann, Walter, *Public Opinion* (New York: Harcourt, Brace and Co., 1922).
Luthans, Fred, Carolyn M. Youssef, and Bruce J. Avolio, *Psychological Capital: Developing the Human Competitive Edge* (Oxford: Oxford University Press, 2006).
Mattl, Siegfried, Carina Lesky, Vrääth Öhner, and Ingo Zechner, eds., *Abenteuer Alltag: Zur Archäologie des Amateurfilms* (Vienna: SYNEMA, 2015).
Mitchell, W. J. T., *Picture Theory: Essays on Verbal and Visual Representation* (Chicago: University of Chicago Press, 1994).
Mitchell, W. J. T., 'What Do Pictures Really Want?', *October*, 77 (Summer 1996), pp. 71–82, doi:10.2307/778960.
Mitchell, W. J. T., *What Do Pictures Want? The Lives and Loves of Images* (Chicago: University of Chicago Press, 2005).
Mitman, Gregg, and Kelley Wilder, *Documenting the World: Film, Photography, and the Scientific Record* (Chicago: University of Chicago Press, 2016).
Mitman, Gregg, and Kelley Wilder, 'Introduction', in *Documenting the World: Film, Photography, and the Scientific Record*, ed. by Gregg Mitman and Kelley Wilder (Chicago: University of Chicago Press, 2016), pp. 1–22.
Neveu, Érik, 'Les sciences sociales doivent-elles accumuler les capitaux? À propos de Catherine Hakim, Erotic Capital, et de quelques marcottages intempestifs de la notion de capital', *Revue française de sciences politiques*, 63, 2 (2013), pp. 337–358, http://www.jstor.org/stable/43124237.
Odin, Roger, ed., *Le film de famille: Usage privé, usage public* (Paris: Méridiens Klincksieck, 1995).
Orgeron, Devin, Marsha Orgeron, and Dan Streible, eds., *Learning with the Lights Off: Educational Film in the United States* (New York: Oxford University Press, 2012).
Ory, Pascal, *La Belle Illusion: Culture et politique sous le signe du Front Populaire, 1935–1938* (Paris: Plon, 1994).
Ostherr, Kirsten, *Medical Visions: Producing the Patient through Film, Television, and Imaging Technologies* (Oxford: Oxford University Press, 2013).
Poels, Géraldine, *Les trente glorieuses du téléspectateur: Une histoire de la réception télévisuelle des années 1950 aux années 1980* (Bry-sur-Marne: INA, 2015).
Powell, Larson, and Robert Shandley, eds., *German Television: Historical and Theoretical Approaches* (New York: Berghahn, 2016).
Rabeharisoa, Vololona, and Michel Callon, *Le pouvoir des malades: L'Association française contre les myopathies et la recherche* (Paris: Les presses de l'ecole des mines, 1999).
Rabinbach, Anson, *The Human Motor: Energy, Fatigue, and the Origins of Modernity* (New York: Basic Books, 1990).

Reagan, Leslie J., Nancy Tomes, and Paula A. Treichler, *Medicine's Moving Pictures: Medicine, Health, and Bodies in American Film and Television* (Rochester: University of Rochester Press, 2007).

Reckwitz, Andreas, 'Habitus oder Subjektivierung? Subjektanalyse nach Bourdieu und Foucault', in *Pierre Bourdieu und die Kulturwissenschaften: Zur Aktualität eines undisziplinierten Denkens*, ed. by Daniel Šuber, Hilmar Schäfer, and Sophia Prinz (Konstanz: UVK, 2011), pp. 41–62.

Reckwitz, Andreas, 'Practices and their Affects', in *The Nexus of Practices: Connections, Constellations, Practitioners*, ed. by Allison Hui, Theordore R. Schatzki, and Elizabeth Shove (London: Routledge, 2017), pp. 114–125.

Reinecke, Christiane, 'Der (damalige) Geschmack der Bourgeoisie: Eine historische Re-Lektüre von Pierre Bourdieus "Die feinen Unterschiede" (1979)', *Zeithistorische Forschungen/Studies in Contemporary History*, 14, 2 (2017), pp. 376–383, http://www.zeithistorische-forschungen.de/2-2017/id=5499, accessed 20 September 2018.

Sauvage, Monique, and Isabelle Veyrat-Masson, *Histoire de la télévision française: De 1935à nos jours* (Paris: Nouveau Monde, 2012).

Scheer, Monique, 'Are Emotions a Kind of Practice (and Is That What Makes them Have a History)? A Bourdieuian Approach to Understanding Emotion', *History and Theory*, 51, 2 (May 2012), pp. 193–220, https://www.jstor.org/stable/23277639.

Scheper-Hughes, Nancy, and Loïc Wacquant, eds., *Commodifying Bodies* (London: Sage, 2002).

Shilling, Chris, *The Body and Social Theory*, 2nd ed. (London: Sage, 2003).

Soulages, Jean-Claude, *Les rhétoriques télévisuelles: Le formatage du réel*. (Brussels/ Paris: De Boeck Université/INA [Médias Recherches], 2007).

Strauven, Wanda (ed.), *The Cinema of Attractions Reloaded* (Amsterdam: Amsterdam University Press, 2006).

Thomson, Kevin, *Emotional Capital: Maximising the Intangible Assets at the Heart of Brand and Business Success* (Oxford: Capstone, 2000).

Vignaux, Valérie, *Jean Benoît-Lévy ou le corps comme utopie: Une histoire du cinema èducateur dans l'entre-deux-guerres en France* (Paris: AFRHC 2007).

Weehuizen, Rifka Maria, 'Mental Capital: The Economic Significance of Mental Health' (PhD thesis, Universitaire Pers Maastricht, 2008).

Zimmermann, Patricia R., *Reel Families: A Social History of Amateur Film* (Bloomington: Indiana University Press, 1995).

Zimmermann, Peter, ed., *Geschichte des dokumentarischen Films in Deutschland*, 3 vols. (Stuttgart: Reclam, 2005).

Zimmermann, Yvonne (ed.), *Schaufenster Schweiz. Dokumentarische Gebrauchsfilme 1896–1964* (Zurich: Limmat Verlag, 2011).

About the Authors

Christian Bonah, MD, PhD, is professor for the history of medical and health sciences at the University Strasbourg, member of its Institute of Advanced Studies and principal investigator of the ERC Advanced grant BodyCapital. He works on comparative, social, and material history of health, health products and services, and bodies especially in connection with media and law.
Contact details: bonah@unistra.fr

PD Dr. **Anja Laukötter** is a historian of nineteenth- and twentieth-century European history working in the field of social and cultural history and history of science. She is a researcher at the Center for the History of Emotions at the Max Planck Institute for Human Development and Co-principal investigator of the ERC Advanced grant BodyCapital. Besides other, the main field of her research is the transnational/global history of media, the history of emotions and the history of psychology and pedagogy.
Contact details: laukoetter@mpib-berlin.mpg.de

1. Playing the Doctor, Playing the Patient: The Performance of Health Identities in Live Medical Television, 1958

Timothy M. Boon

Abstract

Using the example of 'Machines for Living' (8 April 1958) from the BBC's 'Your Life in Their Hands' series, I explore doctors' and patients' performances on live medical television. The point is to examine how the grammar and technology of live television provided affordances and constraints to the representation of medicine, here the high-tech medicine of dialysis and heart-lung bypass at Leeds General Infirmary. I use several theoretical lenses to focus attention on the participants' performances, including work by Erving Goffman, Richard Schechner, Espen Ytreberg, Judith Butler, and Paddy Scannell. Although the analysis is tightly focussed on a single programme, it is intended to be generally applicable to the analysis of medical, and indeed non-fiction television of all kinds.

Keywords: performance; live television; dialysis; heart-lung bypass; Erving Goffman; Richard Schechner; Espen Ytreberg; Judith Butler; Paddy Scannell

Your Life in Their Hands (*YLITH*), broadcast from February 1958, was the series that dramatically changed the representation of medicine on British television.[1] The revolutionary character of the series derives from its character as a live outside broadcast, a format that placed a premium on the performances of the on-screen contributors to the programme, the focus of this essay. Its liveness and location required particular kinds of performance that were

1 It is necessary to draw on my previous published work on this programme, but that did not address questions of performance. Please excuse any overlap: Boon, 'Medical Film'.

Bonah, C. and A. Laukötter (eds.), *Body, Capital, and Screens: Visual Media and the Healthy Self in the 20th Century*. Taylor & Francis Group, 2020
DOI 10.5117/9789462988293_CH01

qualitatively different from those asked of participants in films. *Machinery for Living*, broadcast by the British Broadcasting Corporation (BBC) on 8 April 1958 from Leeds General Infirmary (LGI), the ninth programme in the first series, was concerned with the new medical technologies of renal dialysis and heart-lung bypass for cardiac surgery.[2] The programme starts with an introduction from a London studio by 'a physician in the Department of Medicine in a London hospital'. This is followed, within the programme's 30-minute duration, by three main sections broadcast from Leeds, each led by a member of medical staff from the LGI: an introduction about the hospital, a sequence on the artificial kidney, and another on cardiac surgery using the Melrose heart-lung machine. The latter two main sections feature interviews with patients. The programme anchor closes the proceedings with general concluding comments.

By 1958, medicine was already a staple of non-fiction television, part of the roster of serious subjects the BBC considered worthy of coverage, which otherwise included, for example, politics, religion, the arts, science, and current affairs. In selecting the subjects to treat in its output, staff at the BBC also responded to the demands of interest groups. This was the decade in which, for various groups, including doctors, television began to seem to be the best medium to represent many subjects, on account of the audience that could be reached. Professions differed in their pursuit of representation in the medium. The pattern of medical participation in this particular programme was typical of the unevenness of responses of scientists and doctors to television; some embraced it and others rejected it. In the case of medical doctors, as represented by the British Medical Association, their brush with television over this particular series helped define a new approach that, ultimately, brought them closer to the medium, as Kelly Loughlin has shown.[3] At the heart of that dispute were issues of professional confidentiality and the sacredness of the doctor-patient relationship, both tied up with an ethical objection to any activity that could be seen as advertising. In this series, these were treated by giving the doctors anonymity, though not the patients, as we shall see.

Those in charge of non-fiction television in the 1950s were in a crucible of expansion, serving the increase of viewers, seeking to develop new and compelling genres of broadcasting to convey these subjects, approaches that responded to the particular characteristics of the medium. In particular,

2 'Your Life in their Hands: 9: Machinery for Living', *BBC*, http://genome.ch.bbc.co.uk/4efb0bd132364cb396c83fdb33b91fa9, accessed 14 February 2017.

3 Loughlin, 'Your Life'.

they focussed on the fact that virtually everything that was broadcast in that decade was live; so they made a fetish of the simultaneity of the medium.[4] With *YLITH*, we see one of those interactions between available broadcasting technology, subject, and televisual form that is so distinctive of the development of the medium. From the mid 1950s, the BBC's Outside Broadcast Department began to make its own programmes, rather than just providing a service to other departments.[5] Producers were encouraged to develop new types of outside broadcast (OB) programmes, partially because the quantity of OB equipment in the regions had been increased so that the BBC could better cover sports matches; as these mainly took place at weekends, equipment was underused on weekdays. The department began to concentrate on 'built OB' programmes, as participants named them; OB that did not merely transmit existing events—such as the Coronation—into peoples' homes, but that used real venues as television studios for programmes that reported activities authentic to the chosen site. The OB producers Aubrey Singer, with his science series *Eye on Research*, and Bill Duncalf, with *YLITH*, seized this opportunity, taking cameras into labs and hospitals, respectively.[6] For *YLITH*, that meant a live broadcast from a different regional hospital for each week of the series.

Norman Swallow, a senior television producer, expressed the excitement of live television in his 1966 primer *Factual Television*:

> The viewer is watching something which is truly taking place at the very moment of transmission, and no one really knows what will happen. The tension which such a situation produces in the audience is something that was once regarded as one of television's greatest assets, and to pre-record a programme (and thereby eliminate anything that departs from an arranged plan) is to throw this enormous advantage out of the window.[7]

He went on more specifically to comment on cameras watching 'surgeons at work, performing a real operation on a genuine patient'. His view was that 'to transmit such a sequence live is infinitely more effective than to pre-record it, for there is always an added sense of occasion in being present

4 Recording was difficult until videotape recording became widespread, which did not occur before the end of the 1950s. 'Telerecording'—filming from monitors—was problematic, and making programmes on film prior to broadcast was expensive.

5 In 1954, for the first time, the department was listed as a production rather than a facilities department. See BBC Staff Lists (available at BBC Written Archives Centre, Caversham).

6 For *Eye on Research*, see Boon, 'Formal Conventions'.

7 Swallow, *Factual Television*, pp. 147–148.

when something dramatic is actually happening. To be allowed to watch something which took place yesterday or last week is a poor substitute'.[8] This is the technological 'script', if you like—the constraint and affordance of available broadcasting technology.[9]

For the argument here, it is important to understand the particular 'grammar' of live television and how that relates to the programme's subject. First, we should note that live television (TV) linked on-screen performers to viewers in a simultaneous form, with no opportunity for second takes to produce better results. Second, whereas in film-making sequences are constructed at the editing bench after the event from multiple shots, in live TV, the structure of the programmes is made by a director working at the time of transmission, instructing a vision mixer to cut between the signals coming from two or more cameras. TV cameras in the late 1950s were large and had to be wheeled around ('tracked') to change shots (and they did not generally have zoom lenses until somewhat later than 1958). Programme planning featured detailed choreography of where the programme's participants, as well as the cameras not switched to the broadcast output, would need to move to be able to supply the programme's next shot. Within this grammar, certain conventions were already well established by the late 1950s; for example, one camera might hold a medium close-up on an individual, whereas another might be a 'two-shot' including, perhaps, an interviewer and an interviewee. Cameras would often alternate, guided by headphone-instructions from the director, between 'wide shots', close-ups, and shots of visual material, including, in our programme's case, several animated diagrams constructed by the specialist prop-maker Alfred Wurmser (Figure 1.1).[10] These intricate devices, for which there seems to have been only one supplier, were cardboard models with moving parts, operated by their maker during the programme, often with a handheld pen pointing out salient details, to illustrate the words of the speaker.

Part of the language of live TV, especially before the widespread use of videotape (which became commonplace in the 1960s), was the incorporation of pre-prepared sequences shot and edited on film, and played in using a telecine machine at the appropriate moment. Producers saw these as part of

8 Swallow, *Factual Television*, p. 148.

9 Akrich, 'De-Scription'.

10 The diagrams are described as 'Wurmsers' in the surviving script, transcribed in Turney, 'Disease', pp. 246–251. See Neil, 'Alfred Wurmser'. In a *Panorama* broadcast in 1956, there is a sequence showing Wurmser and one of his diagrams: http://youtu.be/2G36AaMDFdM?t=6m36s, accessed 5 February 2018.

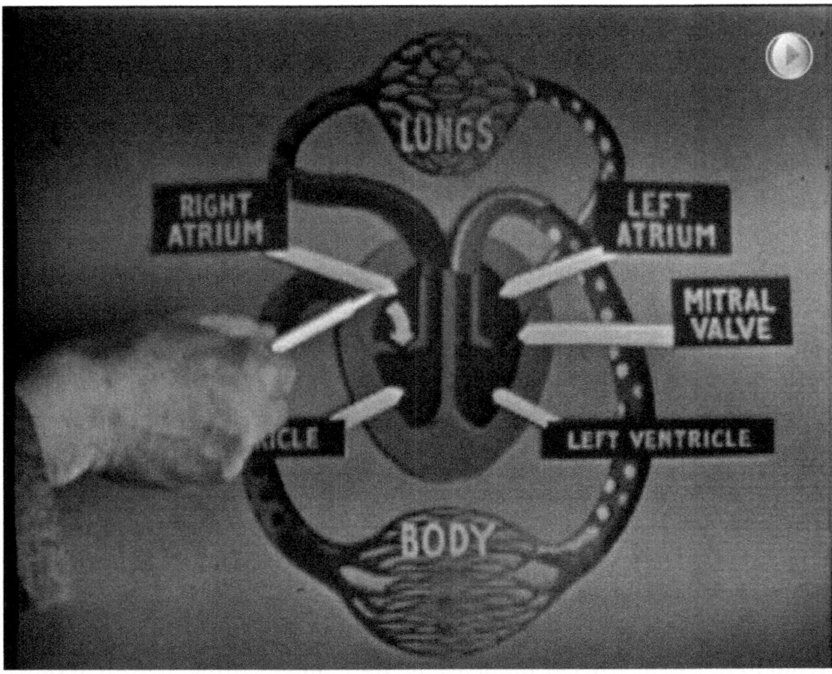

1.1. Alfred Wurmser's working diagram of the circulation. © BBC 1958.

the interpretive armoury of live television, not in any way as a failure of live technique; often, these would show outside scenes, or detailed explanatory sequences that had to be filmed and edited before the programme.

All these aspects were common to studio and outside broadcast programmes, but the latter had extra complications because they were staged at venues that might only have very constricted spaces for presentation, discussion, and camera movement. Unreliability of equipment, much of which, at that time, relied on valves rather than the more reliable transistors, could also be a factor; it was not unusual for a programme planned to use three cameras in different parts of the OB location to have to make do with two.

This analysis is concerned with the performances of human participants in the selected programme, on the argument that what doctors, patients, directors, cameramen, vision mixers, and the rest actually did in the making of the programme constitute its communicative enterprise. My aim is to follow the 'performative turn' to establish a kind and level of analysis that can be tested and extended.[11] To be sure, usage of the term

11 See, for example, Licoppe, 'Performative Turn'.

'perform' has been very broad and various indeed, extending as wide as Annemarie Mol's suggestion within Actor Network Theory that we can think of 'a reality that is *done* and *enacted* rather than observed'.[12] In this essay, using a selection of the performance literature most relevant to my subject matter, I draw on work on performance from sociology, and theatre, literature, and gender studies that has long been influential, but which has, up to now, had little impact on our understanding of medical and science television. Erving Goffman's sociology of the presentation of self in everyday life deployed a swathe of theatrical metaphors to describe the performed nature of everyday interactions. Richard Schechner, anthropologist and theoretician of theatre, focussed more on the nature of deliberate performances, including the relations between the performer and the part performed. The literature scholar Stephen Greenblatt historicized early-modern 'self-fashioning'. Judith Butler, coming from an entirely different background in philosophy, has argued that gender is the product of iterative performances in a discursive sense. Each of these approaches is considered below as a means to interrogate and highlight what the doctors and patients are actually doing in this programme. I do not assume that 'performance' has the same meaning in each of these analyses; rather, my aim is to reveal their potency in interrogating what goes on in television.

The Performance of *Machinery for Living*

In commencing our analysis, the most basic point is to acknowledge the particularity and constructedness of the account of high-tech medicine *Machinery for Living* presents. Beyond noting and recovering the enacted and spatial performances of camera operators, vision mixers, and directors, there is much to be explored about the on-screen performances within this particular programme. *Machinery for Living* consists very substantially of a series of appearances on camera of speaking individuals, mainly men, of differing professional and class statuses. The televisual grammar of the time (whose basic features I have summarized above) required people to do things on-screen so that content could be conveyed; I am defining these actions as performances. A simple but telling example of this basic point is provided by the programme's second sequence, the continuity shot that Ray Lakeland, the director in Leeds, had at the switchover from the

12 Mol, 'Ontological Politics', p. 77, emphasis in original.

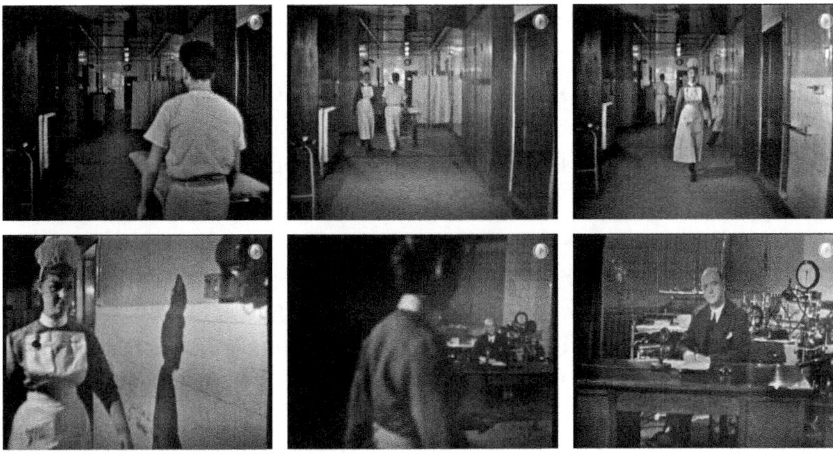

1.2. Establishing shot. © BBC 1958.

anchorman in the London studio to the Outside Broadcast action at the hospital (Figure 1.2):

> A hospital porter walks down a hospital corridor pushing a wheeled stretcher past and away from the camera. A nurse emerges from a side turning and walks towards the camera, which 'tracks back' keeping her in vision and turning to the right to look in as she enters a room; in the room we see a professor sitting at a desk. The vision mixer switches to a second camera that holds him in medium close up.

The shot does the work of reinforcing that this is an OB from a hospital, establishing the medical space of the programme, with visual cues such as the hospital architecture and staff uniforms as key signifiers. But we should note that the porter and nurse did not just happen to be in the line of sight of the cameras shortly after half past nine that evening, and it is no coincidence that the professor was sitting there; all were asked to perform these actions by the director to enable a televisual move between the anchorman's introduction, and the professor's setting of the scene in Leeds. In other words, real people in television are asked to play versions of themselves for the sake of, and within the constraints of, televisual narrative and technique. Medical staff are 'playing doctor', and their subjects are, equally, 'playing the patient'. Furthermore, the pressures of live television force different kinds of performance than those in film, in part because of the lack of opportunity to re-take to perfect the contribution, and in part because of the director's requirement to deliver consecutive performances, often amounting to 30 minutes in total length.

Recognizing these appearances as performances is not simply *post hoc* theorization, as is clear from contemporary discussion. The *British Medical Journal*, in pouring scorn on *YLITH*, found fault with the necessity for performance:

> Though the anonymity of the doctors is being preserved—for what that is worth in this publicity-seeking age—their colleagues may well think *it is demeaning for doctors and nurses to appear as mummers* on the television screen in order to provide entertainment for the great British public.[13]

The pejorative use of the term 'mummer' to describe the activities of the medical figures on-screen is potent: It is clear that contemporaries knew that appearing on television required non-actors to provide a performance fitting to the medium.[14]

Equally, the use of the term 'performance' is a commonplace of production correspondence between programme makers and participants; for example, James McCloy wrote to the neurologist William Grey Walter in May 1957 after the programme *A Question of Science* that 'I would like to thank you for the sympathetic way you adapted yourself to the situation and for the authoritative performance you gave'.[15]

Paddy Scannell summarizes the ways in which camerawork conventions go beyond establishing a spatial sense of the venue (here, the LGI) to enable the viewer to locate the participants in relation to each other and to themselves:

> TV camera angles and movements clearly generate implicatures [implied meanings]—about, for instance, the status of the relationship between speaker(s) in the studio and viewers in their homes. The camera monitors the faces of speakers and hearers in displayed television talk for corroborative evidence of participants' personality, state of mind and alignment (or otherwise) with what's going on. In this the camera behaves as we all do in what Erving Goffman calls 'face engagements' and acts, on our behalf, to produce effects of co-presence.[16]

13 'Disease Education by the B.B.C.', p. 388, emphasis added.

14 A point which Karpf, *Doctoring the Media*, p. 51 also mentions.

15 James McCloy to William Grey Walter, 1 May 1957, TVART1 William Grey Walter, BBC Written Archives Centre, Caversham, pp. 57–65, here p. 60.

16 Scannell, 'Introduction', p. 6.

By such techniques, television directors enable talk to do its work of conveying content. As Scannell argues, '[t]he talk that goes out on radio and television is recognizably [...] intended for and addressed to actual listeners and viewers'.[17] Citing Barthes, he argues that 'the *grain* of the voice gives rise to inferences about the speaker, and changes in voice are an important means of creating implicatures. Voice is the irreducible mark of the spoken, of its physical, embodied presence'.[18] Unlike other televisual and filmic formats where off-screen commentary was favoured, in live TV such as *YLITH*, the requirement for talk to convey content also entailed the presence of people on-screen to do the talking—a visual as well as an aural presence. These televisual performances therefore necessarily feature 'the age, appearance, sex and dress of participants; the manner and style of how they talk to each other'. All of these reinforce the constructed reality of the programme; they 'give rise to warrantable inferences about the nature of the event there taking place, the character and status of the participants and the relationship of event and participants to viewers or listeners'.[19]

Playing the Doctor

To move from generalities to specifics, there are three kinds of human performance within *Machinery for Living*: by the 'physician in the Department of Medicine in a London hospital', Dr. Charles Fletcher,[20] who was the 'anchorman' for the series; by the medical staff (all unnamed in the programme; see below), including Sir Ronald Tunbridge (Professor of Medicine at Leeds),[21] Dr. Frank Parsons (the leading dialysis doctor based at the Infirmary), the lecturer in medicine, Dr. Brian McCracken, and the cardiothoracic surgeon Geoffrey Wooler;[22] and by the four patients who appear in the programme, Mr. Gudor, 'Delice', Mrs. Mitchell, and Mrs. Lawless.

17 Scannell, 'Introduction', p. 1. Similarly, Ytreberg, 'Ideal Types', p. 760: in media studies, researchers 'have shown how the self-presentation and social interactions of persons in the broadcast media involves certain standardized behaviours appropriate to communicating with an absent party'.

18 Scannell, 'Introduction', p. 6, emphasis in original. The terminology of 'implicatures' derives from the linguistic pragmatism of Levinson, *Pragmatics*.

19 Scannell, 'Introduction', p. 6.

20 Booth, 'Obituary'.

21 https://library.leeds.ac.uk/special-collections-explore/4091 between 1946 and 1971, accessed 23 July 2018.

22 All identified by Turney, 'Disease', pp. 192–232.

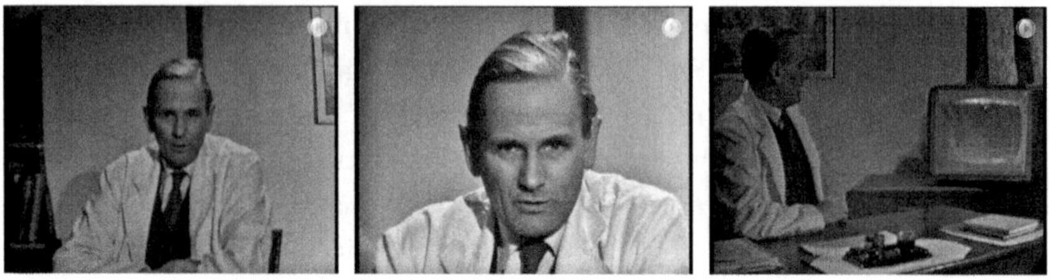

1.3. Charles Fletcher, anchorman, introduces the programme. © BBC 1958.

Let us begin with Fletcher's performance. After the opening titles and signature music against a shot of a nurse filling a syringe, the vision mixer switches to a medium close-up of Fletcher seated at a desk, dressed in a white coat open to reveal a shirt and tie and waistcoat implying a three-piece suit. A bookcase is just visible to the left and a painting to the right, suggesting—according to an old iconography—the learned physician.[23] Christopher Booth's obituary suggests that '[t]all and distinguished in appearance, and with thespian qualities, Charles Fletcher was perhaps a natural choice for television'.[24] As Fletcher speaks directly to the camera, probably from cue cards, about the importance of medical teamwork, then introduces the 'two beautiful mechanical devices' that are to be the topic of the programme, the camera technique underscores his authority by tracking into a close-up, only tracking out again to enable him to appear very briefly on a second camera in a two-shot with a monitor showing the outside broadcast feed from Leeds (Figure 1.3).

The emerging grammar of non-fiction live television often entailed the use of anchormen, the role that Fletcher fulfils here. Paul Fox, editor of the current affairs programme *Panorama*, explained around this time that:

> [T]he personal contact between the programme and its audience is vital, and I am equally sure that the best way to establish the proper kind of contact is by means of a visible personality, someone who has down the years become something of a family friend, a regular visitor to the sitting room, a man whose words are respected and whose very presence has become (and I doubt I rate it too highly) a guarantee of integrity and common sense.[25]

23 'There were a number of pictorial conventions for representing a man who thought. Setting was one: a study-like environment, the possession of books and so on'; Jordanova, *Defining Features*, p. 41. See also Lawrence, 'Medical Minds'.

24 Booth, 'Obituary'.

25 Quoted in Swallow, *Factual Television*, p. 63, who gives no further citation.

Fletcher's televisual familiarity was already established, as he had appeared (even if, again, anonymously) in the 1957 psychiatry series *The Hurt Mind*.[26] Fox's language of respect, integrity, and common sense, encoded in Fletcher's introductory sequence, amounts to a core set of characteristics of expert performance, often linked to authority, as Espen Ytreberg, in a valuable 2002 analysis, argues:

> [For broadcasters,] an important means of communicating [...] public legitimacy is through persons of authority. Among other things, broadcasting is about converting institutional legitimacy into conventions of self-presentation, focused particularly round functions like hosting and anchoring.[27]

For the producers of *YLITH*, it was important that the anchor be identified as coming from a relevant professional background, in this case medicine, unlike the cases of *Panorama* or *Monitor*, for example, where television people—respectively Richard Dimbleby and Huw Wheldon—fulfilled this function.[28] Ytreberg refers to 'the dictates of professional codes such as those of established journalism, which converts a need for trustworthiness and solidity into a measure of restraint and neutrality in self-presentation'. This, in turn, is converted into performance tropes: 'speech, other sound production, mimicry and gesticulation are all subject to a certain rule-bound conventionalization in broadcast media'.[29] Just as, in Ytreberg's account, the professional codes of journalism are significant to the establishment of the ideal types of television performance, so it is clear that other kinds of period-specific professional code associated with the medical profession—and with patienthood—were essential to the kinds of medical performance found in our 1958 programme. The social conventions and expectations of the participants in this programme, as in others, framed the conditions of possibility for the representation of medical practice it contains. John Turney has summarized the constraints that medical participants placed on their involvement in the series:

> The programmes were carefully structured to allay professional concerns and, in particular, to avoid any adverse effect on the doctor-patient

26 This programme is discussed in Long, *Destigmatising*, Chapter 6.
27 Ytreberg, 'Ideal Types', p. 759.
28 Similar assumptions about the importance of having a scientist-anchorman for *Horizon* preoccupied a closely related set of producers five years later; see Boon, 'Televising of Science'.
29 Ytreberg, 'Ideal Types', p. 760.

> relationship. Thus: doctors appearing in the programmes were not named; reference to diseases was kept to the minimum necessary for an understanding of the treatments shown; descriptions of symptoms that might give rise to anxiety were avoided; the availability of other treatments or that treatments were not necessarily suitable for all was acknowledged.[30]

These constraints set the terms of the doctors' performances, leading to the same conversion of a 'need for trustworthiness and solidity into a measure of restraint and neutrality in self-presentation'[31] in the on-screen performance.

With regard to doctors' anonymity, the *Radio Times* billing simply stated, as we have seen, that 'the series is introduced by a physician in the Department of Medicine in a London hospital', without naming the anchorman Dr. Charles Fletcher, and the programme's titles include only a generic acknowledgement of the medical staff, who are left unnamed.[32] They list only key television production roles. Despite his being unnamed, with audiences therefore having no way of knowing, for example, that he was educated at the elite private school Eton, the received pronunciation of Fletcher's voice would immediately have identified him as a member of the upper professional classes.[33]

Tunbridge, introduced by Fletcher as 'the professor of medicine in the university department of medicine', sitting at the desk, speaks to the camera, glancing to his left (probably unsure of which camera to address). Behind him in the shot is a miscellany of clinical equipment. He outlines the history of the LGI before proceeding to a description of the human circulatory system, which is illustrated by one of Wurmser's diagrams. He moves on to introduce the artificial kidney and the artificial heart and lung.

Tunbridge introduces Parsons as 'the assistant director of the medical research unit in the urological department'. The camera pans right, and Parsons walks into the shot, towards the camera. Sitting down on a stool in front of the dialyser, he explains the 'complex' function of kidneys in simple terms. In a lecturing style, and probably reading from cue cards, he briefly delimits his concerns with acute kidney failure; he explains how, in these cases, waste materials can accumulate in the blood. 'To illustrate this point,

30 Turney, 'Disease', p. 229.

31 Ytreberg, 'Ideal Types', p. 760.

32 Transcribed at 'Your Life in their Hands: 9: Machinery for Living', *BBC*, http://genome.ch.bbc.co.uk/4efb0bd132364cb396c83fdb33b91fa9, accessed 14 February 2017.

33 Booth, 'Obituary'.

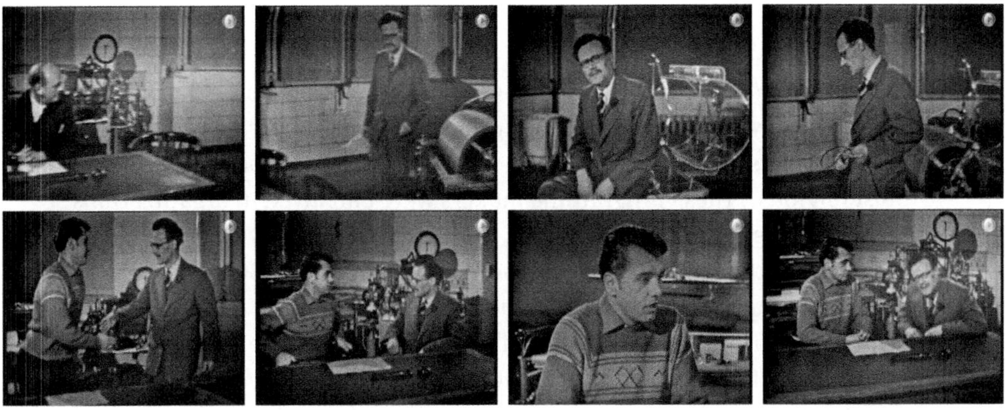

1.4. Tunbridge introduces Parsons; Parsons explains dialysis; Parsons 'interviews' Mr. Gudor. © BBC 1958.

I would like to introduce to you a patient, Mr. Gudor.' During these words, he stands up, and walks to his right, curling up the microphone lead as he goes, offering his hand in a handshake, the camera following in a pan. They both sit down at the desk, by now vacated by Tunbridge, and begin a short interview. Only at this point is there a vision cut to a second camera showing a one-shot of the patient. The second half of Tunbridge's exposition and all of Parsons's explanation has been covered by a single shot, with movements, lasting two minutes and 25 seconds (Figure 1.4). Returning to the right, Parsons explains the function of the machine, once more making use of an animated diagram (shot, again, with a separate camera) and a sample of the cellophane tubing used as the machine's dialysis membrane. He introduces a 'doctor from the department of medicine' (Brian McCracken), who concludes the exposition of the machine's function, including interviews with Delice, 'a little girl who was treated on this machine several months ago' and Mrs. Mitchell, whose dialysis, filmed three weeks before, is shown in two edited film insets that he explicitly introduces. All the medical performances are confident, if varying in ease in their address to camera and in the required movements within the hospital room serving as a temporary studio.

To go a little deeper into the nature of these performances, we can refer to the 'ideal types' of television broadcaster that Ytreberg has identified in discourse on television. Although his purpose is to propose a four-fold classification of television broadcaster into paternalists, bureaucrats, charismatics, and avant-gardists, only the middle two terms are helpful to our discussion here. (The last type, marked by eschewing restraint and neutrality, only emerged much later in the 20th century.) But Ytreberg also quickly moves to dismiss the 'paternalist' type as '[p]art theoretical concept, part analytical tool and part derogatory term', pointing out that 'the image of the paternalist has frequently been invoked to characterize a kind of patronizing elitism'.[34] Instead, he proposes an alternative, 'the bureaucrat' type: 'The traditional figure of the public service programme maker bore a string of resemblances to that of the ideal-typical bureaucrat. Most obviously these programme makers were employed in organizations that had close formal affiliations with the state and were structured according to the principles of state bureaucracies.'[35] The BBC was evidently one such organization. Ytreberg quotes Richard Sennett to describe the kind of performance involved in fitting this ideal type, exactly as we see and hear from the medical performers in *Machinery for Life*, arguing that '[s]elf-control [...] appears as a strength, a strength of calmness and above-the-storm which makes telling others what to do seem natural. [...] In reacting to this dominance those in need can come to perceive autonomous figures as authorities'.[36] He suggests that: 'A restraint of individuality and emotions communicates the power of formalized professional expertise.'[37]

Of the 'charismatic' type, who come beyond paternalists and bureaucrats in Ytreberg's taxonomy, he states:

> The broadcasting 'personality' exudes a personal charm that functions to soothe and reassure the audience. It produces feelings of intimacy and rapport [...]. The audience is invited to believe in what the charismatic says because the charismatic communicates his or her personal belief in it so intensely. [...] Its formal qualities have been extensively elaborated; the use of informal modes of speech, the expressive manners, the extensive conversationalization approaching the patterns of everyday, unmediated interaction.[38]

How do the medical doctors' performances in *YLITH* relate to this? We witness in Fletcher's and McCracken's performances something in common with both the 'bureaucrat' and the 'charismatic' mode of television appearance, and, with Tunbridge and Parsons, perhaps a more unalloyed 'bureaucrat'. Scannell's basic point about dress is pertinent here: Unlike Fletcher, where medical authority is reinforced by his white coat, in the case of the doctors from the hospital, three-piece suits and ties are the order of

34 Ytreberg, 'Ideal Types', p. 761.
35 Ytreberg, 'Ideal Types', p. 763.
36 Sennett, *Authority*, p. 86, quoted in Ytreberg, 'Ideal Types', p. 763.
37 Ytreberg, 'Ideal Types', p. 763.
38 Ytreberg, 'Ideal Types', p. 765.

the day for their television appearance. We see them in scrubs or lab coats for the film inserts of the dialysis and use of the heart-lung machine. It is as though the medical doctor, garbed as 'off duty', is in a position to talk *about* his practice, whereas, in scrubs, he is limited to enacting medical practice.

In all three cases, we see an intensified version of the performance of self that was described by the sociologist Erving Goffman in his 1959 *Presentation of Self in Everyday Life* using a range of theatrical metaphors to convey the performed nature of interactions in everyday life.[39] In that work, he was concerned with using the language of theatre to demonstrate 'the constructed nature of identity, the self as a presentation or performance designed to be appropriate to the circumstances and settings in which it is produced in the presence of others'.[40] Speaking of the 'expression' of a participant in an encounter and the 'impression' received, he also distinguished between an expression given voluntarily, and that 'given off' involuntarily. Both are visible in the televisual performances of all the participants in *Machinery for Living*. That is to say that the bearing and relative ease of the differing performances (the impressions 'given off') are as significant to the impression received by the viewer as those 'given' by the participants' deliberate and controlled speech, and the choreographed and rehearsed movements within the programme's improvised studio. Another of Goffman's distinctions in *The Presentation of Self* is also at play here; as viewers, we experience the 'front stage' of the performance, but, at some level, we know also there to be a 'backstage' that is not presented to us.[41] As Steven Shapin asserts in his application of Goffman's *The Presentation of Self* to questions of trust in science, '[i]ndividuals present themselves to others as persons of a certain kind, likely to behave in certain ways, and, in so doing, request others actively to accept them as that kind of person. Trust in self-presentation is essential to interaction'.[42]

Richard Schechner, theorist of performance, distinguished his study from Goffman's as focussing specifically on 'the doing of an activity by an individual or group largely for the pleasure of another individual or group'.[43] Schechner describes the kinds of transformations that occur in such theatrical performances; most powerfully, he suggests that the performer is both 'not himself' (in the sense that he is playing a part) and

39 Goffman, *Presentation of Self*.

40 Brand and Scannell, 'Talk, Identity and Performance', p. 201.

41 Winkin and Leeds-Hurwitz, *Erving Goffman*, pp. 46–47.

42 Shapin, *Social History of Truth*, pp. 1–14, quotation p. 14.

43 Emigh, 'Liminal Richard', p. 170. This quotation comes from Schechner, *Performed Imaginaries*, p. 43.

'not not himself' (because it is only he who delivers the performance).[44] This describes well the level at which the medical doctors are working in the programme: both authentically performing to deliver content that they are particularly qualified to provide, but within a highly artificial set of conventions that requires a particular style of performance. The medical doctors in the programme can be seen to be performing at these two levels: in the Goffmanian sense of playing the doctor as they might in any off-camera clinical interaction with a patient, and in a Schechnerian performance for the pleasure of, or at least to inform, the distant television viewer.

There is a resonance here with the work on early-modern self-fashioning initiated in 1980 by Stephen Greenblatt.[45] In the sixteenth century, Greenblatt argues, self-fashioning came to be linked to 'manners or demeanor, particularly that of the elite; it may suggest hypocrisy or deception, an adherence to mere outward ceremony; it suggests representation of one's nature or intention in speech or actions'.[46] As Peter Burke has argued, Greenblatt's analysis went beyond Goffman's assumption that there is a fixed self behind the façade and replaced it with a reconstructed, even invented, self.[47] Richard Kirwan has also developed Greenblatt's concern with singular figures such as Thomas More and William Shakespeare to incorporate self-fashioning into the analysis of less prominent individuals, in his case, early-modern university scholars:

> [I]ndividuality was seldom a feature of the more pedestrian self-fashioners [who] sought to advertise their social merits by conforming to the image of a social type or category. In their self-fashioning they followed or imitated the representational models preferred by their peer-group. More than anything they were eager to demonstrate the extent to which they belonged to an elite rather than to mark themselves out as charismatic individuals.[48]

By analogy, this is helpful to our analysis in helping us to distinguish that part of the doctors' performance in *YLITH* that specifically conveys membership of a profession,[49] in this case, medicine, and those aspects or cases (perhaps, to an extent, Fletcher's) that are about creating a more

44 Schechner, *Between Theater*, p. 6; Gouyon, 'You Can't Make'.

45 Greenblatt, *Renaissance Self-Fashioning*.

46 Greenblatt, *Renaissance Self-Fashioning*, p. 3.

47 Burke, 'Representations'.

48 Kirwan, *Scholarly Self-Fashioning*, p. 9.

49 The notion of self-fashioning has also been deployed in the history of science, notably by Jan Golinski ('Humphry Davy') and, more recently, Heather Ellis (*Masculinity*).

singular individual performance not entirely constrained by membership of the wider group of medical doctors, bordering on the kinds of celebrity that television has particularly enabled.

It is also possible to see these performances in a further 'performative' sense that derives from the work of Judith Butler. This study of 'performativity' should not be confused with the sociology of Goffman or the anthropologically inflected theatre studies of Schechner, nor yet the new historicism of Greenblatt, as Butler has defined herself as working in a different tradition 'wandering [...] between literary theory, philosophy, and social theory'.[50] Writing in *Theatre Journal*, she comments that '[p]hilosophers rarely think about acting in the theatrical sense, but they do have a discourse of "acts" that maintains associative semantic meanings with theories of performance and acting'.[51] This discourse, in her work, develops the philosophy of John L. Austin on 'performative utterances' into a formulation that performativity is 'that reiterative power of discourse to produce the phenomena that it regulates and constrains'.[52] Austin distinguishs between 'illocutionary' speech acts that bring about certain realities, as, for example, when judgements are pronounced by a judge, and 'perlocutionary' utterances from which effects follow only when certain other kinds of conditions are in place. In relation to the latter, she argues: 'a politician may claim that "a new day has arrived" but that new day only has a chance of arriving if people take up the utterance and endeavor to make that happen. The utterance alone does not bring about the day, and yet it can set into motion a set of actions that can, under certain felicitous circumstances, bring the day around'.[53]

> With respect to illocutionary utterances, those realities brought into being depend upon a speech act, but the speech act is a reiterated form of discourse, so we would be mistaken to overvalue the subject who speaks. The judge learns what to say, and must speak in codified ways, which means that the codification and ritualization of that discourse precedes and makes possible the subject who speaks.[54]

50 Butler, 'Performative Agency', p. 148.

51 Butler, 'Gender Constitution', p. 519. The *Theatre Journal*, in the same issue, contained an editorial by Sue-Ellen Case ('Comment') clarifying its scope: 'The readership and authorship of articles far exceeds previous disciplinary bounds to include those in anthropology interested in performance, those in art history who work on performance art, and those in the other language departments who work on international theatre.'

52 Butler, *Bodies That Matter*, p. 2.

53 Butler, 'Performative Agency', pp. 147–148.

54 Butler, 'Performative Agency', p. 148.

If this is true of the illocutionary utterances of the judge, then it must also be true of the formulaic language of differential diagnosis in doctor-patient relations.[55] Furthermore, Butler's point must also be true of the perlocutionary utterances of the participants in our programme. We may say that the performative reiteration of a range of perlocutionary speech acts produces the authority of medicine.

Butler most famously developed her analysis, which can be seen to suggest a specific discursive mechanism for social constructionist accounts of reality, as a feminist account of the constitution of gender, especially in the case of women, elaborating Simone de Beauvoir's statement that 'one is not born, but, rather, *becomes* a woman'.[56] Butler's account applies equally to the constitution of masculinity:[57] it is through repeated perlocutionary utterances that the masculine characteristics that Ytreberg and Sennett align with 'bureaucrats'—namely restraint, neutrality, 'self-control', calmness, and being above-the-storm—are constituted.[58] This can help us understand the account of medical relations encoded in *Machinery for Living*, especially that the authority of medicine in the programme is not only class-based, but also gendered. This perspective enables us to separate the part of the doctors' performance that was specific to television and that which—where Butler is with Goffman—was an everyday part of the enactment of their professional role. But, whereas, with Goffman, the performances of everyday life are to be understood sociologically within the frame of theatrical performance metaphors, with Butler, we can see that television frames reiterative discursive enactments that are already the embodiment of professional activity, specifically around class, gender, and the tropes of speech and bearing that denote and reproduce medical authority.

We may also use this interpretation to speculate on the sources of the particular kinds of performance that doctors deliver on television as being in the doctor-patient consultation, in the lecture hall of a teaching hospital,

55 David Armstrong ('Doctor-Patient Relationship') has illuminated the potency of differing general practice tropes in his investigation of the patient's view.

56 Quoted in Butler, 'Gender Constitution', p. 519, emphasis in original.

57 Butler's account follows Simone de Beauvoir's citation of Merleau-Ponty's 'claims that the body is an "historical idea" rather than a "natural species"' as support to her assertion 'that "woman", and by extension, any gender is an historical situation rather than a natural fact'; Butler, 'Gender Constitution', p. 520.

58 Here, we see an echo of Steven Shapin's assertion that 'a personal identity has to be continually made, and is continually revised and remade, throughout an individual career in contingent social and cultural settings'; Shapin, *Social History of Truth*, p. 127.

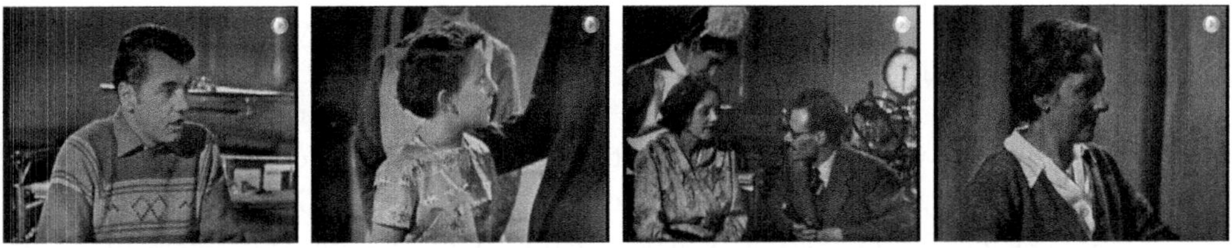

1.5. The patients in the programme: Mr. Gudor, the child Delice, Mrs. Mitchell, and Mrs. Lawless. © BBC 1958.

in the conference hall of the academic medical specialist, in the gender relations of the home. It would certainly be worth pursuing this point further, but, within the scope of this essay, there is no room.

Playing the Patient

It is significant that the patients—Mr. Gudor, the child Delice, Mrs. Mitchell, and Mrs. Lawless (Figure 1.5)—by contrast with the medical staff, *were* named in the programme. It is not clear whether these were their real or substituted names. We may suspect that the doctors' anonymity reinforces their authority, whilst the naming of the patients underlines their lower status as the objects of that authority. The inclusion of real patients on television was highly unusual for the period; their presence on live television was certainly rare, if not exactly unprecedented.[59]

Patients were present in the programme in two ways: as mute bodies—one undergoing dialysis, the other in a demonstration film of the heart-lung machine 'as it would be used in an operation'.[60] Both had been shot, contrary to Swallow's description, three weeks in advance so as to be able to feature patients as post-treatment witnesses to their treatment, which is the second way in which the viewer encounters them. The BBC Archive file for this programme is mainly silent on the recruitment of the patients to appear in either way. But there were certainly contingencies relating to the portrayal that affected their representation. Not only did the final programme differ substantially in detail from the script taken to the operating theatre,[61] but events on the ground forced changes in the programme: two of the patients whose operations were filmed in March 1958 for this programme died within

59 Anne Karpf mentions that the 1957 psychiatry series *The Hurt Mind* featured recovered patients; Karpf, *Doctoring the Media*, p. 50. It's not clear to me whether this was filmed or live.
60 Tunbridge in a link sequence between the film and the programme's final interview.
61 Reproduced in Turney, 'Disease', pp. 231, 246–251.

the week, and it was decided that it would be improper to use the footage.[62] The literal script had to be altered.

In all four of the patient sequences, we witness their performances in the same range of ways that are visible in the doctors' performances. Let us take the example of the conversation between Dr. Parsons and Mr. Gudor. Parsons's first question—'How long have you been in this country?'—marks Gudor as an immigrant. Next, he is asked when he first came to the hospital (at which point there is a cut to a medium close-up on him), and whether he remembers much about it. Then with a cut to a two-shot, Parsons explains why it's unsurprising that Gudor cannot remember; a motorcycle accident had caused skull and pelvis fractures, a concussion, cessation of normal kidney function, and partial paralysis in his right leg. This description of Gudor's medical condition is delivered via a 30-second static two-shot, whilst Gudor listens and looks around, avoiding the camera. In response to a question from Parsons, Gudor replies that he lives in Halifax. Back in two-shot, in a 40-second sequence, Parsons explains Gudor's transfer after six days to the LGI. 'By this time, his waste materials in his blood had accumulated to extremely dangerous levels, and we were able to remove these from his blood by means of the artificial kidney.' Gudor is asked how he feels now, whether he can get about, about his paralyzed leg, whether he has been discharged from the hospital in Halifax, and whether he is receiving any further treatment. He is held in a medium close-up whilst he answers the questions briefly. The interview closes with Parsons getting up, saying: 'It's very kind of you to come along tonight and to see you looking so well.' Throughout, though Gudor is the most assertive of the patients featured, it is Parsons who describes his condition and the treatments; Gudor is constrained by the format, reproducing the medical social reality of 1958, to listen whilst he is described, and to give brief, deferential answers to questions about the more prosaic aspects of the aftermath of his accident.

Similar patterns of deference are seen with Delice, Mrs. Mitchell (the one patient featured both in the insert film and in the live programme), and Mrs. Lawless. Each has their condition described, whilst sharing the shot with the doctor doing the explaining. Each is asked what they recall and how they now feel. All are deferential to the doctors, the women's diction and manner is, in each case, shy. Mrs. Lawless had undergone open-heart surgery the previous July; her interviewer is her surgeon, Geoffrey Wooler. Here again, in two-shot, Wooler gives an account of her condition and treatment as the object of his surgical practice: 'In July 1957 I operated on her using the Melrose heart-lung machine and I was able to improve the function of her mitral valve.' He asks

62 File T14/1,833, BBC Written Archive, Caversham.

her (cut to medium close-up): 'Now Mrs. Lawless, how ill were you before this operation?' She hesitates, nervously; he prompts: 'Were you very ill?' She answers that she was bedbound. She is asked 'do you feel any better now?', to which she replies briefly and deferentially, 'yes, thank you very much.' We may note that the quality of these patient performers was evident to some viewers at the time, as is clear from the audience report for the programme: 'There were occasional complaints to the effect that the introduction of patients merely "wasted time". "They contribute nothing to the programme. They all look bewildered. They slow down the pace, upset the balance and embarrass both doctors and audience", a photographer alleged.'[63]

It is possible to apply the analytical tools proposed for the doctors' performances to understand the patients' performances, too. Within the setting of the improvised studio, all of the patients are presented static and seated, whist both Parsons and McCracken move from standing to seated. The child is partially shown in a special lower-angle shot, reinforcing the doctor's greater height. Following Scannell, we may note the differential in the formality of clothing: Gudor's patterned pullover and open-necked shirt, Delice's specially purchased dress, Mrs. Mitchell's dressing gown, Mrs. Lawless's shirt and cardigan. Here, it is the contrast with the more formal dress of the medical men that begins the work of marking the patients as being of lower status than their interlocutors. We may recall here Richard Sennett's comment, quoted by Ytreberg, that '[i]n reacting to this dominance those in need can come to perceive autonomous figures as authorities'.[64]

We may safely speculate, following Goffman, that the impression the patients 'give off' conveys more to the viewer than the impression they deliberately give. In a Butlerian sense, their deference is perlocutionary, constituting objecthood to medical authority on the basis of a separately existing class differential. This class dimension combines with the power relations of gender to reinforce the observable female deference to male authority, which we may take as a product of Butlerian performativity. Following Schechner, the patients are the ones delivering their performances, but the circumstances of the performance make them 'not themselves' at the same time as it is *they* who deliver the performance. Of our interpretive frames, only the Greenblattian self-fashioning is absent, eclipsed by the patients' status as the objects of medical treatment.

63 File 9/7/33, Audience Research 1958, BBC Written Archive. Audience research worked via panels of viewers, who 'scored' the programmes, giving an 'audience appreciation' score (in this case a high 83) and qualitative data of the kind quoted here. See Silvey, *Who's Listening*.
64 Sennett, *Authority*, p. 86, quoted in Ytreberg, 'Ideal Types', p. 763.

These components of patient performance are, to an extent, products of the ways in which television was developing in the late 1950s. John Corner has written of the 1956 ITV series *Look in on London*:

> The element of class confrontation (often signalled by dress as well as by speech) tends to be made more obvious by the style of interview representation, which uses continuous question and answer sequences and extensive 'two-shot' framing to elicit and present the information rather than the variety of more oblique, post-shoot devices which might now be used in the development of occupational or personal themes.[65]

Conclusions

My intention in this essay has been to demonstrate the potency of understanding what people do in television programmes as varieties of performance, understandable using the many kinds of analytical tool that have developed under the broad heading of the 'performative turn' in the humanities and social sciences. For the purposes of the account here, the particular medical subject matter of high-tech therapeutics is not especially significant, but for the possibility that the extremity of the medical conditions necessitating their use might have served to exaggerate the class and gender relations on show. In that sense, it would be valuable to compare other medical programming from the time to check that what we see here isn't an artefact of the particular subject matter. More valuable would be to draw comparisons across time, not least because 1958 falls early in post-war society's turn to the psychological, which includes, of course, Goffman's analysis of performance and the introduction, with Michael Balint, of psychoanalytical self-consciousness into general practice.[66] In that sense, we can expect sample programmes from later decades to have called forth differing kinds of performance, just as doctor-patient relations in general have, up to a point, been affected by the social revolutions of the 1960s and, especially, their sequels in the patient activism of the Human Immunodeficiency Viruses (HIV) era and the diluted celebrity culture of the age of social media.

It would be contrary to the spirit of this essay to assume that *YLITH* could provide a transparent window onto the doctor-patient relations of the late

65 Corner, 'Interview', p. 45.

66 Balint, 'Doctor'; Armstrong, *Political Anatomy*.

1950s. All the same, it is worth noting that, of the three models articulated by Szasz and Hollender in 1956—activity-passivity, guidance-cooperation, and mutual participation—all the interactions seen in *Machinery for Living* belong in the first category, which is

> analogous to the parent-infant relationship [...] this model is not an interaction, as the person being acted upon is unable to actively contribute. The patient is regarded as helpless requiring the expert knowledge of the doctor, and treatment is commenced 'irrespective of the patient's contribution and regardless of the outcome'.[67]

Kirsten Ostherr's *Medical Visions*, in considering the 'production of the patient'—as its subtitle promises—considers in a single gaze imaging technologies and visual media, including television.[68] My concern here has been less with medicine than with television or, at least, with how television achieves its effects; how the 'grammar' of the medium, at a specific point in its development, required doctors and patients to do particular kinds of things in front of the camera by way of communication about the new capacities of high-tech medicine. The question of how performances by doctors and patients (including fictional representations) 'produced patients' is complex and elusive. Programmes such as *YLITH* must have contributed to this, but to explore how, precisely, must be the work of another essay.

Works Cited

Films, Television Programmes, and Recordings

Eye on Research, series, BBC, 1957–1962.
The Hurt Mind, produced by Andrew Miller Jones, BBC, 1957.
Look in on London, ITV, 1956.
Machinery for Living, Your Life in Their Hands 9, directed by Tom Millett (London) and Ray Lakeland (Leeds), BBC, 1958.
Monitor, BBC1, 1958–1965.
Panorama, BBC1, 1953–.
A Question of Science, BBC, ca.1955–.
Your Life in Their Hands (*YLITH*), BBC, 1958–1964, 1980–1986.

67 Szasz and Hollender, 'Contribution', p. 60, quoted in Kaba and Sooriakumaran, 'Evolution'.
68 Ostherr, *Medical Visions*.

Books and Articles

Akrich, Madeleine, 'The De-Scription of Technical Objects', in *Shaping Technology/ Building Society: Studies in Sociotechnical Change*, ed. by Wiebe E. Bijker and John Law, trans. by Geoffrey Bowker (Cambridge, MA: MIT Press, 2003), pp. 205–224.

Armstrong, David, 'The Doctor-Patient Relationship: 1930–80', in *The Problem of Medical Knowledge: Examining the Social Construction of Medicine*, ed. by Peter Wright and Andrew Treacher (Edinburgh: Edinburgh University Press, 1982), pp. 109–122.

Armstrong, David, *Political Anatomy of the Body: Medical Knowledge in Britain in the Twentieth Century* (Cambridge: Cambridge University Press, 1983).

Balint, Michael, 'The Doctor, His Patient, and the Illness', *The Lancet*, 265, 6866 (2 April 1955), pp. 683–688, doi:10.1016/S0140-6736(55)91061-8.

Boon, Tim[othy], 'Formal Conventions in British Science Television, 1955–1965', *Actes d'Història de La Ciència i de La Tècnica*, 7 (2014), pp. 51–69, doi:10.2436/20.2006.01.184.

Boon, Timothy, 'Medical Film and Television: An Alternative Path to the Cultures of Bio-Medicine', in *The Oxford Handbook of the History of Medicine*, ed. by Mark Jackson (Oxford: Oxford University Press, 2011), pp. 617–634.

Boon, Timothy, '"The Televising of Science Is a Process of Television": Establishing Horizon, 1962–1967', *British Journal for the History of Science*, 48, 1 (March 2015), pp. 87–121, doi:10.1017/S0007087414000405.

Booth, Christopher, 'Obituary: Professor Charles Fletcher', *The Independent*, 23 December 1995, http://www.independent.co.uk/news/people/obituary-professor-charles-fletcher-1527104.html, accessed 30 December 2017.

Burke, Peter, 'Representations of the Self from Petrarch to Descartes', in *Rewriting the Self: Histories from the Renaissance to the Present*, ed. by Roy Porter (London: Routledge, 1997), pp. 17–28.

Brand, Graham, and Paddy Scannell, 'Talk, Identity and Performance: The Tony Blackburn Show', in *Broadcast Talk*, ed. by Paddy Scannell (London: SAGE, 1991), pp. 201–226.

Butler, Judith, *Bodies That Matter: On the Discursive Limits of 'Sex'* (New York: Routledge, 1993).

Butler, Judith, 'Performative Acts and Gender Constitution: An Essay in Phenomenology and Feminist Theory', *Theatre Journal*, 40, 4 (December 1988), pp. 519–531, doi:10.2307/3207893.

Butler, Judith, 'Performative Agency', *Journal of Cultural Economy*, 3, 2 (July 2010), pp. 147–161, doi:10.1080/17530350.2010.494117.

Case, Sue-Ellen, 'Comment', *Theatre Journal*, 40, 4 (December 1988), http://www.jstor.org/stable/3207887.

Corner, John, 'The Interview as Social Encounter', in *Broadcast Talk*, ed. by Paddy Scannell (London: SAGE, 1991), pp. 31–47.

'Disease Education by the B.B.C.', *British Medical Journal*, 1, 5067 (15 February 1958), pp. 388–389, doi:10.1136/bmj.1.5067.388-a.
Ellis, Heather, *Masculinity and Science in Britain, 1831–1918* (London: Palgrave Macmillan, 2017).
Emigh, John, 'Liminal Richard: Approaches to Performance Studies', in *The Rise of Performance Studies: Rethinking Richard Schechner's Broad Spectrum*, ed. by James M. Harding and Cindy Rosenthal (London: Palgrave Macmillan, 2011), pp. 162–176.
Goffman, Erving, *The Presentation of Self in Everyday Life*, repr. ed. (London: Penguin, 1990).
Golinski, Jan, 'Humphry Davy: The Experimental Self', *Eighteenth-Century Studies*, 45, 1 (Fall 2011), pp. 15–28, https://www.jstor.org/stable/41301612.
Gouyon, Jean-Baptiste. '"You Can't Make a Film About Mice Just by Going Out into a Meadow and Looking at Mice': Staging as Knowledge Production in Natural History Film-Making', in *Staging Science—Scientific Performance on Street, Stage and Screen*, ed. by Martin Willis (London: Palgrave Macmillan, 2016), pp. 83–103.
Greenblatt, Stephen, *Renaissance Self-Fashioning: From More to Shakespeare: With a New Preface* (Chicago: University of Chicago Press, 2005).
Jordanova, Ludmilla, *Defining Features: Scientific and Medical Portraits, 1660–2000* (London: Reaktion Books, 2000).
Kaba, R., and P. Sooriakumaran. 'The Evolution of the Doctor-Patient Relationship', *International Journal of Surgery*, 5, 1 (February 2007), pp. 57–65, doi:10.1016/j.ijsu.2006.01.005.
Karpf, Anne, *Doctoring the Media: The Reporting of Health and Medicine* (London: Routledge, 1988).
Kirwan, Richard, ed., *Scholarly Self-Fashioning and Community in the Early Modern University* (Farnham: Ashgate, 2013).
Lawrence, Christopher, 'Medical Minds, Surgical Bodies: Corporeality and the Doctors', in *Science Incarnate: Historical Embodiments of Natural Knowledge*, ed. by Christopher Lawrence and Steven Shapin (Chicago: University of Chicago Press, 1998), pp. 156–201.
Levinson, Stephen C., *Pragmatics* (Cambridge: Cambridge University Press, 1983).
Licoppe, Christian, 'The "Performative Turn" in Science and Technology Studies', *Journal of Cultural Economy*, 3, 2 (July 2010), pp. 181–188, doi:10.1080/17530350.2010.494122.
Long, Vicky, *Destigmatising Mental Illness?: Professional Politics and Public Education in Britain, 1870–1970* (Manchester: Manchester University Press, 2015).
Loughlin, Kelly, '"Your Life in Their Hands": The Context of a Medical-Media Controversy', *Media History*, 6, 2 (2000), pp. 177–188, doi:10.1080/13688800020008628.
Mol, Annemarie, 'Ontological Politics: A Word and Some Questions', *Sociological Review*, 47, 1 suppl. (May 1999), pp. 74–89, doi:10.1111/j.1467-954X.1999.tb03483.x.

Neil, 'Alfred Wurmser', *The Lost Continent: Exploring the Art and History of British Animation*, 25 November 2011, http://ukanimation.blogspot.com/2011/11/alfred-wurmser.html, accessed 23 July 2018.

Ostherr, Kirsten, *Medical Visions: Producing the Patient through Film, Television, and Imaging Technologies* (Oxford: Oxford University Press, 2013).

Scannell, Paddy, 'Introduction: The Relevance of Talk', in *Broadcast Talk*, ed. by Paddy Scannell (London: SAGE, 1991), pp. 1–13.

Schechner, Richard, *Between Theater and Anthropology* (Philadelphia: University of Pennsylvania Press, 1985).

Schechner, Richard, *Performed Imaginaries* (London: Routledge, 2015).

Sennett, Richard, *Authority* (New York: Knopf, 1980).

Shapin, Steven, *A Social History of Truth: Civility and Science in Seventeenth-Century England*, 2nd ed. (Chicago: University of Chicago Press, 1995).

Silvey, Robert, *Who's Listening: The Story of BBC Audience Research* (London: Allen and Unwin, 1974).

Swallow, Norman, *Factual Television* (London: Focal Press, 1966).

Szasz, Thomas S., and Marc H. Hollender, 'A Contribution to the Philosophy of Medicine: The Basic Models of the Doctor-Patient Relationship', *AMA Archives of Internal Medicine*, 97, 5 (May 1956), pp. 585–592, doi:10.1001/archinte.1956.00250230079008.

Turney, John, 'A Disease and Its Device: The Introduction of Dialysis for Acute Renal Failure, with Particular Reference to Leeds, UK, c.1945–c.2000' (PhD diss., University of Manchester, 2013).

Winkin, Yves, and Wendy Leeds-Hurwitz. *Erving Goffman: A Critical Introduction to Media and Communication Theory* (New York: Lang, 2013).

Ytreberg, Espen, 'Ideal Types in Public Service Television: Paternalists and Bureaucrats, Charismatics and Avant-Gardists', *Media Culture and Society*, 24, 6 (2002), pp. 759–774, doi:10.1177/016344370202400602.

About the Author

Tim Boon, Head of Research & Public History for the Science Museum Group, is a historian and curator of the public culture of science. His published research—including the books *Films of Fact* (2008) and *Material Culture and Electronic Sound* (co-edited with Frode Weium, 2013) as well as more than 50 papers—is mainly concerned with the history of science in documentary films, television, museums, and, latterly, music.
Contact details: Tim.Boon@ScienceMuseum.ac.uk

2. The BBC's *Children in Need* Telethon: The Currencies of Compassion

Karen Lury

Abstract

This chapter illustrates how the BBC's *Children in Need* telethon is informed and legitimated by different currency models as part of its aesthetic strategy. It demonstrates how these *televisual* currencies may be directly aligned with other kinds of *medical* currency models emerging within the economy of the UK's National Health Service. Through close textual analysis of the programme and a related analysis of medical currency models proposed and piloted in relation to the NHS, it is argued that the 'aestheticization' of currency models provided by the programme reflects an ideological shift in the representation of medical care on public service television, in line with the ideology of neoliberalism and the incremental colonization of 'financialization' into all aspects of contemporary society.

Keywords: telethon; financialization; currency models; charity; child/children; textual analysis; public service television; campaign film; *Children in Need*

What follows is a brief description of a fifteen-minute sequence from the live broadcast of the *Children in Need* telethon, first transmitted at approximately 9.30 p.m. on British Broadcasting Corporation 1 (BBC1) on Friday 13 November 2015. This is an annual broadcast for the benefit of children who are ill, disabled, or living in poverty.

The colours in the television studio theatre are luminous—the predominant colour scheme is made up of purples, pink, and gold—and, at the start of this sequence, the television camera pans rapidly in, over a seated, cheering audience, to focus in on the presenters, Dermot O'Leary and Fearne

Bonah, C. and A. Laukötter (eds.), *Body, Capital, and Screens: Visual Media and the Healthy Self in the 20th Century*. Taylor & Francis Group, 2020
DOI 10.5117/9789462988293_CH02

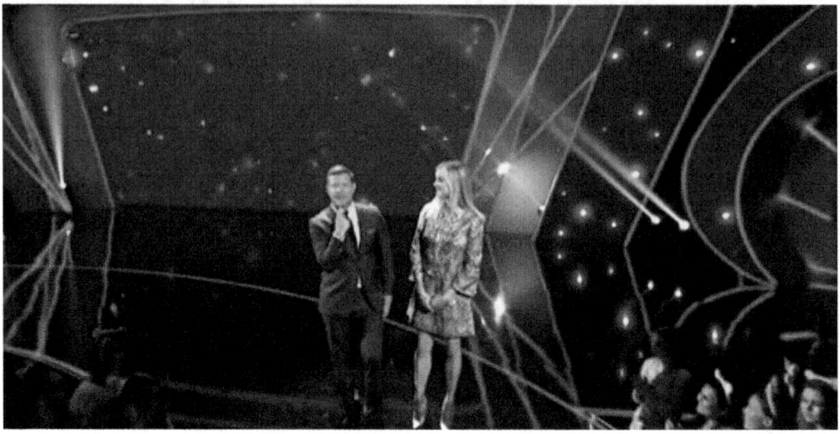

2.1. Dermot O'Leary and Fearne Cotton, *Children in Need*, 13 November 2015, BBC1.

Cotton (Figure 2.1).[1] They stand at the front of the stage, speaking both to the in-studio audience and the viewing audience at home. Framed by two large video screens, they are dressed formally—Dermot in a designer leisure suit and Fearne in a sparkly special occasion dress. Pausing to make a short, improvised joke in which they poke gentle fun at the presenter of the previous live segment, the actor Shane Richie, Dermot and Fearne then direct the viewers' attention to the next segment, a live outside broadcast.[2] In this heavily trailed stunt, the BBC's Radio 1 presenter, Scott Mills, will abseil from the top of the *ArcelorMitall* Orbit—a huge, red, metal structure, designed by Anish Kapoor, and one of the few landmarks remaining from the London 2012 Summer Olympics. Supported by another well-known children's television presenter and 'action woman', Helen Skelton, Mills successfully completes the abseil.[3] The event culminates with cheers from a small crowd of spectators at the scene and an explosion of fireworks as Mills reaches

1 Dermot is a television presenter no doubt familiar to millions from the United Kingdom's version of *The X-Factor* and, previously, the reality show, *Big Brother*. Fearne Cotton has been on British television since she was a teenager, initially presenting *The Disney Club* on the commercial channel Good Morning Television (GMTV) and later presenting the BBC's now-defunct popular music programme, *Top of the Pops*.

2 Richie, who is well known on British television as both an actor and presenter, had been fronting celebrity interviews from the 'Queen Vic'—the fictional public house well known from its location within the heart of Albert Square and the 'home' of the BBC's long-running soap opera *Eastenders*. In the soap opera, the Queen Vic pub was once owned and run by Richie's character, 'Alfie Moon'.

3 Skelton is well known in the UK context from her appearance on the BBC's long-running children's show *Blue Peter* and is regarded commonly as an action woman for her successful completion of various adventurous stunts, some of which were for another charity telethon also

the ground. The tension and excitement that is generated for the television audience by this stunt is amplified by the added (non-diegetic) sound of tense, rhythmic music and the rapid cutting of a series of close-up shots of Scott's open-eyed expressions of fear, interspersed with an additional series of quick cut-aways to Skelton, who offers breathless and enthusiastic support. Throughout the stunt, a ribbon videographic runs across the bottom of the television screen, urging viewers to 'Support Scott' by donating money to Children in Need. Once the abseil is completed, the programme returns to the studio, with both Dermot and Fearne warmly congratulating Mills for his bravery and applauding his endeavour as a significant part of the evening's fundraising. The next segment is then introduced by both presenters who are now framed in a mid, rather than long shot, and who stand directly in front of one of the video screens. While suggesting that the next film is 'incredibly sad', they urge viewers 'to please stay with us' as the well-known Scottish actor David Tennant is about to introduce us to an 'incredible couple' who have suffered a terrible loss. This introduction then leads to a short campaign film, made about Robin House—a children's hospice in Scotland—which details the medical history and deaths of two young children, although it is the support offered by the hospice to their parents that is the focus of the film. When we return to the television studio, Dermot is standing alone by a video screen with his arms crossed and his hand to his mouth. His voice cracks with emotion when he states that, as he was only asked 'at the last minute' to stand in for the regular presenter of the telethon, this means that he—like the television viewer—'had not seen the film until this evening' and that he is seeing these scenes 'as you see them at home'. Seemingly on the verge of tears, he once more commends the 'incredible couple' featured in the film for their bravery, and he urges the viewing audience, once again, to donate, reading out the direct telephone line and the internet address for charitable donations, which are now displayed on the screen behind him (Figure 2.2). He then directly hands over to Fearne, who is standing some distance away, at the centre of the stage. At first, she speaks in a serious tone, reflecting the intense emotion previously expressed by Dermot. However, as she continues and introduces the next segment, which will bring into the studio the celebrities and children involved in another extended stunt—the 'Rikshaw Challenge'—she allows the excitement in her voice to overcome her initial sombre tones, and her intonation rises when she warmly introduces another pre-recorded video sequence, in which each of the 'inspirational'

broadcast by the BBC *Sports Relief*. This included a 150-metre tightrope walk between chimneys at London's Battersea power station in 2011.

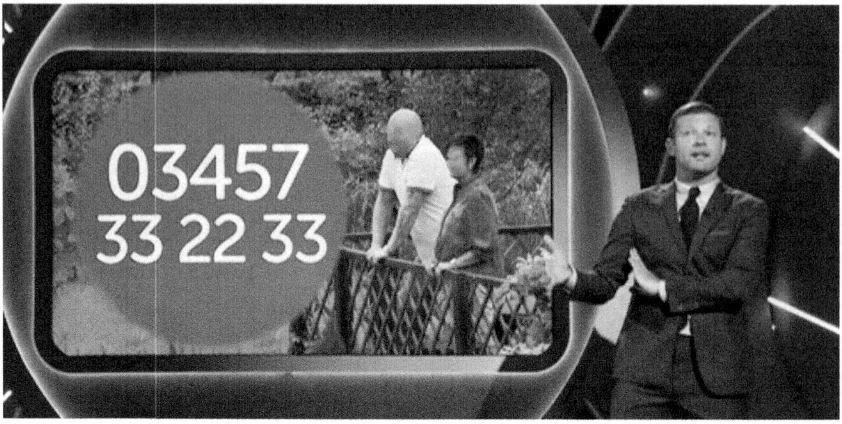

2.2. Dermot O'Leary, *Children in Need*, 13 November 2015, BBC1.

young riders involved in the challenge are identified, all of whom have, she observes, previously been supported by projects 'funded by Children in Need'.

This sequence is not exceptional. As a television broadcast, the programme, which has been running for over 35 years, is both familiar and predictable for British audiences, and, as such, it is frequently regarded by critics and perhaps by many of the television audience as banal. Yet, its incorporation of the live and recorded, the serious and silly, and the necessary emotional turbulence this engenders, actually suggests this is a programme of extraordinary complexity. It is certainly controversial, as this conflicted response from a reviewer for the *The Guardian* newspaper suggests:

> Children in Need might be hard to sit through. Usually that's the whole point—as a television programme, it exists purely to destabilise you with such an unrelenting volley of conflicting emotions that you end up flinging money at it in a kind of sobbing fugue state.[4]

Children in Need—as its title suggests—provides funds for a variety of different children's charities, many of which are involved in the care and support of severely ill children and their families. Originating in 1927, via an annual radio appeal, it was initially broadcast by the BBC on Christmas Day. Christmas, of course, represented a suitably emotive and appropriate time for such an appeal. It is a particularly resonant period within the British context, as it is so closely aligned with the Dickensian framing of

4 Heritage, 'Children in Need'.

Christmas as a time for charity and inclusive good deeds. The figure of 'Tiny Tim' from the Dickens's novella *A Christmas Carol* (1843), looms large in the popular imagination, as a concrete representation of the 'deserving sick' and the poignant figure of the plucky, yet tragically disabled child. From the 1970s, the appeal was led by the BBC's hugely popular radio and television personality, Sir Terry Wogan. A move to a telethon format in 1980 seems to have been, in part, a response to the transmission of a successful charity telethon from a rival independent broadcaster within the London area, Thames Television.[5] *Children in Need* is now usually scheduled by the BBC for the third Friday in November—so, whilst it is no longer scheduled on Christmas day itself, its place in the calendar means that it has become established as a kind of secular advent to the BBC's Christmas season of television programming.[6]

The *Children in Need* programme, like other telethons, is an evening-long event, incorporating a variety of celebrity sketches and musical performances. Its format differs slightly from other telethons as it devotes a lot of screen time to illustrating the fundraising efforts of the 'great British public'[7] as well as focussing on a variety of stunts associated with different BBC programmes (e.g. *The One Show*'s 'Rikshaw Challenge') and radio channels (e.g. Scott Mills's abseil and BBC Radio 2's celebrity auctions.) These fundraising events—whether by celebrities or 'ordinary people'—are often humorous in nature, involving dressing up, or may otherwise be regarded as 'silly' (such as the waxing of male chest and leg hair, or when BBC newscasters attempt a song and dance routine). Alternatively, stunts can

5 North American television has also been broadcasting charity telethons since the 1960s, the best known of which is the Muscular Dystrophy Association (MDA) telethon presented by the comedian Jerry Lewis. For more on the US version of the charity telethon, see Longmore, *Telethons*.

6 Wogan presented the BBC's telethon for 35 years but, in 2015, he was forced to pull out at short notice due to ill health, and Dermot O'Leary was the main host for that year. Wogan died in January 2016 and, from November 2016, *Children in Need* has presented a 'fundraiser of the year award' in Wogan's name. Now led by another experienced and popular presenter/broadcaster, Graham Norton, the live programme and associated events continue to raise large amounts of money—over £50 million in 2017.

7 The 'great British public' is a commonly used term relating to national identity; frequently employed by British television presenters and politicians, it refers to the notion that, in times of crisis, the 'British public' will act together for the greater good. In popular memory, this is largely associated with the apparent response to the 'Blitz' bombing of cities in the Second World War. In recent tabloid newspaper reporting, the 'great British public' has re-merged as a way of eulogizing the public's response to terrorist events. An amusing analysis of the term is presented by the British comedian David Mitchell: https://www.youtube.com/watch?v=SdVnEbHZjzo, accessed 24 July 2018.

be endurance- or challenge-orientated, including dares (parachute jumps, abseils), sponsored walks, runs, or silences. In many of these activities, fundraising is associated with exhibiting or testing the fundraiser's own body, so that the activity of the fundraiser and, by implication, the television audience, is not simply to donate money but to make themselves (temporarily) exceptional, visible, and active. Such exhibitionism is, of course, appropriate for a charity that needs to secure content that is entertaining, but, in a more complicated sense, the fundraisers' bodily alignment with the 'vulnerable bodies' of the 'children in need' is also significant. Children who are to be recipients of the donations may be seen to be exceptional through their visible disabilities and medical histories; equally, they may be understood to represent endurance or face significant challenges through their suffering, whether this is a result of accident, illness, or economic deprivation. As a result of their fundraising exertions, able-bodied children and adult fundraisers may also experience and exhibit either (temporary) exceptionality or undergo challenges and feats of endurance, suggesting that the donors and recipients of the charity are, at least briefly, aligned.[8] Indeed, the emphasis on participation and the relationship between 'us' (donors) and 'them' (as recipients) has become increasingly blurred by the inclusion of disabled children who participate in the 'Rikshaw Challenge' and, from 2016, by the presence of Ade Adepitan, a television personality and Paralympic sportsperson, as one of the co-presenters for the in-studio broadcast. While the increasing visibility and participation of disabled presenters and children in the broadcast may be seen positively (in terms of representation and agency) it nonetheless obscures the self-exploitation inherent to the programme. From this perspective, the programme presents a rather unfortunate coincidence in which disabled or 'needy' children provide their labour—free of charge—to raise funds they themselves need. As such, they are not only representatives of the deserving poor or sick ('Tiny Tims') but are asked to perform or establish their (monetary) value to the television audience.

Despite its wide-ranging and, frankly, rather peculiar content, in the context of UK public-service broadcasting, *Children in Need* is as much

8 The alignment of the fundraisers' and recipients' bodies is similar to the 'productive turn' described by Timm Knudsen and Stage in *Global Media*. However, aspects of their argument suggest that that this 'productive turn' is largely beneficial for those involved. As will become evident, I am less certain that these 'new constellations' really offer new possibilities and agree with their more cautious conclusion that 'the accusations of narcissism that are levelled at all forms of charity are not refuted once and for all by the productive turn'; Timm Knudsen and Stage, *Global Media*, p. 85.

a part of the annual British 'broadcast calendar' as the Wimbledon Tennis Championships or the opening of Parliament. In terms of charitable programming in the UK, it is similar to, and, in terms of celebrity activity and international profile, possibly overshadowed by other charity broadcasts such as *Comic Relief*.[9] Channel 4 has also, since 2012, screened another regular telethon, *Stand Up to Cancer*.[10] *Children in Need* therefore appears as one among several different kinds of charity programmes on British television. It differs from other British telethons, in part, because of its longevity—*Comic Relief* has only been running biannually since 1985 and *Stand Up To Cancer* had its first broadcast in 2012—but it is also unique in the exclusive focus on children and its provision of funds only for children from the UK. The appeal to the viewer in terms of empathy and compassion is therefore not in relation to the 'distant other' or the starving child familiar from a range of international charity appeals, nor does it ask for medical research funding, which is the primary focus of *Stand Up to Cancer*.[11] Rather, the *Children in Need* (previously *Children in Need of Help*) appeals for British children who are impoverished, or who may be suffering from a range of medical or psychological challenges, including bereavement, mental illness, physical disability, or serious life-limiting conditions. The complex needs of the children and the various services they are dependent on mean that many of the children are recipients, not just of charitable support, but a variety of different medical services. The charity and the broadcast itself are therefore implicated in the complex evolution of the British care system and related medical provision offered by the UK's National Health Service (NHS).

The purpose of this chapter is to illustrate how the programme is informed and legitimated by different currency models and to demonstrate how these televisual currencies may be directly aligned with other kinds of currency models emerging within the economy of the NHS. The use of the term currency here adapts contemporary sociological theories, which argue that everyday life is now increasingly determined by the way in which social and emotional practices—in this instance, medical care, sentimental

9 *Comic Relief* is a private charity, founded in 1985 by the British film-maker and writer Richard Curtis, as a response to the huge success of *Band Aid/Live Aid* in 1984/1985. While Comic Relief and its associated 'sister charity' *Sports Relief* are both regularly broadcast on the BBC they—unlike *Children in Need*—are not part of the BBC itself. While both *Comic Relief* and *Sports Relief* provide some funding for UK charities and groups, much of the funding is focussed, like *Band Aid/Live Aid*, on international concerns. For more information, see their website https://www.comicrelief.com, accessed 25 July 2018.

10 For more on *Stand Up to Cancer*, see Charlesworth, 'Stand Up to Cancer'.

11 In relation to the concept of the 'distant other', see Boltanski, *Distant Suffering*.

valuation, and philanthropy—are being assigned numerical values, and, in a related manner, embedded into the processes of 'financialization'. As Catherine Happer explains, the concept of financialization not only describes the current political economy as shaped by financial markets, but it also 'incorporates an emphasis on the "naturalisation" of finance and [...] refers to the way in which aspects of everyday experience are quantified and interpreted in financial terms'.[12]

In any national context, medical care obviously depends upon financial systems and budgets in order to operate: However, my concern here is the way in which the UK's system—the NHS—whose constitution confirms that the system is comprehensive and, in most instances, 'free at the point of use', increasingly organizes and legitimates budgetary decision-making in relation to the principles of financialization. The 'naturalization' of financialization that Happer refers to is an ideological shift within the larger context of neoliberalism and is, I suggest, unsurprisingly mirrored in different aspects of the television broadcast which has had long-term and substantial links both to a range of different private charities and to the NHS itself. Whilst I am not claiming that there is deliberate collusion here, what could be understood as the programme's 'aestheticization' of financialization reflects an ideological shift that may have real consequences for the British public's perception as to how and why decisions are legitimated in relation to the resources made available for a range of medical and social needs.

There are a variety of ways in which currency models operate both within and alongside the broadcast.

1. Television viewers' donations of money are the most explicit way in which currency (in the form of pounds donated and raised) is made visible. As is customary in the telethon, throughout the evening, these donations are represented by a running total—a 'totalizer'—that is displayed and announced at key points in the programme. The totalizer establishes that the stunts and skits produced by celebrities and ordinary people are effectively paid for—the labour of the participants is given a specific and visible monetary value (Figure 2.3).[13]

12 Happer, 'Financialization', p. 438.

13 This aspect of the programme is perhaps not as explicit now as it was in the earlier years of the programme's history. However, the crude nature of this exchange can be seen in a stunt that was replayed in the *Children in Need: 50 Greatest Moments*—a special programme of highlights from the different broadcasts that was screened in 2010 to celebrate the show's 30th anniversary. In the clip, from 1983—in a stunt that is framed as Wogan's particular 'favourite'—Joanna Lumley (a well-known British actor/presenter) volunteers to 'take her dress off' if money is pledged to

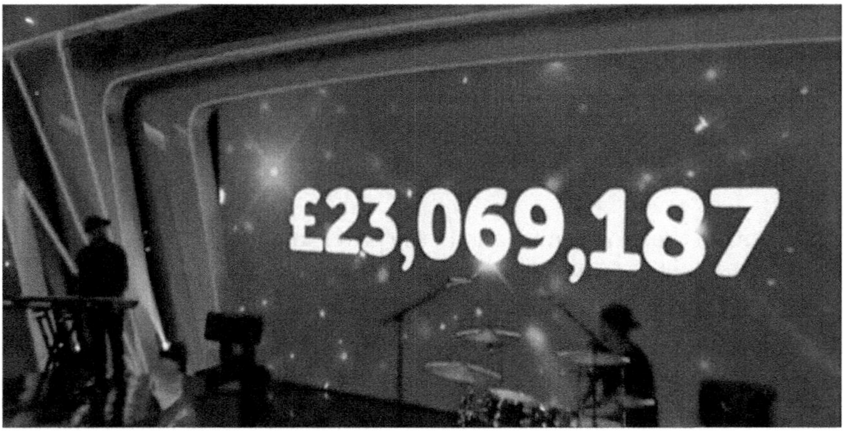

2.3. The 'Totalizer', *Children in Need*, 13 November 2015, BBC1.

2. Elsewhere within the programme, a currency of sorts can also be recognized as the manifestation of the (usually less than explicit) contract between the BBC and its national audience, in which the illusion of a 'nation'—a holistic, caring entity—is self-consciously generated and sustained by the programme's continued attempts to include as many different regions and individuals as possible. This is significant because it allows the BBC not only to defend and sustain the concept of 'one nation', but also to align this concept, and thus the BBC, with the NHS as a highly valued institution and as part of the make-up of a British national identity.[14]
3. Within the campaign films, the repetition of a familiar narrative structure establishes that there is another kind of currency at work in the programme. Each film organizes segmented instances of heightened emotional content to derive a specific monetary response (a donation) from the viewing audience. As I will explain, these moments within the films may be directly compared to Laura Grindstaff's conception of the 'money shot' in other genres of film and television.[15]
4. Another relevant model of currency exists outside the broadcast itself, and relates to financial planning within the NHS. This currency is

the programme. As the clip later reveals, enough money appears to be donated and she duly strips to her underwear on camera.

14 The sacrosanct status of the NHS within British national identity is very much a focus of contemporary media coverage, and its place within a shared 'national fantasy' was also made evident by its presence in the opening ceremony for the 2012 Olympic Games. See Bryant, 'National Art'.

15 See Grindstaff, *Money Shot.*

> dependent on the recorded data of individual medical needs, which are then rationalized and calculated as numerical values ('health care units'). These 'health care units' as currency may then be employed as a way to forecast and rationalize healthcare funding for patients, including children with life-limiting conditions.

Thus, within the programme and in the provision of healthcare in the UK, these different kinds of currency establish an economy through which the dying and deaths of children may be assigned a specific monetary value. In effect, representations of dying and dead children function for these currencies as their 'gold standard'.[16]

The BBC's Currency: One Nation = One BBC

The Children in Need charity's staff are BBC employees but they are not programme makers. Whether the BBC's production teams who make the campaign films, or who supervise the live broadcast at the various regional centres, are paid for their labour is undisclosed. However, the charity's website states clearly that the celebrities and professional hosts are not paid for their work, although the programme must provide an opportunity to raise profiles and publicize forthcoming films, programmes, and music. As an umbrella organization, Children in Need does not run any charitable activities itself; rather, it awards grants and support to a wide range of other smaller charities across the UK, in the 'name of the BBC'. The charity thus has a national status but allocates money locally. In that sense, it reflects the broadcasting model of the BBC itself. It offers a specific example of how local provision (such as television for regional audiences) may be embedded in a national broadcast, asking audience members to recognize themselves as both 'local' and 'national'. As a public-service broadcaster, the BBC is still currently funded by a universal licence fee paid by everyone in the UK who accesses BBC content either through television screens or via digital platforms. This means that, in order to sustain its financial position, the BBC must constantly negotiate and reaffirm its position and value as a *national* broadcaster but, at the same time, remain sensitive to diversity and the various individuals within the regions and nations that make up its audience.

16 The 'gold standard' refers to the now-abandoned financial system through which individual currencies were valued—or guaranteed—in relation to each other via the price of gold.

In a 1986 report on the programme (commissioned by the BBC's Director of Public Affairs), the authors, Geoff Buck and Johnny Wilkinson, make two key comments that reinforce how this mixture of the local and national makes the programme particularly significant for the BBC. Commenting on the benefits for the BBC, they reflect on the way in which the programme enables the BBC to bring the 'network' (that is the London centre of operations) and the regions and 'nations' (BBC Wales, Scotland, and Northern Ireland) together, suggesting: 'It was indeed an occasion in which all parts of the BBC domestically were involved, and normal territorial distinctions were forgotten.'[17]

At the same time as bringing the various parts of the BBC together, the report argues that the programme also serves as a live event that could bring together the viewing audience as a national community—perhaps suggesting it was an occasion in the British context that could only be matched by a royal wedding. The conclusion of the Director of Public Affairs (DPA) report suggests:

> The importance of the appeal from a social point of view cannot be overestimated. People throughout Britain, who do not belong to a church, a political party, or a national or local organisation, can get involved and identify with it as individuals and feel part of a national community.[18]

This national community is still very much evoked in the contemporary programme—for example, a regular stunt is the children's choir, in which groups of children across the United Kingdom are brought together at different regional production centres and sing together 'live' so that one song bridges the transition to the different children at different locations across the various parts of the country—from Wales, to Scotland, to the North East and Northern Ireland. The apparent technological and operational challenge this presents, with its successful execution clearly dependent on all the different production personnel in the different BBC regions working together, pays dividends both for the reputation of the BBC—revealing it to be a national and expert broadcaster—as well as for the community-building aspect of the programme itself.[19]

17 Buck and Wilkinson, 'Report', p. 5.

18 Buck and Wilkinson, 'Report', p. 3.

19 This practice—an attempt by the BBC to construct an imaginary 'national community'—is obviously very much in line with Benedict Anderson's notion of the nation as an 'imagined community'; see Anderson, *Imagined Communities*.

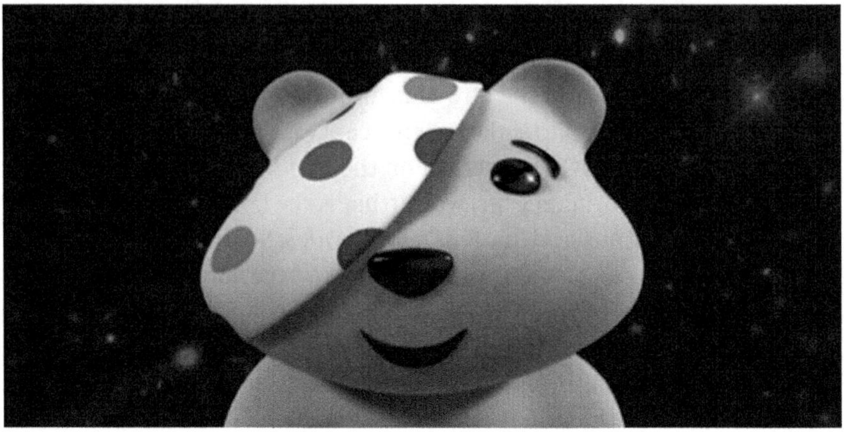

2.4. Pudsey, *Children in Need*, 13 November 2015, BBC1.

Yet, in practice, the relationship between the network and regions and nations has often been more problematic. In the BBC Archives, a considerable number of papers demonstrate the way in which other parts of the BBC felt that they were excluded or marginalized by the demands of the producers in London.

In a letter to Keith Clements, who was then Head of Broadcasting at the BBC, John Adams, the Scottish producer of *Children in Need* in 1990, comments on the mismanagement of what was clearly meant to be a nationally unifying stunt—a series of different instances in which the 'Pudsey special' (Figure 2.4), a train travelling over the course of one day, beginning in Edinburgh (Scotland) to Cardiff (Wales) would climax with the arrival of the train at Paddington in London in the evening.[20]

> My AFM (Assistant Floor Manager) tells me that it took as much effort to organise the departure of the train and its brief stop in Edinburgh as it did to organise the rest of the events that evening. She and many others worked 21 ½ hours that day beginning at 05.30. But should we have asked severely disabled kids to get out of their beds at 04.30 just to get on a train to be paraded before the camera? We certainly got a good one-and-half minute piece of it which we showed early in the evening.

20 'Pudsey'—a yellow teddy bear—has been the trademark 'mascot' of the charity since the mid 1980s. He can be seen throughout the programme either as someone dressed in a 'Pudsey' costume or as an animated character. Different kinds of Pudsey merchandise—T-shirts, headbands, and small teddy bears—are also available from October each year in stores around the UK and online.

> The failure, however, of the arrangements to send a package from the train PSC crew from Cardiff down the line to London meant that the rest of the UK did not see the start or the passage of the train, only its arrival in Paddington. And it was the arrival of the train that threw the 22.45 opt out; so, I think questions have to be asked about the wisdom of that whole enterprise.[21]

Initially, as this quotation suggests (with its reference to the 'opt out' meaning a return to the BBC Scotland live broadcast at 22.45), earlier versions of the broadcast programme incorporated extensive live coverage from what might be understood as 'the national within the national' broadcasters (such as Wales, Northern Ireland, and Scotland but not smaller regions such as the Midlands). In Scotland, the majority of the broadcast time for the first 30 years of the programme's history was managed locally, with a return to the 'network' (or the London studio) only occurring for high-profile celebrity performances and sketches. However, as the quote above suggests, this was difficult to manage and caused increased friction, rather than enhancing the relationship between the BBC's 'territories'. It is perhaps not surprising that, from 2010, the programme reverted to a model in which the majority of the programme is broadcast and managed from London, with shorter segments produced by its regions/nations. Thus, despite the programme's attempt to be 'inclusive' and incorporate activities across the nation, production constraints mean that the London operation remains dominant, going against the grain of the BBC's recent attempts to diversify and 'spread' its production base.[22] In recent programmes, such as the 2015 broadcast, attempts to re-establish some sense of this diversity were reflected in the way in which aerial shots were used in interstitial sequences to emphasize how different towns and regions are all included in the fundraising activity (Figure 2.5).

Despite the ultimate dominance of the London-based production studio and personnel, the programme continues to present a very careful managing and orchestration of diversity, locality, and identity in terms of image and representation. In doing so, it establishes the illusion of a *national* caring community, which simultaneously sustains the illusion of a *national* viewing audience. This is particularly useful to the BBC within a contemporary

21 Letter from Johan Adams to Keith Clements (1 January 1990), *BBC Written Archives' Centre*, archive ref: SC140/1041/1 (26348109).

22 For example, the BBC moved its production of Sports, Children's, and Breakfast television to Salford (near Manchester) in 2011.

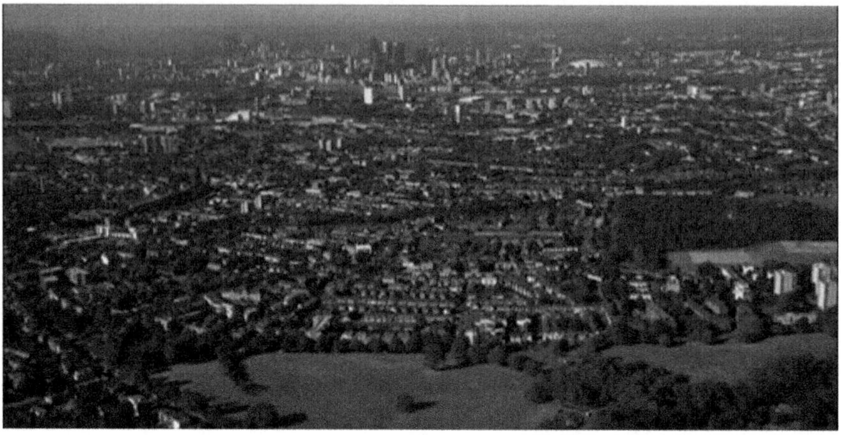

2.5. 'From Morecambe to Milton Keynes', image from interstitial sequence, *Children in Need*, 13 November 2015, BBC1.

context in which television programming and audiences are increasingly spread across numerous digital platforms and independent providers. The continuing success of the programme sustains an illusory national audience, and thereby shores up the currency that underpins the financial basis for the BBC.

Confirming the BBC as a national institution promotes its strong alliance with what is often regarded as its sister institution, the UK's National Health Service. And, like the BBC, while the NHS is still attempting to provide universal provision for all, it offers quite different kinds of medical care locally and intra-nationally. For example, a recent focus of newspaper headlines has been the emergence of what has been called a 'postcode lottery'—a term referring to the fact that certain kinds of care may only be offered in particular parts of the country.[23] As the development and increasing utilization of a 'health care currency' demonstrates, funding for particular kinds of health provision are rationalized to local, and increasingly personalized, models of healthcare funding. In relation to *Children in Need*, the national audience conjured into existence via the broadcast generates the illusion of a national community and a nation state, which allocates funding on the basis of 'need'. This operates within a particular context in which the needs of the child—because of the child's apparently sacrosanct status in current political and social discourses—comfortably supersedes the needs of other (here invisible) individuals, such as the elderly, even though, in many instances, the entanglement of intergenerational care,

23 See, for example, Press Association, 'Postcode Lottery'.

for both young children and ageing (grand)parents, is a central aspect of many families' experiences.

This sleight of hand causes some issues for the programme. As indicated, several of the charitable organizations included by the programme are the children's hospices and their films, which necessarily focus on the stories of severely ill, dying children. These films provide some of the most compelling content and depict some of the most deserving recipients of charity. However, while their campaigns are usefully emotive and dramatic, their recognized 'value for money'—that is, the return on the money invested in terms of emotional or sentimental recompense for the viewer—is such that it might be a surprise for the audience to learn that children's hospices are not entirely funded by the NHS and are, in fact, institutions largely funded via charitable donations. For example, the hospice featured in a 2015 campaign film—Robin House (part of the children's charity, Children's Hospice Association Scotland)—currently receives approximately 19 per cent of its funding from the NHS, including some smaller grants for specific activities from the Scottish government.[24] Although Dermot does explain to viewers that Robin House is dependent for 70 per cent of its financing from charitable donations, in the short film about the hospice, what is and isn't funded by these charitable donations is not clearly explained, as this would obviously distract the audience from the individual stories of the children and the film's intent to generate pathos and sentiment in the viewer. In relation to the overarching ethos of the programme, too much information regarding what is and isn't funded would also impact the meaning and integrity of the gratitude expressed by the celebrities, presenters, families, care workers, and children throughout the evening (Figure 2.6). If the thanks they express were more overtly understood to be, in part, for activities and actions that are or should be supported by the NHS—which is funded through taxation—then this would undermine the integrity of the programme. This is because the programme depends upon the notion of charity, as a series of individual and temporarily collective actions, as an acceptable mode of funding for those most in need. By directing the audience's attention away from the evolving patchwork of state and philanthropic funding that is the reality of social care and healthcare provision in the UK, the programme avoids representations of 'children in need' that might be regarded as political.

24 For figures related to NHS funds (restricted) and charitable funds, see Children's Hospice Association Scotland, *Annual Report*, p.16.

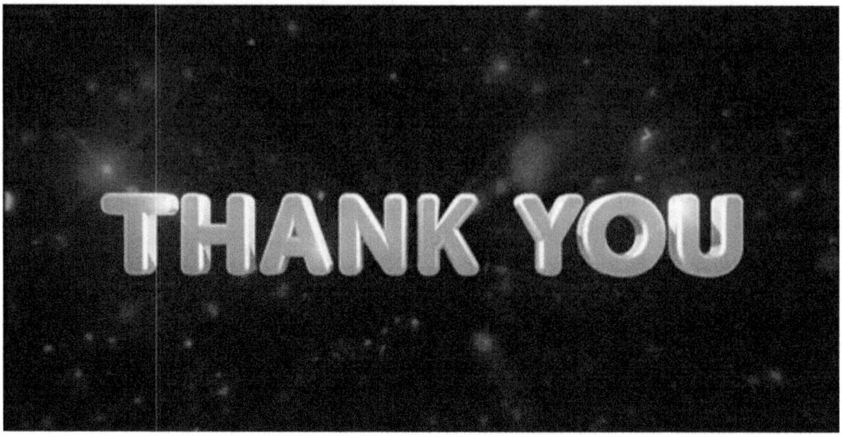

2.6. *Children in Need*, 13 November 2015, BBC1.

Currency as Aesthetic Strategy: The Campaign Films

Aside from the wider context of the programme and the currency that underpins the financial basis of the BBC itself, it is also possible to identify a currency at work in the campaign films.

Campaign Film (1): 'Robbie and Rosie's Story', Robin House, Scotland

In the 2015 film concerning Robin House (located near Balloch in Scotland), the audience is witness to tragedy—the loss of two children by the same parents, Mark and Ann. Their children, Robbie and Rosie, are both diagnosed with the same hereditary life-limiting condition—Infant Battens Disease. The short film is introduced via a direct address from the Scottish actor David Tennant, and it provides details of Robbie and Rosie's lives from the appearance of their initial well-being to their deterioration and ultimately their death. The hospice, its grounds, activities, and staff are clearly presented as essential to the children's lives and to the continuing resilience of the parents. The short film consists of montages of family photographs of Robbie and Rosie, an interview with Mark and Ann during which they relate the narrative of their births, diagnoses, illness, and death, and other sequences which show Ann visiting one of the bedrooms in the hospice used by Rosie at the time of her death, as well as other kinds of activity involving children and staff at the hospice (Figure 2.7).

After relating the suffering and death of Robbie and Rosie, the story is concluded with a happy ending—of sorts—as we witness in the final reveal

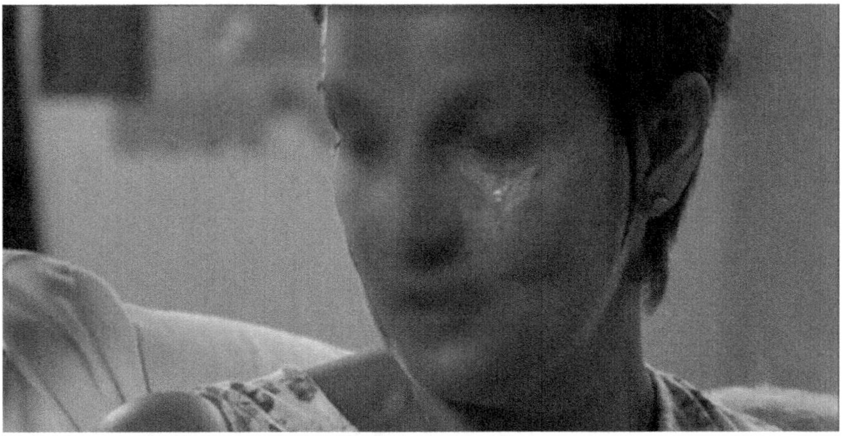

2.7. 'Robbie and Rosie's Story', from *Children in Need*, 13 November 2015, BBC1.

that Mark and Ann have been able to have two other children (Ruby and Roxy), who are not carriers of the defective gene which caused the life-limiting condition of their siblings. The children do not speak to the camera but are seen playing and interacting with Mark and Ann in the gardens of the hospice. Unsurprisingly, details as to how the beautiful, healthy daughters must have presumably been conceived after extensive screening and medical intervention are not discussed. In the breakdown of the narrative in Table 2.1, we can see that the segmentation of the film provides specific instances through which the audience will anticipate and then experience moments of intense emotion, such as Ann's tears as she recalls the death of Rosie at the hospice.

Campaign Film (2): 'Vanessa's Story', Great Ormand Street Hospital and the 'Raise a Smile' Foundation, London

Broadcast in November 2017, 'Vanessa's story' details the short life of a young girl suffering from neuroblastoma, a rare and aggressive form of cancer. The film is introduced and narrated by the British actor Olivia Coleman. We first meet Vanessa (in a short sequence recorded in 2012) when she has already been diagnosed with cancer (Figure 2.8).

From there, we are taken through a relatively compressed montage indicative of her various treatments and are provided with two key instances of charitable intervention, in the form of visits from two different female singers from the 'Raise a Smile' foundation who engage with and facilitate Vanessa's love of singing. We hear Vanessa singing short sequences from a couple of keenly emotional songs—'On My Own' from the West End musical, *Les Miserables* and ABBA's 'Thank you for the Music' (Figure 2.9).

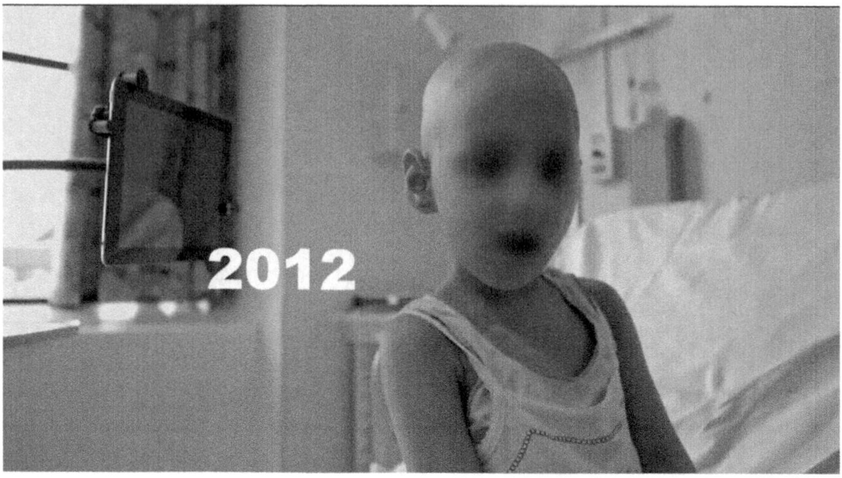

2.8. 'Vanessa's Story', from *Children in Need*, 17 November 2017, BBC1.

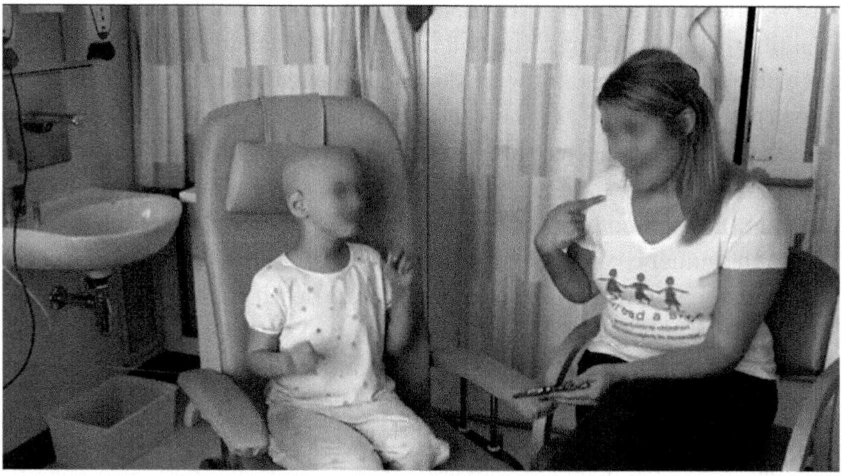

2.9. 'Vanessa's Story', from *Children in Need*, 17 November 2017, BBC1.

At another point in the film, we see her threading beads onto a necklace with her mother, and the voice-over informs us that each bead represents a new procedure in her care. Vanessa and her mother explain that the four large blue beads on the necklace refer to the four times she has lost her hair over the course of her treatment. Most of the filming takes place in hospital. Vanessa explains at one point that, while she lives in the hospital, her sisters live at home and we see her share a family meal with them via FaceTime or Skype on a computer screen in Vanessa's hospital room. Towards the end of the film, we are told that, in the summer of 2017 (therefore, three of four months before the television broadcast), Vanessa is offered one last trial treatment and we witness her hair being shaved (again in hospital). We are then told that, as this treatment fails, on 5 September 2017, two months before the broadcast of the telethon, Vanessa leaves the hospital. We then witness—on what appears to be a handheld camera—Vanessa singing and dancing in school uniform in a classroom context (it is not made entirely clear, however, when or where this footage is taken). An intertitle—a black background with the text in white—then informs us that Vanessa died 'the next day' (on 6 September 2017). The film concludes with a brief sequence in which we return to the previously seen, handheld footage of Vanessa in her school uniform. Vanessa moves in close to the camera, smiling.

Palliative Care Currency: A Developing Model

Having established the segmented narrative structure of the campaign films (Tables 2.1 and 2.2), we can now compare these with a proposed template for a 'specialist palliative care currency' for children with life-threatening conditions. While this template is in development, the model it articulates aligns directly with the kinds of funding models preferred by the current government, as evidenced in the following recent debate in the House of Lords, where, after a series of interventions, the Conservative Parliamentary Under-Secretary of State, for the Department of Health, Lord O'Shaughnessy, responded:

> The noble Baroness, Lady Walmsley, asked about care currencies. She was quite right about the tendency to jargon in this area; it is described as a specialist palliative care currency model, I am afraid, so it is worse than she feared. But the idea is a good one—she highlighted the importance of it—which is to provide a level of transparency and certainty on the kind of funding that will follow. It will not be precisely payment by results or payment by outcome, because of the importance of the charitable sector, but it will provide greater transparency and certainty on the funding of hospices. We aim to publish that shortly.[25]

In Figure 2.10, we can see that, as an exemplar, a child (a boy aged eleven years) has been diagnosed with neoplasms. His care, or the story of his

25 House of Lords, 'End of Life Care', column 1852.

Sequence	1	2	3	4	5	6	7	8
Phase duration (min.)	00.00–00.20	00.20–01.09	01.09–01.52	01.52–02.57	02.57–03.15	03.15–03.55	03.55–04.08	04.08–04.50
Voice Over (VO) **Audio Visual** (AV)	AV: David Tenant direct to camera: 'every child should have a future'	AV: Photographs of healthy looking baby VO: Robbie's diagnosis of Infantile Battens disease, Rosie's birth 11 January 2005	AV: Close up of parents. 'It was bad news' VO: Rosie also has the disease AV: Parents: 'End of the world really'	AV: Pictures of Robin House—respite care for children with life limiting conditions. AV: Activities Director: 'Children come here to live'	VO: 'Robbie died.' 'He was six'	VO: 'What was to come with Rosie.'	VO: 'Her time came' AV: Ann in bedroom at Robin House: 'she passed'	AV: Moving on—Ann leaves bedroom to garden beyond VO: 'Meet someone else too: Ruby and Roxy.'
Phase of Illness	Stable	Diagnosis	Unstable	Stable	Death	Stable	Death	

Table 2.1. Segmentation of the film 'Robbie and Rosie's Story', from *Children in Need*, 13 November 2015, BBC1.

Sequence	1	2	3	4	5	6
Phase duration	00.00–00.30	00.30–02.58	02.58–04.30	04.30–05.37	05.37–05.48	06.00
Voice Over (VO) **Audio Visual** (AV)	AV: Olivia Coleman: 'You would give everything to make your child well'	VO: 'countless painful procedures' '800 days in hospital' AV: beads on necklace = abacus	VO: 'seriously ill' '10 million times happier' AV: Sings 'On my own'	VO: 'new trial treatment' 'every day counts' AV: Sings 'Thank you for the music'	VO: 'leaves hospital for the last time' AV: dancing with school friends	AV: White font on black screen 'Vanessa died'
Phase of illness	Diagnosis	Stable/Unstable	Unstable	Deteriorating	Dying	Dead

Table 2.2. Segmentation of the film 'Vanessa's Story', from *Children in Need*, 17 November 2017, BBC1.

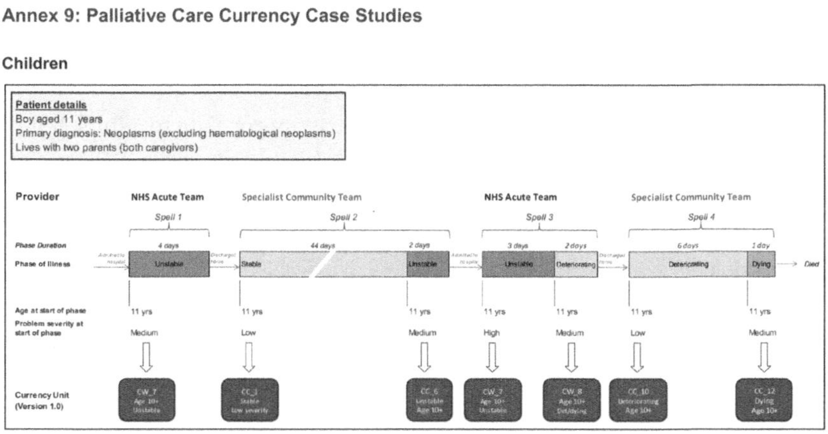

2.10. Annex 9: Palliative Care Currency Case Studies from NHS England, *Guidance*, p. 39.

illness, is then mapped and segmented into spells and phases during which he is under the care of particular types of nursing provision, either the 'NHS acute team' or the 'specialist community team'. It is likely that this 'specialist community team' will include provision from the children's hospice, which, as already noted, is largely dependent on charitable funding. One of more phases (days) of his illness and treatment are bundled into these 'spells' of care. Each phase of care begins with a calculation of the extent (low/medium/high) of his 'problem severity'. This rises or falls dependent on the perceived stability of the child (which, in itself, is guided by a number of related factors such as pain, physical symptoms, psychological and spiritual problems, carer and/or family concerns). These factors are then rationalized to estimate and award a value to the currency units that are associated with each spell of care the child receives. In this instance, the report explains: 'Currency is the word that is given to a consistent unit of healthcare which can form the basis of payment for that service.'[26] As an example of how the currency model is usually most effective, the report references a routine procedure such as a tonsillectomy. In other words, the currency model is most effective when the medical intervention has a clear procedure and defined outcomes and it is not, as might be the case in relation to an individual child with a life-limiting condition, potentially skewed by a wide range of social, medical, and psychological complexities. Within an associated report—*Guidance for Using the Children's Palliative Care Currency*—in which pilot studies were

26 NHS England, *Guidance*, p. 4.

executed in relation to both adult and child contexts of palliative care, this is acknowledged:

> There's not a one size fits all—The language is appropriate to adults, but less so for children's. A child's trajectory is likely to be very different, even in 2 children with the same condition. However, specialist palliative care, adult oncology patients' journeys can be very similar (and almost textbook).[27]

The deep contradiction here, of course, is that the notion of currency is premised precisely on the fact that, whatever vagaries there may be in their initial quantification, numerical values (the units of currency) are meant to represent robust, objective, and scientific evidence as opposed to discursive or qualitative values that are seen to represent evidence that is dangerously subjective, variable, and anecdotal.

At the time of writing—and from the discussion evident in these recent reports—it is acknowledged that more work (and, of course, given the ideology underpinning the enterprise, more data collection) needs to be done. Equally, there appears to be no real-world context in which the virtual currency being promoted here has been in use so far. As the reports evidence, it has been piloted but not yet mandated. As yet, then, this specific healthcare currency has not been used as way of pricing and allocating funds within the NHS.

Nonetheless, the language of both reports suggests that it will ultimately be adopted: Throughout each report, the need for the currency is emphasized with the promise that it will provide robust evidence for discussions between 'providers and commissioners' and that it will 'provide the evidence base to support discussions on payment'.[28] Clearly, the model speaks directly to the current ideology of neoliberalism: an ideology that derives its legitimacy via the data-driven—and extraordinarily complex—models of both personalization and financialization. As such, the 'health care currency' is likely to remain a focus in the current context where the allocation of NHS funds (how much, for whom, and where) is under intense scrutiny.

As should be clear from the examples given above, the various campaign films shown across the *Children in Need* telethon have—in part due to their

27 NHS England, *Guidance*, p. 25. This is one of two guidance documents to support the *Development of a New Approach to Palliative Care Funding—Final Report 2015/16 Testing*, made available to organizations who wish to use the currencies to support commissioning of Specialist Palliative Care services for adults and children.

28 NHS England, *Guidance*, p. 11.

ubiquity and familiarity—also established a very similar kind of currency model. The segmented narratives of the campaign films depend upon agreed (or tried and tested) units that are understood to have a particular weight in relation to their meaning and sentimental value and certain 'sequences' in the campaign film might be aligned with the 'spells' of care that feature in the NHS currency template. That is, each 'sequence' in the film provides a familiar co-incidence of sound and image and this will prompt a specific response, or estimation of its monetary value, just as each 'spell' of care is identified as having a specific numerical value in the NHS currency. As I have described, in the most typical examples, some of the film will be taken up with a photomontage of happier days, although the audience will anticipate the moment when a melancholic song plays as the child inevitably deteriorates. This is the point at which the camera often moves in closer to capture the tearful testimony of parents and siblings, or where we watch as the parents embrace the ailing child on their lap, or stroke their hair or hands as they lie in a hospital or hospice bed. There may also be instances in which the child is appealing directly to the camera, looking through the 'fourth wall' of the camera lens to the audience at home. These 'units' of high emotion—such as tears, lip wobbles, resigned expressions, moments of tender touching, hair stroking, cuddles, or direct eye contact—are not so dissimilar from the moments described by Laura Grindstaff, in her study of US 'reality chat shows' as the 'money shot'. The 'money shot' is the moment when the television cameras successfully capture an instance of extreme emotional outrage or upset from guests.[29] *Children in Need* viewers who are prompted to donate money in relation to the films' empathetic cues—sequences in which emotions run high—are acting in response to the successful execution of these narratives' 'money shots'.

What I have deliberately underplayed in my summary analysis of both films is their sincere emotional content. Undoubtedly, the audience's emotional responses will be amplified by the use of music, familiar domestic snapshots, and the use of close-ups, as well as the inclusion of the sometimes tearful but brave testimonies of the children's parents and siblings. These are real children and real families. My analysis is not intended to belittle the suffering of these particular children or to cast doubt on the intentions of the parents, caregivers, charity workers, or film-makers. It does not undermine my argument to insist that each film depends upon the very real and individual personalities and situations of the families and

29 The term 'money shot' is also used in relation to the capturing of male ejaculation in pornography.

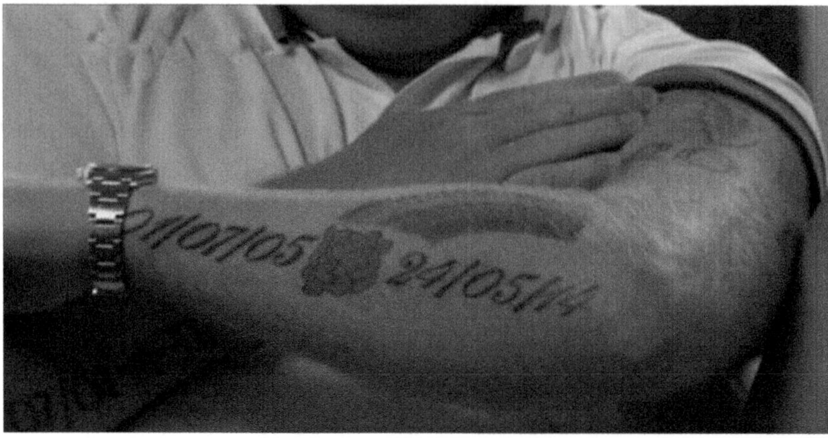

2.11. 'Robbie and Rosie's Story', from *Children in Need*, 13 November 2015, BBC1.

children involved. In terms of the ethics of the films and the question of the children's consent, in the first film discussed, from 2015, due to the fact that they have died before filming and the nature of their condition, it is unlikely that either Robbie or Rosie could have given any kind of informed consent as to their inclusion in the broadcast. It is evident that their parents, who speak lovingly for and about them, are fully committed to the telling of their children's stories and are determined to affirm the value of Robin House not only for the children they have lost, but also for their own resilience, as well as the mental well-being of their living daughters. This is further confirmed by a short sequence at the end of this film, during which Mark—the father—discusses his tattoos (Figure 2.11). These large tattoos, which take up each forearm, include the names, the date of the births, and the date of the deaths of Robbie and Rosie. He states, somewhat defiantly, that people are often curious about his tattoos but then are often disturbed or bemused that he has included both their dates of birth and the date of their deaths. 'They are my children' he says, and 'I like talking about them'.

Equally, in the second film I have analysed, Vanessa, who is, in most of the sequences, chatty, alert, and articulate, appears entirely comfortable with being filmed and engages directly—through eye contact as well as through singing and talking—with the film-makers, and she presumably recognizes that there will be additional viewers for her story. Vanessa and her family are unique: Evidently, and, as we are told by Coleman, Vanessa is 'special'. However, I can't help finding an uncanny co-incidence in terms of form, content, and ideology in Vanessa and her mother's attempt at making a coherent narrative out of the 'one after another' of Vanessa's successive medical treatments. The beads on her necklace, referred to earlier, are both touching and touchable,

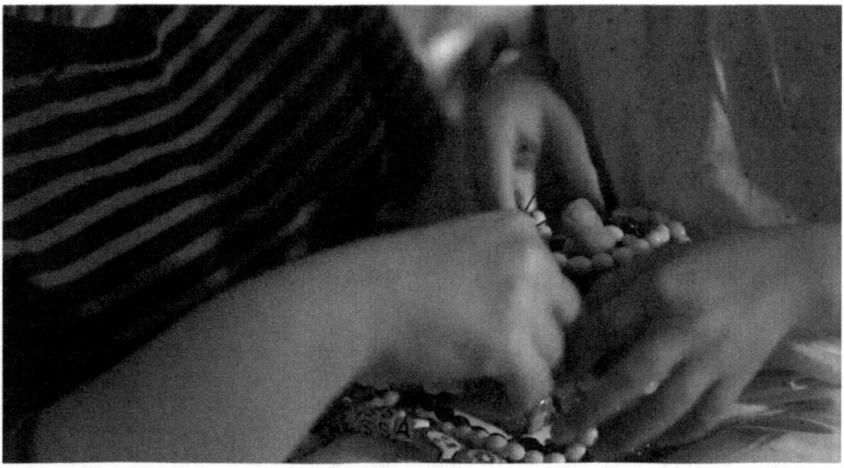

2.12. 'Vanessa's Story', from *Children in Need*, 17 November 2017, BBC1.

feminized reminders of what were painful and ultimately unsuccessful medical procedures; at the same time and, in the context of my argument, they might also recall beads on an abacus, representing the calculations, numbers, and currency underpinning Vanessa's life story (Figure 2.12).

However sensitive we may want to be to these specific individuals, we cannot escape the sense in which these terminally ill children are incorporated into a broadcast, which is simply one more programme in a long history of similar broadcasts that actively formats their individual life stories into a monetized narrative economy.[30]

Conclusion

Telethons and their related campaign films are implicated in dismaying assumptions about disability, illness, and the way in which medical care

30 It is beyond the scope of this chapter, but it is worth noting that several British charities have also adopted an explicitly financialized model of legitimating their worth—the Social Return on Investment (SROI) analysis—which 'calculates the social, economic and financial benefits' apparently generated from a £1 donation. For example, a recent SROI analysis was conducted by the consultancy firm Rocket Science for 'The Yard'—a Scottish charity providing an adventure play service for disabled children. (The charity has also featured on *Children in Need*.) Using evidence from interviews, 'outcomes mapping workshops', and choice modelling, it was calculated that, for every £1 invested or donated, the overall 'social return' (in terms of time saved, medical care not required, other care services not requested because of the services) for 'The Yard' could be valued at £20.50. See The Yard, *Social Return on Investment*, p. 4.

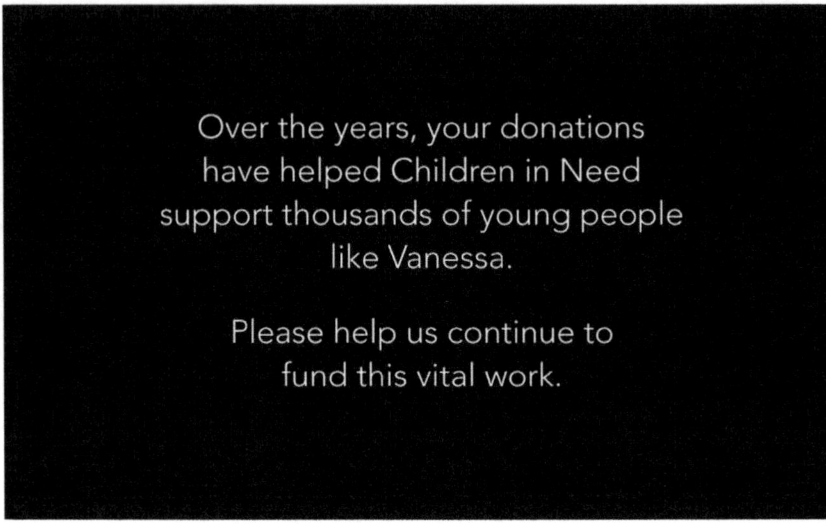
Over the years, your donations
have helped Children in Need
support thousands of young people
like Vanessa.
Please help us continue to
fund this vital work.

2.13. 'Vanessa's Story', from *Children in Need*, 17 November 2017, BBC1.

should be managed and financed in contemporary Western society.[31] In this chapter, however, my purpose was to focus on the significance of financialization and to unpack the mechanics of and units of exchange within the various models of currency at work within the *Children in Need* broadcast. The first currency model I identified—represented most explicitly by the graphic 'totalizer' representing the incremental amounts of money raised over the evening—is an isolated, meaningless number whose value is asserted primarily in relation to the numerical amount that was raised in previous years. While there may be information provided as to how many children the money has helped (another instance in which numbers are used to 'prove' value), these figures are often very general ('thousands') and there is no wider context given for the money (How many children are not helped?) and no suggestion that funding might be more appropriately derived from taxation, despite the fact that the care supported is understood to be 'vital' (Figure 2.13).

For the BBC, the programme conveniently shores up another currency model (the universal licence fee), which is dependent on the BBC's promise to bring individuals together as 'one' national audience. This alliance between the audience and the nation is bolstered by the programme's promotion of active participation and exhibition by fundraisers. Interestingly, in the policy document by Buck and Wilkinson cited earlier in the chapter, reference is

31 See Longmore, *Telethons*.

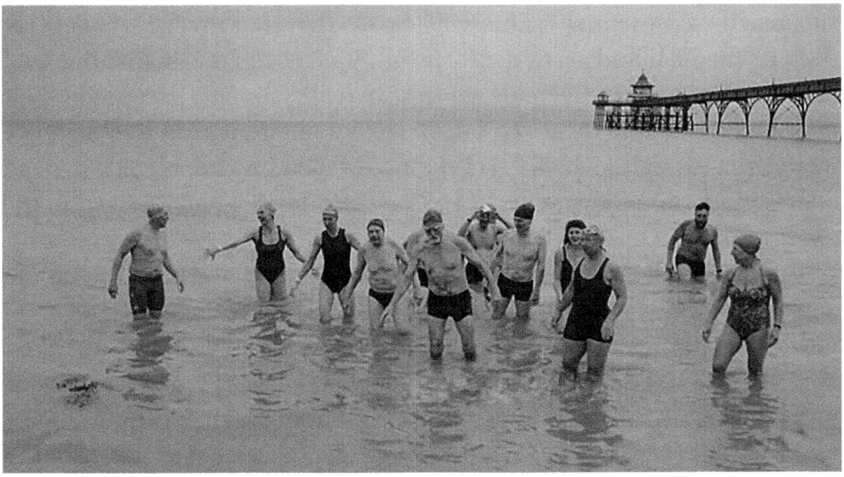

2.14. 'Wild Swimmers', *One-ness ident*, dir. Martin Parr, 2017, BBC1.

made to the policy at that time of branding of the BBC as 'One BBC'. In 2017, this concept was reimagined as 'One-ness'. Current idents for the channel exemplify the participatory aspects of this concept as they picture a variety of different community groups undertaking various activities, including aerobics, wild swimming, and urban skating (Figure 2.14).

Embedded within the live programme, but necessarily distinct from the pantomime antics of the various stunts that make up the rest of the broadcast, there are a number of pre-recorded charity films that exhibit powerful instances of human suffering. These films are carefully framed, segmented narratives that may also be understood to represent another kind of currency model. However unappealing it may sound, the charity films are undoubtedly carefully organized to provide a series of 'money shots' designed to provoke particular kinds of emotional response and thus donations from the viewing audience. Finally, the currency model of the charity campaign films may then be directly aligned with the 'specialist palliative care currency' currently being piloted as a funding model for the NHS in relation to the care of severely ill children. The narrative segmentation and progress of the dying child in terms of their representation within the medical and broadcast currency models might appear inevitable—in both models, after all, the child dies. However, the significance of their alliance is because the currency model is dependent on the equivalence of 'money' to 'value'. As Mary Poovey argues, the construction of a currency is problematic because money's 'very nature dictates that its value depends on a gap between its material form and the ground of the value it supposedly represent[s]'.[32] This 'gap' means that the currency model—in both its medical and aesthetic forms—requires the rationalization and homogenization of individuals who are, in reality, unique in terms of their personalities and medical and social needs. Equally, within this currency model, the extent to which certain kinds of medical care already depend on charitable donations is disguised, just as it is underemphasized in the *Children in Need* broadcast itself.

My focus on currency models has allowed me to illustrate the way in which financialization increasingly underpins the aesthetic strategies of medically significant narratives such as the telethon, that would otherwise appear to provide a context in which the television audience is encouraged to demonstrate unabashed empathy rather than conduct empirically rational valuations as to who is, or isn't, deserving of medical and social care. The increasing colonization of financialization into the wider culture is in line with shifts elsewhere in the charitable sector, as Eve Chiapello observes:

> When someone decides to give some money to a charity, or when a local authority decides to award a grant to some social actor, there is always some form of valuation beforehand. First of all, the decision must be made to provide support, and then how much. This valuation operation is what is gradually becoming financialised.[33]

What *Children in Need* demonstrates is how financialization, or what Chiapello terms as the 'financialisation of valuation' may also be an *aesthetic strategy* at work within the broadcast itself. The audiovisual operation of the broadcast, and its various generic borrowings, from light entertainment, reality talk shows, pornography, and documentary, illustrates the way in which medical, televisual, and economic discourses are increasingly aligned.

Works Cited

Films, Television Programmes, and Recordings

Big Brother, Endemol/Channel 4, 2000–2010.
Children in Need, BBC 1980–.
Children in Need: 50 Greatest Moments, BBC, 2010.

32 Poovey, *Genres*, p. 62.
33 Chiapello, 'Financialisation of Valuation', p. 25.

Eastenders, BBC, 1985–.
The Disney Club, Disney/GMTV, 1993–1998.
The One Show, BBC 2007–.
The X-Factor, SyCoTV/ITV, 2004–.
Top of the Pops, BBC, 1964–2006.

Books and Articles

Anderson, Benedict, *Imagined Communities: Reflections on the Origins and Spread of Nationalism*, rev. ed. (London: Verso, 2006).

Boltanski, Luc, *Distant Suffering: Morality, Media and Politics*, trans. by Graham Burchell (Cambridge: Cambridge University Press, 2005).

Bryant, Christopher G.A., 'National Art and Britain Made Real: The London 2012 Olympics Opening Ceremony', *National Identities*, 17, 3 (2015), pp. 333–346, doi :10.1080/14608944.2014.990958.

Buck, Geoff, and Johnny Wilkinson, 'Report for Director of Public Affairs on the Children in Need Appeal' (1986), *BBC Written Archives' Centre*, archive ref: R78/2/633/1(10084125).

Charlesworth, Diane, 'Stand Up to Cancer 2012 and 2014: The Medical Telethon as UK Public Service Broadcasting in a Neo-Liberal Age', *Critical Studies in Television*, 11, 2 (2016), pp. 217–229, doi:10.1177/1749602016645750.

Chiapello, Eve, 'Financialisation of Valuation', *Human Studies*, 38, 1 (2015), pp. 13–35, doi:10.1007/s10746-014-9337-x.

Grindstaff, Laura, *The Money Shot: Trash, Class and the Making of TV Talk Shows* (Chicago: University of Chicago Press, 2002).

Happer, Catherine, 'Financialisation, Media and Social Change', *New Political Economy*, 22, 4 (2017), pp. 437–449, doi:10.1080/13563467.2017.1259301.

Heritage, Stuart, 'Children in Need: We'll Miss Terry Wogan but We're in Safe Hands with Dermot O'Leary', *The Guardian*, 13 November 2015, https://www.theguardian.com/tv-and-radio/tvandradioblog/2015/nov/13/children-in-need-well-miss-terry-wogan-but-were-in-safe-hands-with-dermot-oleary, accessed 24 July 2018.

House of Lords, 'End of Life Care', 14 March 2017, *House of Lords Hansard*, vol. 779, https://hansard.parliament.uk/Lords/2017-03-14/debates/9E00B6E2-F0D6-4D3B-A788-A48A8B3FA95D/EndOfLifeCare, accessed 25 July 2018.

Longmore, Paul K., *Telethons: Spectacle, Disability and the Business of Charity*, ed. by Catherine Kudlick (New York: Oxford University Press, 2016).

NHS England, *Guidance for Using the Children's Palliative Care Currency*, 22 March 2017, https://www.england.nhs.uk/wp-content/uploads/2017/03/guidance-using-childrens-palliative-care-currency.pdf, accessed 25 July 2018.

Press Association, '"Postcode Lottery" Revealed in NHS Care', *The Guardian*, 8 September 2016, https://www.theguardian.com/society/2016/sep/08/postcode-lottery-revealed-in-nhs-care, accessed 25 July 2018.
Children's Hospice Association Scotland, *Annual Report and Accounts, 2016–17: For the Year Ended 31 March 2017*, https://www.chas.org.uk/about-us/our-vision/our-publications, accessed 27 August 2018.
Poovey, Mary, *Genres of the Credit Economy: Mediating Value in Eighteenth- and Nineteenth-Century Britain* (Chicago: University of Chicago Press, 2008).
Timm Knudsen, Britta, and Carsten Stage, *Global Media, Biopolitics and Affect: Politicizing Bodily Vulnerability* (New York: Routledge, 2015).
The Yard, *Social Return on Investment: Technical Report 2016/17*, by Clare Hammond with Clara Mascaro and Michael Brown (June 2017), https://www.theyard-scotland.org.uk/Handlers/Download.ashx?IDMF=362f08f6-6049-4d98-b60f-9c9b0cce5ba4, accessed 26 July 2018.

About the Author

Karen Lury is Professor of Film and Television Studies in the School of Culture and Creative Arts at the University of Glasgow. She has published in film and television studies, with a particular focus on the representation of the child in film and in relation to children's media more generally. She is currently co-editing a critical anthology for Bloomsbury, entitled, *Discourses of Care: Media, Medicine and Society* and is a longstanding editor of the international film and television studies journal, *Screen*.
Contact details: Karen.Lury@glasgow.ac.uk

3. Let's Talk about S...: The Influence of *Cinéma Vérité* on Sex Education in French National Television around 1968

Christian Bonah

Abstract

Studying the French audiovisual mediascape the contribution asks when and how the issue of sexuality and sexual education surfaced on TV. As direct cinema *micro-trottoire* techniques met sex education they challenged classical talk shows. Thereby they reframed who could be a speaking subject in front of the TV camera. Contrasting official TV shows used in a systematic fashion as principal primary source the contribution moves on to look at school television and amateur videos, used as counter-archives. How did these multiple screens differ in informing or educating about sexuality? Their comparative and integrated analysis emphasizes how intimate, ordinary, and 'real' self-exhibition in intimate confessional scenes and unscripted street interviews became key portraits and tropes situated on the fence between exploring and exploiting.

Keywords: sex education, television, France, 1970s, direct cinema, school television, ORTF, contraception, birth control, abortion, sexuality

Between late February and early May 1968, four news reports from regional centres for televised news (Centre d'actualités télévisée, CAT)[1]— which had been created in a half-hearted attempt to decentralize and democratize Gaullist television in 1964–1965 by the Minister of Information, Alain Peyrefitte—reported on an unusual event, far from the usual regional, political, or sports news. Barely two months before the heady days of May 1968, a

1 Lafon, *Histoire de la télévision régionale*, pp. 66–80.

Bonah, C. and A. Laukötter (eds.), *Body, Capital, and Screens: Visual Media and the Healthy Self in the 20th Century*. Taylor & Francis Group, 2020
DOI 10.5117/9789462988293_CH03

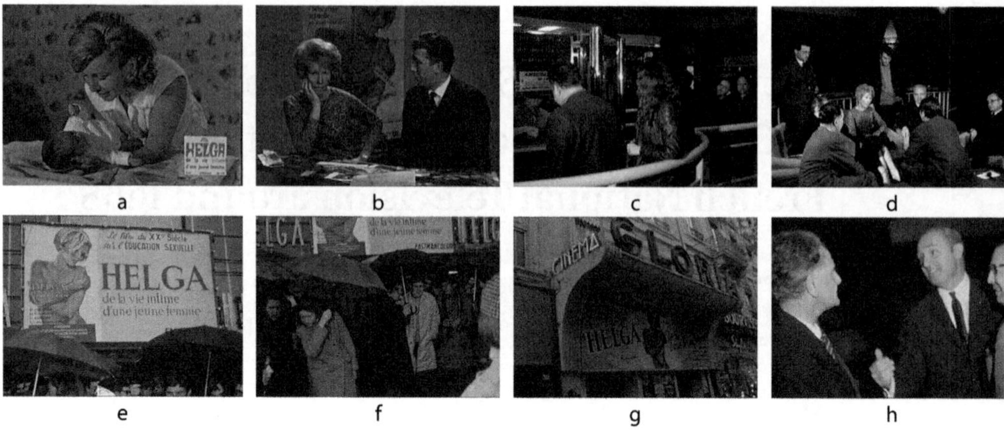

3.1. a/b: *Cinéma: Sortie du film Helga*, Nord actualités télé, 29 February 1968, 02:45 minutes; c/d: Magazine: *Le problème de l'éducation sexuelle*, Provence Actualités, 29 February 1968, 06:33 minutes; e/f: *'Helga'*, Limousin actualities, 22 March 1968, 15 seconds; g/h: *Le film Helga à Lyon*, Rhône Alpes actualités 2 May 1968, 26 seconds (source: INA Archives).

cinematic event received television news coverage from Lille to Marseille, Limoges to Lyons. French television news reported on large crowds gathering in front of cinemas, spectators fainting, and politicians and officials viewing and discussing a particular film. At the centre of it all was the commercial theatrical screening of the recently released French adaptation of the West German sex education film *Helga: The Intimate Life of a Young Woman* (1967).[2]

It all began with a two-and-a-half-minute report televised by the Lille regional news. The report included a studio interview with the gynaecologist Marie-Andrée Lagroua Weill-Hallé appearing at the beginning of the French *Helga* adaptation.[3] Dr. Lagroua Weill-Hallé was one of the founders of the French family-planning organization La Maternité heureuse in 1956 (after 1960, known as MFP) who, since 1960, had been establishing birth control centres throughout France, despite the legal barriers posed by the then standing 1920 law. The news report opens with a maternal scene featuring a newborn from Helga's intimate life, then moves to a studio discussion (Figures 3.1a–3.1h). The tone of the interview is set by Dr. Lagroua Weill-Hallé, who states that the film has much to offer young audiences on the subject of procreation. Praising the film as 'sound, precise and clear', the interviewer raises the question of an age restriction for viewers, but concludes that, as a father and educator, he is grateful that the producers had created such an

2 *Helga: Vom Werden des menschlichen Lebens* (UK poster title: *Helga: The Intimate Life of a Young Woman*), directed by Erich F. Bender, RINCO-Film (Munich), released on 22 September 1967. On *Helga*, see: Schwarz, 'Helga (1967)'; Schwarz, 'Vom Jahrmarktspektakel'; Winkler, 'Biology, Morality and Gender'; Laukötter, 'Politik im Kino', pp. 413–430.

3 Le Naour and Valenti, *Histoire de l'avortement*, pp. 207–214.

informative, well-made film. On the same day, a six-and-a-half-minute news report from Marseille broadened the discussion, with Dr. Lagroua Weill-Hallé again the focus. At the studio were a school physician, a representative of a French family-planning organization, a social worker, a representative of the state orphan service, and a general practitioner. The Catholic Church was absent, and the unanimous conclusion was that the film was informative and that it stimulated further questions and discussion about issues in sex education. Three weeks later, *Limousin News*, providing footage for the national Parisian Office de radiodiffusion television française (ORTF) office, took a different perspective. Their sequence switched from the erotically suggestive and provocative *Helga* film billboard (featuring the saucy subtitle 'The Intimate Life of a Young Woman' and a drawing of the naked upper body of a woman covering her breasts, providing an interplay between erotic teasing and sex education) to the back of an ambulance rescuing a young woman who had fainted, to the predominantly male audience crowded in front of the cinema (Figures 3.1e–3.1f). News reports thus oscillated between addressing the issue with frankness and visually suggesting that it went too far. Lastly, on 2 May 1968, the *Lyons CAT* half-minute news short reported on *Helga* with jazz music in the background, stressing that the film was the subject of heated debate and that the Member of Parliament and author of the recently approved French oral contraception legislation, Lucien Neuwirth, had attended a screening.[4]

Commissioned by the West German Federal Ministry of Health and the Federal Agency for Health Education (Bundeszentrale für gesundheitliche Aufklärung, BZgA), the film *Helga* was part of a series of initiatives introduced by Minister of Health Käte Strobel between 1966 and 1969 to raise public awareness of the need for sex education.[5] Her campaigns for nationwide sex education were founded in her conviction that sex education needed to be talked about and illustrated without inhibition. 'Without inhibition' meant circumventing traditional forms of moralizing education by developing curricula with information on the biology of sex, postnatal care, and adolescent psychology. Rather than disguising moralizing lessons as education, this new form of sex education provided essential

4 Lucien Neuwirth (1924–2013) was the French right-wing politician who successfully drafted and promoted the law carrying his name that authorized oral contraception and legalized birth control in France on 28 December 1967. Le Naour and Valenti, *Histoire de l'avortement*, pp. 217–224; Marks, *Sexual Chemistry*; Chauveau, 'Les espoirs déçus'.

5 See the contribution by Anja Laukötter in this volume. See also Winkler, 'Biology, Morality and Gender', pp. 142–189; Schwarz, 'Vom Jahrmarktspektakel'; Herzog, *Sex after Fascism*; Laukötter, 'Politik im Kino', pp. 413–430.

biological and psychological information to young people and included nudity and other explicit content. However, *Helga* remained centred on heterosexual partnerships and nuclear family values and avoided scenes of sexual intercourse and direct promotion of birth control. Adapted for foreign countries like France, Spain, the United Kingdom, and the United States, the erotic, sensualist overtones of the film were ambiguous. They catered to box-office sales and commercial distribution. They teased with commercialized sex. At the same time, their erotic titillation was used as a vehicle to get broader swathes of society to view a film that was part of a rather traditional public-health campaign anchored in family values and teaching about biological reproduction.[6] By early 1968, the female body had become a form of visual erotic capital in the competitive marketplace of the film industry.[7]

This vignette underscores three points. First, it was before May 1968 that the issue of sexuality and sex education surfaced in the French audio-visual public sphere, despite the fact that, since the 1920s, there had been a longstanding political, religious, and legal condemnation and repression of contraception and abortion.[8] Second, it points to the manifold links between cinema and television in France (as in Germany): TV reported on the cinematographic event, direct cinema influenced sequences of *Helga*, and the German original of *Helga* had been conceived initially as an educational (school) film including (school-)TV broadcasting before it was progressively and, in a later stage, transformed into a commercially distributed feature.[9] Historical accounts of visual sources should therefore address television history within this wider visual context of an ecology of viewing practices. Third, it highlights that television news reports on *Helga*'s release in France primarily took the format of studio discussions that staged debates amongst doctors, social workers, and politicians, who played the role of the public.[10] A central concern for this chapter is that, beyond the intimate content, it was the question of who could speak in front of the camera that was challenged in France in the late 1960s when *micro-trottoire* met sex education.

6 For the new imperatives of audiovisual health campaigns since the 1970s, see the contribution by Berlivet in this volume.

7 Hakim, *Erotic Capital*; Neveu, 'Les sciences sociales'.

8 The 1920 law (31 July 1920) against 'provoking' [promoting] abortion and contraceptive propaganda was followed on 27 March 1923 by a law declaring abortion illegal; Le Naour and Valenti, *Histoire de l'avortement*, pp. 160–164.

9 Paci, *Entre promesse et menace.*

10 See the contribution by Timothy Boon in this volume.

Still, the film *Helga* is an example of how sex education films of the 1960s broke with the old schemes that preferred moralizing and shocking as their techniques and sexually transmitted disease as their topic. While depicting a new constellation of biological bodies and adolescent psychology, many traditional and/or reactionary elements dominated educational screens, including nuclear families, marriage, and the avoidance of issues like abortion and contraception.[11] Novelty was not only expressed in explicitness of information, but also in a renewed take on the old tension between eroticism and education. But was that all? In order to testify to the difficulty of talking openly about sex education, *Helga* features a scene in which a reporter pretending to conduct a survey asks passers-by for their experiences with sex education and contraception. The climax of these interviews comes when an interviewee slaps the reporter when he asks her if she takes the pill. These kinds of direct cinematic techniques—made possible by lighter cameras and direct sound recording—became normal in sex education films of the 1960s, positioning their insights as authentic and in touch with social reality.[12] Of course, the technical possibilities of film do not automatically imply accurate representation, and audiovisual production remains a question of approach, framing, narration, and intention. What did interviews display and who spoke in them, from what point of view, to say what and how?

This chapter analyses how state-controlled television in France contributed to and reported on a series of social, political, and legal events that crystallized in 1967 with the legalization of oral contraceptives and culminated in the battle for the decriminalization/legalization of abortion through the Simone Veil law, which was adopted on 29 November 1974. Further, the Fontanet Act (*circulaire Fontanet*) of 1973 rendered sex education obligatory in French schools.

Our approach may be framed as neither history 'of', nor history 'with' but rather history through visual sources of a given period and place. Accordingly, official TV shows are primarily used in a systematic fashion and as principle primary source. Secondly, they are read against other audiovisual sources, used as counter-archives, including amateur film and school television, to explore avenues for reading audiovisuals and the history revealed by contrasting framings in a shared audiovisual mediascape.[13]

11 Schaefer, *Bold*; Eberwein, *Sex Ed*; Bonah and Laukötter, 'Introduction'; Laukötter, 'Politik im Kino'; Winkler, 'Biology, Morality and Gender'.

12 Winkler, 'Biology, Morality and Gender', pp. 142–189.

13 Amad, *Counter-Archive*.

The connection between bodies, capital, and TV screens can be traced as follows. Gary Becker argued in 1962 that human capital is the embedding of a resource in a person to influence future real capital.[14] Erotic capital can be seen as a subtype of symbolic capital based on a bodily materiality associated with its aesthetic, visual, physical, social, and sexual attractiveness.[15] The 1960s was a decade of rising press, television, and film investment in erotic capital. Yet (visual) productions and performances were deeply dividing society as the intimate subject of sexuality had been morally, religiously, and politically loaded and occulted for a long time. Profound changes in Western societies around the sexual revolution of the 1960s have to be acknowledged. They raise the question of how concomitant multiplying audiovisual forms mirrored, participated in, or resisted these changes. Our central hypothesis is that the empirical analysis of the television-related mediascape from 1950 to 1975 in France does not testify to a major investment in erotic body capital. Rather, it engages with the invention of an early form of television of intimacy that is characterized by its engagement with direct cinema and its preoccupation with exploring social situations, conditions, and consequences of male conservative sexual domination by interviewing ordinary citizens. The transition from silent extras to directly speaking to real, ordinary persons gave screened bodies a sociologically and politically critical role at a time when French television was not yet a commercial industry that produced real capital. And, we argue that, in the outcome, ironically, sex education and critically engaged TV productions paved the way for reality television of the 1990s with unknown individuals, purportedly unscripted real-life situations, and their intimacy-revealing confessional sequences.[16]

Sexual Revolution, Television, and Markets in France

Sex information and education varies from country to country. At the same time, it was influenced by broad transformations of views on sexuality in Western countries in the 1960s and 1970s, commonly referred to as the 'sexual revolution'. This included the liberalization of sexual behaviours; the acceptance of premarital and extramarital sex; the destigmatization

14 Becker, 'Investment in Human Capital'.

15 Hakim, *Erotic Capital*, p. 15.

16 Hill, *Reality TV*; Biressi and Nunn, *Reality TV*.

of homosexuality; the decriminalization of abortion, contraception, and pornography; and a revolt against conservative morals. As a consequence, issues related to sexuality lost, in part, their status as unmentionables and became widely debated in public spaces. Discussions took place in books, journals, fiction films, and documentaries on television and in school education, and were often framed as a 'question of civilization'.[17] As a contemporaneous TV magazine suggested, 1960s France seemed to be at the intersection of two approaches, midway between a Northern 'hygienic tradition', in which nudity and sexuality were culturally accepted and seen as an 'almost natural extension of gymnastics', and an 'oriental mystical tradition where sexuality as initiation and voluptuary techniques' were confidential and taboo.[18]

Historical research on the 'sexual revolution' in the West has contended that it involved a complex and ambiguous transition and that it remains questionable if the attractiveness of sexual liberty *per se* can explain the success of the revolt/revolution.[19] Furthermore, historical research has highlighted interconnections between the sexual revolution and the exploitation of sexuality and nudity in post-1950 consumer culture's advertising, marketing, and mass media. The marketing of desire, medical and technical innovations of the early 1960s, and especially the pill helped dissociate reproduction from sexuality, and political activism for women's rights and the liberalization of abortion and contraception played an important role, too. It is thus difficult to discern causes from effects clearly. In France, significant steps included early French emancipation literature, such as Françoise Sagan's *Bonjour tristesse* (1954), which portrayed the loss of virginity; Simone de Beauvoir's *Les Mandarins* (1954), which contained a description of the sexual act beyond pornography; and eroticized films like Roger Vadim's drama *And God Created Woman* (1956), which depicted Brigitte Bardot as a lascivious, sexually uncontrollable female. All these cultural events paralleled mass-media productions that fed into the omnipresence of sexual imagery. All this stood in stark contrast to previous eras, when legal regulations prohibited public mention of contraception, sexually explicit visuals, and detailed

17 'on en fait un problème de civilisation'; 'A propos de l'éducation sexuelle', *Zoom Magazine*, 13 February 1968, 53:51.

18 'civilisation hygiénique', 'où la gymnastique paraît avoir pour prolongation la sexualité', 'allons vers l'Orient, vers l'Inde [...] une tradition mystique où la sexualité est présentée comme quelque chose qui correspond à une initiation [...] aux techniques voluptueuses', 'A propos de l'éducation sexuelle', *Zoom Magazine*, 13 February 1968, 55:22.

19 For different national contexts, see Bänziger et al., *Sexuelle Revolution*; McLellan, *Love in the Time*; Herzog, *Sexuality in Europe*; Cook, *Long Sexual Revolution*.

biological information about reproduction and sexual organs.[20] The pill and pornography were cast between capitalist consumption society and counterculture. Thus, pertinent questions for an analysis of the connection between the sexual revolution and audiovisual media include: Who could address the subject? What were the themes chosen? And in what visual public sphere did they address which audiences?

The years between 1950 and 1974 were marked by industry-based therapeutic innovation, the epidemiological transition, increasing life expectancy, the rise of chronic disease, and the golden age of the European welfare state.[21] These shifts had important consequences for sex education film and television. With the advent of penicillin, venereal diseases disappeared from the screen in the 1950s, and with the therapeutic revolution, the contraceptive pill stepped on the stage. Launched in 1960 for menstruation disorders but rapidly used for contraceptive purposes, first by married women, and, after the late 1960s, by single women, putting the pill on-screen remained difficult given legal and societal restrictions. But, as a contemporaneous French observer put it, these health transitions meant that the prolongation of adult life, coupled with the extension of school education, 'postponed youth's entry into the working world, [creating] a dissociation of youth's biological and social maturity'.[22] In other words, there was a time lag between when youth were biologically capable of reproduction and when their economic situation 'enabled' them to cope socially with choosing a partner and having children.

The move from sexual hygiene to sex education films in the 1960s should also be viewed in the context of the history of sex education in 20th-century France. Yvonne Knibiehler has claimed that, between 1860 and 1960, France experienced 'a dark century for sex education in urban environments'.[23] The then prevailing 'conspiracy of silence' has, even today, not entirely vanished.[24] In 1969, one commentator on the situation in France stated that

20 *Information sexuelle* ('Sexual information', RTS, 1970). See the section concerning the film and Figure 3.3.

21 Greene et al., *Therapeutic Revolutions*.

22 'parce qu'elle [la jeunesse] ne travaille pas [encore] de façon productive [...] le décalage entre la maturité biologique et la maturité sociale crée un déséquilibre'; Natanson, 'Education sexuelle', p. 17. All translations by the author unless otherwise stated.

23 'Le XIXe siècle citadin apparaît comme une parenthèse obscure'; Knibiehler, 'L'éducation sexuelle', p. 11.

24 This is illustrated, for example, in a cultural history of sex education in 20th-century Europe in which France is missing; Sauerteig and Davidson, *Shaping Sexual Knowledge*. Nevertheless, see Pavard, 'Contraception et avortement'; Blanchard et al., *Les jeunes et la sexualité*; Hagemeyer, 'Sexualerziehung in Frankreich'.

> if revolt is more brutal in France this is undoubtedly due to the fact that [France] has lived for 37 years under the restrictive law of 1920. Sex education, as contraception, has been admitted only under the premise and condition that it does not interfere with fecundity and even less with the family.[25]

The May 1968 student revolt demonstrated that part of the youth population had forged its own opinion: As a chanson by Antoine poetically put it, 'when the pill would be sold in supermarkets the sexual act could be clearly dissociated from reproduction and procreation'.[26] In 1968, France thus awoke to the fact that sex education needed to be adapted to the 'social realities' of sexuality of the time.

Sex Education on TV before Official Sex Education in France (1960s)

Audiovisual spaces and technologies changed profoundly over the 20th century.[27] The middle of the century is often described as the age of television. With its popular appeal and national characteristics, it pushed on mass media and mass culture.[28] The keen investment in state television by Gaullist France after 1945 seems to be a national specificity that played a key role in sex information television in the period between 1960 and 1975. Pioneered in the interwar period, use and distribution of television extended after the Second World War. In February 1949, Radiodiffusion-television française (RTF) was created; initially limited to Paris, it was expanded to other regions in the early 1950s. RTF began collaborating with the BBC in 1952. By 1954, 1 per cent of households were equipped with a television set; by 1960, it was 13 per cent. As television sets were a household fixture, the audience addressed was the family circle.[29] By 1964, a second TV channel went into operation and

25 'Si la révolte est plus brutale en France, c'est sans doute que nous payons d'avoir vécu pendant 37 ans sous le régime de la loi de 1920. Sa suppression a dû triompher de multiples résistances, et reste assortie de mesuresrestrictives. Comme pour l'éducation sexuelle, les adultes n'ont admis la contraception qu'à la condition qu'elle ne toucherait pas à la fécondité et encore moins à la famille.'; Natanson, 'Education sexuelle', p. 16.

26 Natanson, 'Education sexuelle', p. 16, referring to a line of the 'Les Elucubrations' sung by Antoine: 'Mettez la pilule en vente dans les Monoprix'.

27 Boon, 'Medical Films and Television'; Reagan et al., *Medicine's Moving Pictures.*

28 Poels, *Les trente glorieuses.*

29 Poels, *Les trente glorieuses*; Lévy, 'Les représentations sociales'; Lévy, 'Famille et télévision'.

the RTF became the Office de radiodiffusion television française (ORTF), gaining in autonomy as control by the Ministry of Information decreased and competition increased between channels.[30] This leads us to consider the various formats tested out by TV broadcasts to capture the increasingly turbulent years known as the sexual revolution.

The 1960s were also a period of new forms of cinematic expression and creativity, with the ascent of the *Nouvelle vague* and direct cinema (*Cinéma direct*) and the democratization of film-making, both of the militant and home-movie sorts, that came with the advent of lighter amateur cameras. The chapter seeks to hit upon all these different media by first studying sex education in early television and its links to cinema direct, and then by looking at school television and amateur videos in France, questioning how these multiple screens addressed different ways of informing or educating about sexuality.[31]

An inventory of the French television broadcasts between 1950 and 1980 mentioning sex education amounts to 186 programmes (Figure 3.2).[32]

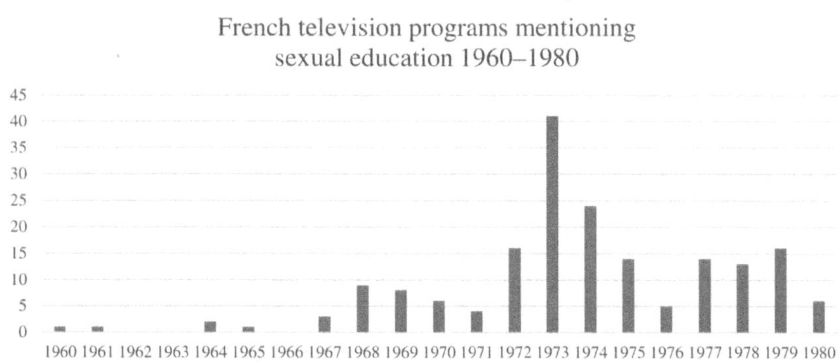

3.2. French TV broadcasts mentioning sex education between 1950–1980.

30 Sauvage and Veyrat-Masson, *Télévision française*, p. 83; Bourdon, *Télévision sous de Gaulle*, pp. 61–75.

31 Delavaud and Maréchal, *Télévision.*

32 Based on a full-text keyword research of 'éducation sexuelle' and 'information sexuelle' between 1950 and 1980 on the Institut national de l'audiovisuel (INA) databank INAMediaPro. For a 1987 inventory of French television broadcasts identifying 105 programmes related to family issues between 1956 and 1986, see: Lévy, *Regards*. Figure 3.2 is based on a full-description keyword search in the INA database (INAMediaPro and Hyperbase) between 1950 and 1980. The search yielded no entries before 1960. Keyword searches in full-text descriptions yielded 186 entries for 'éducation sexuelle' and 125 for 'information sexuelle'. Cross-matching establishes 235 broadcasts. The histogram for 'information sexuelle' is similar to the one displayed in Figure 3.2. Genre variations for 'information sexuelle' search yielded a higher percentage of magazines

Roughly one third concerned TV news (*journal televise*, JT), another third TV shows (*magazines*), and the last third comprised 20 reports, 15 talk shows, 15 debates, 5 sketches, and 6 documentaries. Chronologically, they trace sporadic treatment of the topic until 1967, when there was an increase of coverage of the subject just before the May 1968 student revolt in 1968 and 1969, and an especially rapid rise before and during national debates about the law prescribing sex education courses in public schools in 1972 and 1973. A selection of 12 programmes (see Table 3.1, Appendix) will serve here to establish general trends, while allowing a more detailed analysis of some of the programmes, especially the TV documentaries.

In the 1950s, discussions on the subject of sex and sexuality were absent from French television screens. When marital life was portrayed, it appeared in the context of TV magazines and reports about women either as domestic housewives or as domestic organizers in rural farms. A documentary series produced by Jacques Krier in 1957–1958, *A la découverte des Français* ('Discovering the French'), presented social portraits of families from different backgrounds, ranging from rural farmers to industrial workers. The series often focussed on economic hardships and praised the virtues of the traditional family order. The forms of social engagement depicted are limited to everyday practices, and the people depicted never talk or express themselves.[33]

An exceptional documentary report was 'Le contrôle des naissance' ('Birth control') (1960), an episode of the series *Faire Face* produced by Etienne Lalou and Igor Barrère, conceived as a live show that allowed viewers to call in and ask questions. Using a split screen, the questions were selected by an operator, who relayed them to the host (Etienne Lalou), who then presented them to four guest experts in the TV studio and to the audience. The experts included representatives of the medical profession, the Church, and the National Institute for Demography (INED). Intertwined with the question-response sequences are field reports that harp on the financial and moral hardships brought on by undesired maternity and the health problems caused by multiple pregnancies. There is uneasiness

mentioning 'information sexeulle' (50%), news programs treated 'information sexuelle' less frequently than for 'education sexuelle'. For genres reportages, debates and interviews percentages are equivalent.

33 Marital relationships surface in youth and women's programmes only when questions about the desired number of children are asked. This surreptitiously allows space for mentioning birth control. Sometimes reports on large family awards are coupled with interviews expressing hardship and sacrifices endured by women, thereby pleading indirectly and undercover for birth control measures.

and the unspoken hovering over a consensus-based, controlled expert discourse until the complex programme strategy finally pays off when a female spectator openly enquires about the pill. The host, Etienne Lalou, hardly disguises his excitement as the TV debate tips over. Connecting to a second outside TV studio with a Swiss physician, Dr. Devedville, he was allowed to discuss the progressive Swiss legislation on contraceptives, a fact contrary to existing French TV regulations and censorship. A priest, Father De Lestapie, expressed Catholic opposition to all 'mechanical or automatic means' of contraception. A French physician, a woman who, albeit not officially identified by her name, was none other than the pro-MFP gynaecologist Marie-Andrée Lagroua Weill-Hallé (mentioned above) oddly does not mention the movement for family planning, but willingly acknowledges the medical profession's considerable opposition to contraception and the pill. Even under the watch of state control, the technically challenging, sometimes chaotic format and the ingenious framing of the programme allow the producers to make television into a public space of debate over the abrogation of the repressive 1920 laws prohibiting abortion and the promotion of contraception. The call-ins and the live responses to viewers' questions made it possible for a taboo topic—contraception—to be discussed on television. The presence of the liberal Swiss physician is telling of the outcome that the producers anticipated. On the surface, the talk show addressed reproduction from the perspective of demography and population politics. However, it surreptitiously explored and mobilized techniques used by family social documentaries produced before in order to '*discover the French*'.[34] By interviewing ordinary citizens, the talk show narrows the gap between conventional discourse and social realities, which are translated by television as public opinion. A second episode in November 1961 reported more overtly and directly on the opening of the first centre for family planning in Grenoble. The episode features an interview with a man lamenting the marital problems caused by avoiding pregnancy by abstinence, discussions at the workplace, and a piece on how a Catholic woman reconciled her use of birth control with her religious conscience. As a whole, the episode casts contraception as a social necessity and an urgent social and humanitarian question. The breach was not further exploited before the mid 1960s.

With the transformations brought about by French public television opening a second channel and gaining in autonomy in 1964, surveys and

34 *A la découverte des Français*, documentary TV series by Jean-Claude Bergeret and Jacques Krier, 1957–1960.

enquiries about French society became more present in TV documentaries, reports, and news magazines, especially on the still less-frequented but more liberal second channel. Programmes targeting specific audiences—especially young people—multiplied, as exemplified by *Seize millions de jeunes* ('Sixteen million teenagers'). Beginning in April 1964, the series, produced by Alain de Sédouy and André Harris, explored the social malaise of youth in depth.[35] Whispered secrets and private and intimate matters and feelings are exposed in the series' films, which portray individual histories that neither victimize nor glorify.[36] If this series suggests changes, it was the talk show *Zoom*, also produced by Sédouy and Harris, which targeted a general public, that most substantially benefitted from liberal Jacques Thibau's nomination as second director of ORTF and his incentive to create 'TV magazines that escape central television news control'.[37] With the hiring of directors and producers from outside the ORTF sphere, it became possible to screen broadcasts that scrutinized France's social problems (including strikes, racism, social movements, and juvenile marginality) and critically questioned society and its responsibilities. Thus, it is not surprising that a February 1968 broadcast devoted to sex education openly stated and summarized what had only been hinted at in previous documentaries on the topic of contraception. Enquiries and surveys about ordinary everyday life of the late 1950s were enriched by private words explaining personal choices and the individual conceptions of the human condition. The one-hour programme shifts between six filmed interviews and a discussion on the studio set with Dr. Dalsace and Dr. Verdoux, president and secretary of the family-planning movement, respectively; Dr. Kahn-Nathan, a gynaecologist from the Paris medical faculty; and Dr. Berge, a psychiatrist and psychoanalyst who directed a centre for sexual and affective education (Figures 3.3a–3.3e). The only people not from the field of medicine who are featured are a school principal and teacher and a rural Catholic priest. André Harris, who hosted the show alongside journalist Michelle Bailly, introduces the programme with a serious, dramatic tone, directly addressing the viewers: 'We will talk about the sexual problems of the French tonight.'[38] To ascertain the degree to which ignorance had led

35 Lévy, 'Les représentations sociales', p. 211.

36 For similar productions with emotion-laden content in the GDR, see the contribution by Anja Laukötter in this volume.

37 'qui échappent au contrôle des services de l'actualité télévisée'; Lévy, 'Les représentations sociales', p. 211.

38 'Nous allons parler ce soir des problèmes de la sexualité des Français'; 'A propos de l'éducation sexuelle', *Zoom Magazine*, 13 February 1968, 01:38.

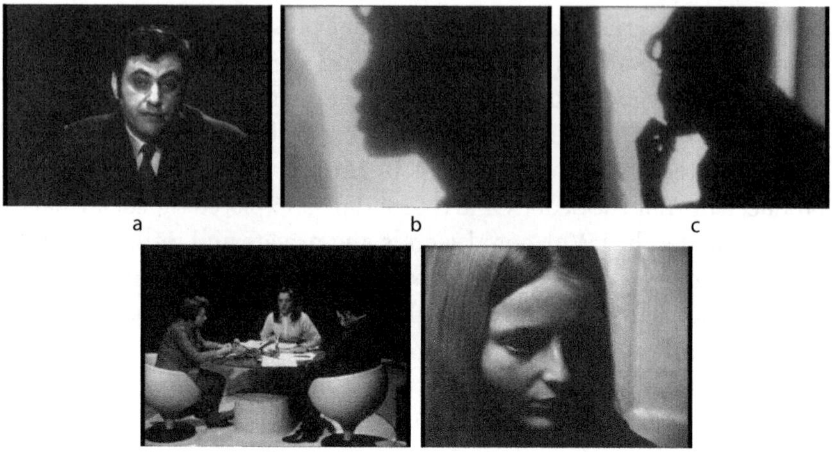

a b c

d e

3.3. 'A propos de l'éducation sexuelle', *Zoom Magazine*, 13 February 1968, ORTF, at a: 01:28; b: 06:09; c: 09:20; d: 10:41; e: 16:47.

to an estimated 300,000 abortions annually in France, the show depicts anonymous testimony from a young single mother. Her interview is filmed as a Chinese shadow in order to protect her privacy and visual identity. Close-up framing underlines the calm and intimate sensitivity of the young woman's inexperience and naivety (Figures 3.3b–3.3c). The interview, visually reminiscent of a confession scene filmed from the side, juxtaposes the moral incrimination (implied by her being filmed in silhouette) with her innocence and lack of education.

A second interview, again filmed close-up and relating 'truths about adolescence', shows a female Catholic gynaecologist and a teenager discussing premarital sex in the doctor's office. The morally rigid doctor gives the young woman a lesson in morality from off set, while the camera scrutinizes the young woman's facial reactions (Figure 3.3e). Some reverse angle shots from below serve to distort the doctor and her authority slightly, which underscore the programme's indictment of the insensitive, reactionary profession. The studio discussion with the secretary of the family-planning movement bluntly picks the sequence apart, concluding that 'the young woman who has not waited for the doctor's advice to have sex should benefit from adequate advice about contraception'.[39] Continuing to debunk stereotypes and received ideas, the magazine/show discusses the question with school

39 'de donner à cette jeune fille qui n'a pas attendu des conseils du médecin pour avoir des rapports sexuelles de lui donner des moyens de contraception'; 'A propos de l'éducation sexuelle', *Zoom Magazine*, 13 February 1968, 20:41.

teachers and a country priest. The discussions focus on two points: On the one hand, they uncover the prevailing ignorance of the discussants, and, on the other, they make clear the ways in which teachers slip sex education into life sciences classes and the fact that the liberal Catholic priest seeks to help parents with sex education. The priest acknowledges on camera that he deals with the subject in catechism straightforwardly. The message is clear: If the Catholic Church had contributed to moralizing and making talking about sex taboo in the past, its servants' attitudes were changing. The final interview sequences counterpose two parental situations: a father, filmed against light hiding his face, admitting failure as his children had never dared to ask him questions about sex education; and a mother with an eight-year-old boy, dialoguing freely with him about menstruation and how children are conceived, developed, and delivered. To conclude the programme and return to the invited expert speakers, André Harris asks them if they think that they themselves had been successful in resolving the problems of sex education with their own children. The centrality of the interviews in the broadcast reverses the hierarchy between field reports and expert comments. Audiovisual intensity and authority resides with the former. Experts are still present, but they only add to the interviewees' testimonies. In contrast to German Democratic Republic (GDR) educational film productions of the same time, Sédouy and Harris were less interested in psychologizing adolescents' love and sexual relationships than in investigating the social causes and consequences of insufficient sex education.[40]

Zoom provided, in February 1968, a meticulous and scrupulous exploration of a social and political question that was on the minds of the entire nation. With classical fixed-camera studio techniques, the programme went a long way not only to capture intimate testimonies of ordinary citizens, but to use them to give direction to the studio discussions. In contrast to prior programmes, Sédouy and Harris's broadcast stirred up a major debate in the written press; in this sense, the television show succeeded in revealing and amplifying latent questions.[41] The show was innovative in that it used intimate and seemingly unstaged testimonies (evidently, they were indeed staged) and juxtaposed them to mutually reinforce a set of individual statements. These technical decisions allowed the programme to visualize and condense changes and demands that, were at the time, still latent. During his presentation, Harris himself stresses the nonconformist point of view of the magazine/show, its intention to end the silence around

40 See the contribution by Anja Laukötter in this volume.
41 Lévy, 'Les représentations sociales', p. 212.

a taboo subject, and the producers' desire to inspire a youth emancipation movement.[42] Beyond simply giving voice to a social issue, *Zoom* opened a new form of enquiry into the ordinary social realities of sexuality in France. It achieved this not through camera techniques, but through the quality and degree of intimacy obtained in the interviews. *Zoom* was more concerned with finding out and broadcasting what citizens—and thereby potential TV viewers—thought rather than telling them what to think. Instead of teasing spectators with erotic, attractive bodies, Sédouy and Harris reveal ordinary peoples' perspectives in a confession-like emotional atmosphere, where bodies are not extras, but are there to convey presence through speech. These socially engaged, documentary-based sequences about ordinary people's experiences produced effects that were rearranged and exploited 20 years later when televisual elements like ordinary, confessional, and intimacy-exposing *cinéma vérité* shots were turned around and exploited for commercial TV reality-show productions.

A distinctive feature of the late 1960s was the advent of questions about how parents should address their children's questions about sexuality. Programmes did not always take the route of provocative nonconformism. In 1969, the ORTF broadcasted another innovative, 14-minute documentary, *Mysteries of Birth* (1969, FR), produced by Marie Claire Patris. Addressing parents, the documentary treats the dreaded question 'Mom, where do babies come from?' Rather than resorting to the staging of a liberal mother and her eight-year-old boy deep in conversation, as *Zoom* had done (and was heavily criticized for) or to the classic didactic approach of adapting an illustrated book, Marie Claire Patris films with discretion the discovery of such a book by two little girls, Ariane and Eve, sitting on their bed. Showing them giggling, reading, and commenting aloud, while, at the same time, interspersing some of the book's images depicting the reproduction of flowers, animals, and humans, the documentary captures well the girls' reception of the book's message. The film also illustrates the girls' state of knowledge before reading the book, which is stranded somewhere between magic and snatches of catechism vaguely associating the Virgin Mary and baby Jesus. This approach used the subjective social observation of what children really knew and thought as a strategy to inform and instruct parents on how to tackle sex education. Again, the camera was turned into a tool for social observation, recording their real presence and real-life spoken exchange. Presenting ordinary individuals and their direct speech became a filmic device deployed to frame and report about the transmission of

42 'A propos de l'éducation sexuelle', *Zoom Magazine*, 13 February 1968, 00:39.

sexual knowledge. Even if this happened on the second channel, which was still limited in terms of viewer numbers, written press—or, for *Helga*, TV news—contributed to amplify messages of such marginal or confidential audiovisuals on a national level.

Counter-Archives 1. Not for the Classroom: The Aborted 1970 Attempt to Include Sex Education in School Television

Paula Amad has recently suggested that the 183,000 metres of film footage gathered by the French-Alsatian banker Albert Kahn between 1908 and 1931 under the name *Les Archives de la Planète* can be used as a counter-archive. They are useful for the manufacture of the product called history in order to provide dissenting views to official, state-generated, and political events centred accounts based on official written and visual archives.[43] Transposing the concept of the counter-archive to the 1960s mediascape implies looking for contemporary visual sources of a private, ordinary, unceremonious nature capable of challenging traditional descriptions of historical events. The counter-archival operation can be understood on two levels. One is related to film's inherent properties as a mechanical device capable of capturing considerable detail, inciting unmanageable and unpredictable curiosities, and suspending common modes of memory and perception, which usually overlook or suppress background information. The other is more concerned with unofficial, vernacular culture and perspectives on ordinary life documented by private, amateur, home, and utility films and audiovisuals. I have chosen three examples of such counter-archival approaches: an extract from the *Canopé School Television Archives*, an experimental TV programme produced by the ORTF research service, and a militant video from amateur-film archives from the Simone de Beauvoir audiovisual centre.

Even before the creation of the RTF, its predecessor *Radiodiffusion française*, established an experimental department for educational television in 1947 that drew on popular education films of the interwar period. Based on the principles of republican and non-confessional popular education, the service was incorporated into the reorganized RTF in 1949. Early on, it established connections to the Ministry of Education (Education nationale), which led to the creation of the independent School Radio and Television Service (Radio Television Scolaire, RTS) in 1963. By early 1960, RTS was

43 Amad, *Counter-Archive*, pp. 1–24 and 164–194, here p. 18.

producing four hours of programming a day; by 1964, it had reached ten. Its productions were for primary, secondary, and professional schools, and it also published the periodicals *Bulletin de la RTS* between 1964 and 1969, and *Media* beginning in 1969. The *Bulletin* only mentions the question of sex education very sporadically in the 1960s. RTS productions followed two formulas: documentaries directed at pupils to complement traditional teaching activities, and productions directed at teachers for their in-service training. Programme coordination and film production was headed by a programme committee composed of education inspectors, researchers, and peer teachers, who all formed work groups organized by school level and discipline. Film production usually took 18 months and films were generally 35mm films reformatted for TV use.

In 1969, the RTS programme committee was confronted by a group of natural science teachers and researchers who complained about the fact that teachers were required to reduce discussions of sex to matters of biology.[44] The programme committee elaborated a project for a broadcast on sex education that was based on a year-long experimental research group of teachers, physicians, psychologists, and specialized educators and addressed four major themes: (1) the body and genital organs, (2) flirting and couples, (3) fecundity and birth, including contraception, and (4) child development from birth to adolescence. The general philosophy of the RTS on the subject consisted of including approaches from psychology and the social sciences in the school curriculum, arguing that moral education should be taught at home. *Information sexuelle* ('Sexual information', RTS, 1970), the first in what was to be a series of five films on sex education called *Entrer dans la vie* ('Entering life'), was produced under the direction of Guy Prébois and with the guidance counsellor Paul Geron. The 28-minute pilot film starts with a classic reference to François Truffaut's first short film, *Les mistons* ('The mischief makers', Les films du carrosse, 1957), showing schoolboys sneaking up on an adolescent girl stopping her bicycle and running to a river to rinse her underpants during menstruation. Replacing Truffaut's original commentary, a voice-over explains that 'today [1970], whereas sexual information seems to be more freely available in the press, film and publicity, youth are not any better informed as the information does not

44 The following account and analysis are based on an interview conducted on 7 May 2018 with Annette Bon, professor at the École normale d'institutrices d'Amiens, who joined RTS in 1966 and became a director of RTS in 1969. She worked until 2004 with RTS' successors, including Office français des techniques modernes d'éducation (Ofrateme), Centre national de documentation pédagogique (CNDP), and Institut national de recherche pédagogique (INRP).

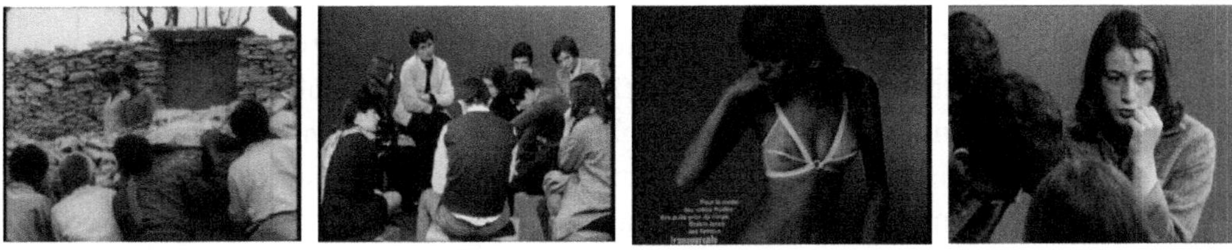

a b c d

3.4. *Information sexuelle* (1970), a: the Truffaut opening scene; b: the TV studio set discussion; c: rock music accompanied by photographic intertitles; d: close-up of one of the students hesitantly contributing to the discussion.

correspond to what they would like to know'. A nod to mainstream cinema, the stated objective of the film was to enquire into young people's desire for knowledge, which would enable film-makers to decide how to respond. With these comments, the setting changes and the viewer sees a group of adolescents between 15 and 17 years of age participating in the project in a TV studio (Figures 3.4a–d).

Even if momentary guidance is provided by a young teacher, their informal discussion takes up a large part of the remaining 26 minutes.[45] Dialogue is hesitant, with long silences and embarrassed laughter, as the teens are nervous about sharing their questions and revealing their ignorance. The intimacy created on the studio set is surprising and owes much to the lengthy preparation of the film with the group. Three cameras in the RTS studio in Bizet allow close-ups and frequent changes of perspective whenever the centre of interest changes. Five one-minute sequences using photographs and pictures suggesting the usual visual (erotic) environment of the adolescents, accompanied by pop and rock music, announce four major themes in this exploratory film. Again, it is the real presence of the pupils with their real bodies, their real words, and their history that brings about pragmatic and far-from-commonplace questions: Can a virgin use a tampon? What is masturbation? Do girls masturbate? Are there consequences? Is virginity important to you? The pill? While the initial instalment offers responses to the questions raised during the group discussion in the form of four further instalments to be used in schools, the project stopped there and further production was cancelled.

Returning to this period, Annette Bon, an RTS director at the time, recalls that, after the first episodes had been produced, the project was stopped on the grounds that 'on these social subjects, things had gone a bit too far in the precise examples mobilized and that that was not necessary for high school

45 For a comparison with Germany, see Verheyen, 'Der ausdiskutierte Orgasmus'; Verheyen, 'Eifrige Diskutanten'.

education'.[46] The cancellation was an exceptional event in the history of the RTS and hints to the strong opposition that the Ministry of Education had with interfering in what many thought should remain a private family affair. So, while the second television channel had opened up new possibilities, developing programming specifically for pupils was still difficult, which clearly held even when the students shown in the film were far from being wild libertines and still valued their virginity.

It is remarkable that the clearly educational film begins not with the message to be transmitted, but rather with a survey of what adolescents want to know. Even if the conception of the programme seems rather basic—simply bringing a group together to discuss a difficult subject in front of the camera—the amount of time devoted to discuss and prepare with the pupils and to construct the subject (one year) as well as the reproduction of a classroom setting were strategic elements used to facilitate the sharing of knowledge, questions, and experiences, which worked, to a certain degree. The rather provocative still images that frame the discussion sequences aim to situate the discussions in their everyday visual environment and testify to the gap between social realities and conventional discourse about sexuality and reproduction. Displaying this gap allows the producers to capture the 'real' state of pupils' knowledge and the questions that concern them. School television adapted to the screen what the Kinsey Report had produced in written form 20 years earlier: an enquiry about beliefs, knowledge, and practices of human sexual behaviour. A Kinsey-like enquiry with and for adolescents on the screen, however, still caused shock and outrage in France, just as the initial Kinsey Report had challenged conventional beliefs and norms.

Counter-Archives 2. Experimental and Militant Film-Making: Direct Cinema, Street Interviews, and Simply Talking about Sexuality

The public and school television broadcasts discussed here have in common their honest intention to sound out citizens' attitudes and opinions about

46 'Sur ces sujets sociaux, les choses sont allées un peu trop loin dans les exemples précis mobilisés et qui n'étaient pas nécessaire pour l'éducation scolaire.' For context, see 'Grand témoin de la radio-télévision scolaire: Annette Bon', 28 November 2012, *Canal U*, https://www.canal-u.tv/video/universite_paris_diderot/grand_temoin_de_la_radio_television_scolaire_annette_bon.11356, accessed 9 August 2018.

sexuality. This came at the end of a decade in which oral contraception had become a social reality and birth control a widely, if not openly, addressed topic. Less and less a purely official voice or a complacent mirror for middle-class spectators,[47] France's experiments in television[48] were extended by a movement that became known as the 'revolution' of direct cinema.[49] 'Direct' meant that the relationship between the film-maker and the filmed subject was to be closer than customary in conventional film production. Camera teams were reduced from tens of technicians to two (camera and sound), as cameras became lighter and could be held by one person on their shoulder. In principle, they filmed anyone, anywhere, anytime. Most important of all, they filmed outside of the studio settings so prominent in what we have analysed thus far. And direct sound gave ordinary people, who previously had only a figurative presence in socially critical films, a voice embodying real words on the screen.

The technical development of the Éclair 16 camera in the early 1960s opened the path for many of the interviews conducted by Sédouy and Harris. But the aesthetic and political movement of *direct cinema* preceded technology and was more than just that. Robert Drew and Richard Leacock filmed *Primary*, covering the election of John F. Kennedy in 1960; Edgar Morin and Jean Rouch produced *Chronique d'un été* in 1961; and, in 1962, Chris Marker produced *Le joli mai*, in which he interviewed Parisians about how they live. These films invented direct cinema before the major technical inventions that pushed the movement further. They also invented man-on-the-street interviews (micro-*trottoire*), deploying them as a political and aesthetic act that could more accurately represent humans as living, talking, social beings.[50] In 1962, Mario Ruspoli produced a film for the research service of RTF, which introduced many studio technicians to direct cinema, ultimately giving rise to what might be called the 'French school of TV documentary'.[51] The direct-cinema movement broke through when Super/Single 8mm cameras came out in 1965. This technology democratized film-making and popularized private, amateur, and home movies, as well as militant cinema. These all transformed visual spaces and often ran counter to established visual, film, and television production, while, at the same time, influencing them.[52]

47 Poels, *Les trente glorieuses*, pp. 43–53.
48 Delavaud and Maréchal, *Télévision*.
49 Comolli and Sorrel, *Cinéma*, pp. 142–152.
50 Comolli and Sorrel, *Cinéma*, p. 146.
51 Comolli and Sorrel, *Cinéma*, p. 147.
52 Odin, *Le Film de famille*; Zimmermann, *Reel Families*.

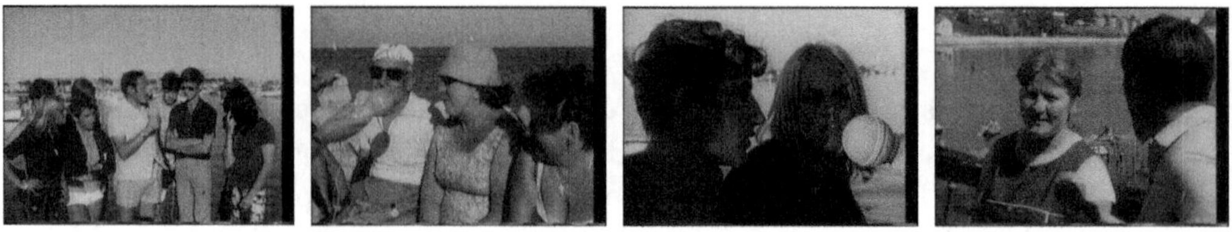
a b c d

3.5. *A propos de la contraception*, Service Recherche ORTF, 1 January 1968, a: the amateur film team and their teacher; b–d: the microphone in hand conducting interviews on Antibes Street and the beach with randomly chosen vacationers on perceptions and opinions of contraception.

In 1967, the research department of the general Radio-Television Française ORTF produced, and broadcast on 1 January 1968, the direct-cinema film *A propos de la contraception* ('Concerning contraception', 1968). In the film, adolescents were not the subject of an experimental television set-up that was designed to educate them, but were instead the producers of an amateur film made during an internship at a film studio. In the introduction to their 32-minute film, they declare that the choice of subject was theirs. The title suggests the shift in perspective: from the above-mentioned 'concerning sexual education', we move to the adolescents' preoccupations with 'concerning contraception'. The group, guided by their cinema teacher, travels along the harbour and beaches of Antibes, filming with a highly mobile Super 8 colour camera. They ask members of the older generation about their sexual liberation and about contraception with the pill. The editing juxtaposes interviews with elderly people, parents, and a group of teenagers, which highlights the points of agreement and disagreement between the generations and individuals (Figure 3.5). But divergences are not as evident as stereotypes might suggest. Nevertheless, the older generation strongly disagrees that a sixteen-year-old girl should go camping with her boyfriend. Contraception is generally viewed with scepticism, which ranges from rumours about birth defects caused by the pill to concerns about its efficacy. Ignorance is widespread. All sides are concerned about the risk of undesired pregnancy, a concern that garners some shocking answers, such as when a young man says that, if a girl he sleeps with becomes pregnant, that's her problem.

Seeking to avoid a biased perspective, the film's objective is to report and to explore individual French citizens' opinions about a widely discussed, yet difficult subject. As young people become the authors of a film that searches for answers to their questions, the cinema internship becomes an experimental setting in itself, portraying society as much as it enquires into contraception. In broadcasting the film, television implicates to a certain degree those who usually are only its spectators or its voiceless subjects at best. In the interns' film, reproduction is not framed as a biological issue, but as a social question and as a question of the younger generation to their forefathers. The young film-makers take advantage of the possibility to film anybody anywhere in order to capture their relationship to the older generation, thus creating an image of social authenticity.

Another blind spot is revealed with our last counter-archival visual source. In 1971, militant amateur film-maker and member of the French women's liberation movement (Mouvement pour la liberation de la femme, MLF) Carole Roussopoulos produced early militant videos with the first portable analogue video system, Sony's Portapak. After filming the first women's demonstration in Paris on 20 November 1971, the video artist produced a visual counter-archive with the title *Y'a qu'à pas baiser* ('Just don't screw') in 1973, in the midst of debates about decriminalizing abortion in France.[53] The 17-minute video is a collage of screenshots from the ORTF second channel INF2 news report from 6 February 1973, which featured an interview with Professor Jérôme Lejeune, a supporter of the anti-abortion movement 'Let them live', who became a leader of anti-abortion physicians in France; he had multiple TV appearances in 1972 and 1973. Roussopoulos, in the fight for the liberalization of abortion, contrasts Lejeune's stigmatizing 'the common market of abortion and the abortionists in white, while the blood of the mother and the foetus are red' with the street demonstration, where she interviews passive bystanders.[54] The title is a quote from an elderly woman who says 'Just don't screw'. The filmed street atmosphere oscillates between scenes of passive support in responses like 'why don't you march with us? I am too old' and scenes like that of a frightened saleswoman and a pharmacist in their boutique hastily blocking the doors. The statement 'just don't screw' is a verbal slap in the face (it is followed by the ennunciation 'and paf') reminiscent of the above-described *Helga* scene with a real slap in the interviewer's face. It is a woman interviewing a woman here (Figure 3.6).

There is little in the sex education broadcasts that have been discussed thus far that links the issue to the French movement for women's liberation, even if the key topics of contraception and abortion were prominent undertones. But the major blind spot Roussopoulos's video shines light

53 *Y'a qu'à pas baiser*, directed by Carole Rousspoulos, France 1971 (17 minutes), Béta SP, Black and White, sound, http://base.centre-simone-de-beauvoir.com/DIAZ-Y-a-qu-a-pas-baiser-510-652-0-1.html?ref=f8a666b0fd993c937c910f29adab34da, accessed 9 August 2018.

54 'Le marché commun de l'avortement et des avorteurs en blanc, alors que le sang de la mère et du foetus sont rouges.' *Interview Lejeune Champetier*, INF2, ORTF, 6 February 1973, 00:01:49, INA MediaPro database identification number CAF96080016.

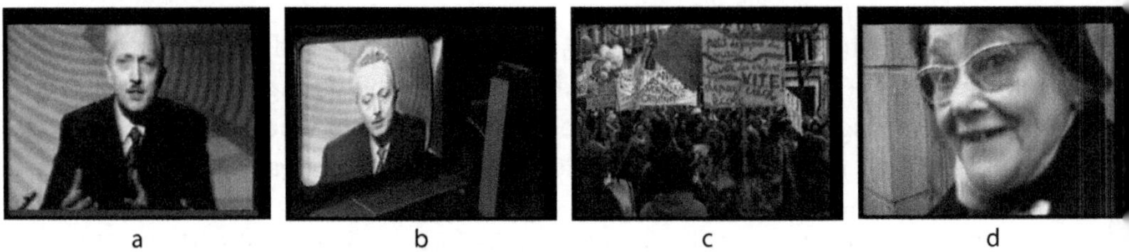

3.6. *Y'a qu'à pas baiser*, Carole Rousspoulos, France, 1971 (17 minutes), Béta SP, black and white, sound, a–b: Professor Lejeune's news appearance; c: the demonstration; d: the elderly interviewee.

on is the way in which it thematizes television not as a neutral media, but as an active stakeholder in the debates about sex education. It makes the militant claim that TV serves the interests of a powerful few. Roussopoulos's montage makes clear that it is Professor Lejeune and the 'Let them live' movement who appear on the public screen. A comparison between the official ORTF news reports of 20 November 1971 and the MLF video has a similar effect: both show the same demonstration, but, while ORTF statically films the demonstration from outside, Roussopoulos films it while marching, her swaying camera intimating her participation in the protest.[55] While she steps out to interview bystanders about their opinions on contraception or abortion, the ORTF report closes with the images of 300 protesters interrupting a marriage service in a church, thus suggesting that MLF posed a threat to fundamental French family values and institutions.

Conclusion

The article has sought to demonstrate that, while mainstream French TV was not entirely silent on the subject of sex education, it was discreet. Yet, even 'confidential' individual productions could put issues on the public stage. As the 1968 *Zoom* broadcast shows, media-to-media amplification, significant spokespersons, and stakeholders in public debates all served to give even individual television productions influence. Although ORTF generally sided with traditional conservatism, surreptitiously criticized the movement for sexual liberation as threatening the family (INF2, February 1973), and even staged a TV trial against the 'invasion of sexuality in everyday life',

55 *Manifestation MLF à Paris*, JT 20H, ORTF, 20 November 1971, 00:01:38, INA MediaPro database identification number I15246536; *Manifestation de femmes à Paris*, JT 20h, ORTF, 20 November 1971, 00:01:40, INA MediaPro database identification number CAF90010438.

television around 1968 was no longer run by a single group of producers and nonconformism was possible.[56]

A systematic analysis of ORTF broadcasts that touched on the topic of sex education between 1950 and 1980 shows two peaks, one around 1968 and a second five years later. Our analysis here has centred on the audiovisual mediascape between 1968 and 1971. Research should be conducted on the second peak of the systematic INA database analysis, but it is beyond the scope of this chapter.

To write history through audiovisuals, our analytical framing has engaged with the archival and counter-archival mediascape of the time. Different framings by different actors and stakeholders provide for a variety of points of view. Mainstream ORTF news, shows, and magazines lambasted the movement for sexual liberation that threatened the institution of the family as the binding force of the nation. At the same time, the new second channel broadcast nonconformist shows that reported on the consequences of the lack of adequate sex education in France, honing in on the barriers that stood in the way, such as parents' difficulties with the subject, a lack of societal acceptance for it, and a lack of professional preparedness for dealing with it. These broadcasts framed the problem in terms of social inequalities rather than in terms of sexuality and its psychology *per se*.[57] When TV engages seriously with what ordinary people or pupils think and do—be this in school television or mainstream TV—it is more pragmatism than politics and ideology that surface, relegating excess and revolt to the sidelines. MLF's activism for women's liberation and equality invested in birth control, contraception, and abortion as causes to be defended and as levers for change. The representations of sexuality in this corpus are not limited to images of biological reproduction. Rather, they are a collection of social representations that depict the complexity of sexuality and its various aspects: as an affair of honour and success, an act of pleasure, a duty, and, finally, as something that needs to be talked about. Many of the films portray a society in which new forms of discussion were coming into being and show that the democratic movements of 1968 exerted a strong effect on the media landscape, thus establishing a link to *cinéma vérité*.

Concluding, it might be of interest to point out some of the links between the man-on-the-street style investigations of ordinary peoples'

56 'L'invasion de la sexualité dans la vie quotidienne', Série *Procès*, ORTF, 25 January 1971, 01:02:07, INA MediaPro database identification number CAF93024168.

57 See the contribution by Anja Laukötter in this volume.

views on sexuality and the wider history of cinema and documentary film. As films move from figuration without words in the late 1950s to direct interviewing in the 1960s, one might ask how interviews and other forms of focussing on individuals' speech in film were more in line with the spirit of May 1968 and its critique of conventional, consensus-based, commonplace ideas. It is tempting here to draw on Pier Paolo Pasolini's film *Comizi d'amore* ('Love meetings') from 1963. In this 89-minute documentary, Pasolini himself conducts interviews with Italians from different social classes, asking them questions about the subject of sex. The first Italian *cinéma vérité* film, it turns out, happened to address the subject of social views on sexuality. Starting with the question that also kicked off one of the French sex education films— 'Where do babies come from?'—Pasolini travels as a 'salesman' throughout Italy, from the beaches close to Rome to industrial Milan, from a stadium in Viareggio to peasants in Bologna and Modane. The outcome of part one is disappointing. Answering a set of general questions about sexuality, the interviewed Italians reproduce conventional stereotypes. Part two of the documentary then changes strategy and asks a blunt question: What about homosexuality? The strategy paid off and answers became more incisive, as people expressed disgust and pity at the supposed limits of 'normality'. Parts three and four of the documentary deal with questions about infidelity, divorce, and the closure of brothels. What Pasolini's film hints at in the context of this contribution is the fact that *cinéma vérité* was about more than just interviewing and that documentation requires reflexivity, construction, and strategy to succeed at capturing its subject. Some of the documentaries discussed above pay tribute to this, in addition to their link to *cinéma vérité* . Last but not least, what *Comizi d'amore* and many of the programmes discussed above have in common is that, when searching for what people think and say about reproduction and sexuality, these documentaries represent portraits of individuals in a society in which people prefer to remain ignorant about factual knowledge about sexuality, even if educational norms were changing. In contrast to educational optimism and belief portrayed in the films analysed above, Pasolini's *Comizi d'amore* is profoundly pessimistic: It portrays workers as more interested in aspiring to become participating members of consumer culture rather than finding love for love's sake, and young couples reproducing the pitfalls of the kind of marriage that their parents were trapped in. Maybe capturing such dissonances is precisely what *cinéma vérité* is about. Technological changes made conducting interviews much easier, but Pasolini's pessimism was joined by TV producers' disenchantment with what, in the rising age of viewer measurements, was considered attractive for mass audiences. Measuring and marketing posed new challenges for TV production. Erotic capital, absent from the TV broadcasts discussed above, became more and more attractive in the rising age of commercial TV and broadcasting intimate confidences, situated on the fence between exploring and exploiting, became another trope of television in the 1980s.[58] Direct cinema's attempts to capture truth and reality influenced TV productions of the future. But *cinéma vérité* required a reflexive stance on decency and dignity when the 'direct' fostered self-exhibition. To abolish distance and, at the same time, to maintain it became part of the right cinematic gesture. In the following decade, it also became a dividing line between TV entertainment and artistic cinema. Commercial TV of the early 1980s generalized erotic capital investment at the same time that intimate, ordinary, and 'real' self-exhibition became a basic feature of reality shows. The body's erotic attractiveness, as well as its reality effect, became two essential resources for commercial television. Interestingly, though, the groundwork for both was laid by the introduction of sex education issues on TV. The irony of our analysis is that, while critically opposing the commodification of (female) bodies on the TV screen, some of the socially engaged, innovative, early French TV productions that explored social inequalities ultimately participated in paving the way for TV's exploitation of confession-like self-exhibition. In the end, the element captured by reality shows that produced real capital was not necessarily the aesthetic attractiveness of the body, but its intimate, ordinary, 'real' presence.

58 Poels, *Les trente glorieuse*, Chapter '1964–1984 histoire d'une déception', pp. 48–61; Laukötter, 'Politik im Kino', Chapter 'Vermessung und Vermarktung', pp. 405–413.

Appendix

English translation of title & original title	Series	Date & duration	Producer	Director	Information
Birth control Le contrôle des naissances	Faire Face Magazine	13 October 1960 01:04:04	RTF Etienne Lalou, Igor Barrère	Igor Barrère	Anchorman: Jacques Sallebert; participants: Alfred Sauvy and Marie Andrée Lagroua-Weill-Halle (physician)
The Grenoble experience (Family planning) L'expérience de Grenoble (planning familial)	Cinq colonnes à la une Magazine	3 November 1961 15:00	RTF	Actualité	Report on the first French family planning centre established in 1961 in Grenoble, informing the public about married life, sexual problems, and birth control
Concerning sexual education A propos de l'éducation sexuelle	Zoom Magazine	13 February 1968 59:52	ORTF Alain Sedouy, André Harris 2nd channel	Jean-Paul Thomas	Report with filmed interviews and TV studio debates on single motherhood, premarital sex, sex education in school, from clergy's point of view
Concerning contraception A propos de la contraception	Film internship	1 August 1968 32:52	Service de la Recherche ORTF cinéastes amateurs	Georges Flament, Jean Paul Alphen	The TV research service organized, in collabora-tion with the Ministry of Youth, an internship with Super 8 cameras doing street interviews in Antibes
First Fair on sexual education Première exposition sur l'éducation sexuelle	JT Evening News	16 December 1969 02:40	ORTF	Journalist: Daniel Cazal	Visit to the first sex education fair
Mysteries of Birth: Tell me Mom, how are children born Les mystères de la naissance: Dis maman comment naissent les enfants	Régie 4	28 October 1969 14:13 28 October 1970 19:17	ORTF	Marie Claire Patris	Rather than make an educational documentary the director discreetly follows two little girls, Ariane and Eve, leafing through a sex education book commenting on what they see and discover

English translation of title & original title	Series	Date & duration	Producer	Director	Information
Jean Richard 'The Kinsey Report' Jean Richard 'Le rapport Kinsey'	La joie de vivre	2 February 1970 05:10	ORTF	Jean Pignol	The comedian Jean Ricard (wearing a doctor's cap) mimics 'The Kinsey Report'
The General States of women, Versailles Les Etats généraux de la femme à Versailles	JT 20H News	20 November 1970 03:53	ORTF	Journalist: Guy Sarthoulet	Report from the first General States of Women organized by the magazine *Elle* and Radio France Inter, Participant: Prime minister Jacques Chaban Delmas (TV reformist)
Chancellor Gauthier: Sexual education Recteur Gauthier: éducation sexuelle	JT 13H News	4 January 1973 03:06	ORTF	Journalist: Dominique Laury	Studio set interview by the journalist Dominique Laury with the chancellor Henri Gauthier in connection with the announced passage of the Fontanet Act, on obligatory sexual information in schools in life science classes. Maintenance of a strict separation between sexual information and education.
A sex education class Cours d'éducation sexuelle	JT Evening News	19 January 1973 02:50	ORTF	Journalist: Rosie Maurel	Short news report on a mixed school class sex information hour following an explanation of embryogenesis by a slideshow
Sexual information in school Information sexuelle à l'école	JT 13H News	18 December 1973 02:05	ORTF	Journalist: Jean Pierre Férey	Pupils leaving school, then the chancellor Henri Gauthier comments on a studio set on the implementation of sex information in school but outside of official school hours.
Jacques Martin: Sexual education on television Jacques Martin: L'éducation sexuelle à la Télévision	Taratata	24 January 1974 02:30	ORTF Jacques Martin	Roger Benamou	The comedian Jacques Martin performs a sketch on the impossibility of sex education on television and ends up doing so in a dark studio under the table

Table 3.1. Overview of the selection of 12 of the 186 TV broadcasts mentioning sexual education between 1950 and 1980 that are analysed in more detail in the text.

Works Cited

Films, Television Programmes, and Recordings

A la découverte des Français, realized and produced by Jean-Claude Bergeret and Jacques Krier, RTF, 1957–1960.

And God Created Woman, directed by Roger Vadim, Éditions René Chateau, France, 1956.

A propos de la contraception, ORTF, 1968.

Chronique d'un été, produced by Edgar Morin and Jean Rouch, 1961.

Comizi d'amore, directed by Pier Paolo Pasolini, 1963.

Helga: The Intimate Life of a Young Woman, directed by Erich F. Bender, RINCO-Film, Munich, 1967.

Information sexuelle, directed by Guy Prébois, RTS, 1970.

'Le contrôle des naissance', episode of the series *Faire Face*, produced by Etienne Lalou and Igor Barrère, 1960.

Le joli mai, produced by Chris Marker, 1962.

Les Archives de la Planète, by Albert Kahn, 1908–1931.

Les mistons, directed by François Truffaut, Les films du carrosse, 1957.

'L'invasion de la sexualité dans la vie quotidienne', Série *Procès*, ORTF, 25 January 1971.

Manifestation de femmes à Paris, JT 20h, ORTF, 20 November 1971.

Manifestation MLF à Paris, JT 20H, ORTF, 20 November 1971.

Mysteries of Birth, produced by Marie Claire Patris, 1969.

Primary, directed by Robert Drew and Richard Leacock, Drew Associates, 1960.

Seize millions de jeunes, produced by Alain de Sédouy and André Harris, 1964–1968.

Y'a qu'à pas baiser, directed by Carole Roussopoulos, 1973, http://base.centre-simone-de-beauvoir.com/DIAZ-Y-a-qu-a-pas-baiser-510-652-0-1.html?ref=f8a666b0fd993c937c910f29adab34da.

Zoom, produced by Alain de Sédouy and André Harris, ORTF, 1965–1968.

Books and Articles

Amad, Paula, *Counter-Archive: Film, the Everyday, and Albert Kahn's Archives de la Planète* (New York: Columbia University Press, 2010).

Bänziger, Peter-Paul, Magdalena Beljan, Franz X. Eder, and Pascal Eitler, eds., *Sexuelle Revolution? Zur Geschichte der Sexualität im deutschsprachigen Raum seit den 1960er Jahren* (Bielefeld: Transcript, 2015).

Becker, Gary S., 'Investment in Human Capital: A Theoretical Analysis ', *Journal of Political Economy*, 70, 5.2 (1962), pp. 9–49, https://www.jstor.org/stable/1829103.

Blanchard, Véronique, Régis Revenin, and Jean-Jacques Yvorel, eds., *Les jeunes et la sexualité: Initiations, interdits, identités (XIXe-XXIe siècle)* (Paris: Autrement, 2010).

Biressi, Anita, and Heather Nunn, *Reality TV: Realism and Revelation* (London: Wallflower Press, 2005).

Bonah, Christian, and Anja Laukötter, 'Introduction: Screening Diseases: Films on Sex Hygiene in Germany and France in the First Half of the 20th Century', *Gesnerus*, 72, 1 (2015), pp. 5–14.

Boon, Timothy, 'Medical Films and Television: Alternative Paths to the Cultures of Biomedicine', in *The Oxford Handbook of the History of Medicine*, ed. by Mark Jackson (Oxford: Oxford University Press, 2011), pp. 617–633.

Bourdon, Jérôme, *Histoire de la télévision sous de Gaulle*, new ed. (Paris: Presses des Mines-Paristech, 2014).

Chauveau, Sophie, 'Les espoirs déçus de la loi Neuwirth', *CLIO: Histoire, femmes et sociétés*, 18 (2003), pp. 223–239, doi:10.4000/clio.623.

Comolli, Jean-Louis, and Vincent Sorrel, *Cinéma, mode d'emploi: De l'argentique au numérique* (Lagrasse: Verdier, 2015).

Cook, Hera, *The Long Sexual Revolution: English Women, Sex, and Contraception 1800–1975* (Oxford: Oxford University Press, 2004).

Delavaud, Gilles, and Denis Maréchal, *Télévision: Le moment expérimental* (Rennes: Apogée, 2011).

Eberwein, Robert, *Sex Ed: Film, Video, and the Framework of Desire* (New Brunswick, NJ: Rutgers University Press, 1999).

Greene, Jeremy A., Flurin Condrau, and Elizabeth Siegel Watkins, eds., *Therapeutic Revolutions: Pharmaceuticals and Social Change in the Twentieth Century* (Chicago: University of Chicago Press, 2016).

Hagemeyer, Elisabeth, 'Sexualerziehung in Frankreich', *Sexualpädagogik*, 3, 3 (1971), pp. 134–145.

Hakim, Catherine, *Erotic Capital: The Power of Attraction in the Boardroom and the Bedroom* (New York: Basic Books, 2011).

Herzog, Dagmar, *Sexuality in Europe: A Twentieth-Century History* (Cambridge: Cambridge University Press, 2011).

Herzog, Dagmar, *Sex after Fascism: Memory and Morality in Twentieth Century Germany* (Princeton: Princeton University Press, 2005).

Hill, Annette, *Reality TV: Audiences and Popular Factual Television* (London: Routledge, 2005).

Knibiehler, Yvonne, 'L'éducation sexuelle des filles au XXe siècle', *Clio Histoire, femmes et sociétés*, 4 (1996), pp. 1–15, doi:10.4000/clio.436.

Lafon, Benoît, *Histoire de la télévision régionale: De la RTF à la 3, 1950–2012* (Bry-sur-Marne: INA, 2012).

Laukötter, Anja, 'Politik im Kino: Eine Emotions- und Wissenschaftsgeschichte des Sexualaufklärungsfilms im 20. Jahrhundert' (Habilitation thesis, Humboldt Universität zu Berlin, 2018).

Le Naour, Jean-Yves, and Catherine Valenti, *Histoire de l'avortement XIXe–XXe siècle* (Paris: Seuil, 2003).

Lévy, Marie-Françoise, 'Les représentations sociales de la jeunesse à la télévision Française: Les années soixante', *Hermès, La Revue*, 1, 13/14 (1994), pp. 205–217.

Lévy, Marie-Françoise, 'Famille et television—1950–1986', *Réseaux*, 13, 72/73 (1995), pp. 177–193, doi:10.3406/xxs.1988.4857.

Lévy, Marie-Françoise, *Regards de la télévision française sur la famille: 105 émissions sélectionnées à travers les archives 1956–1986* (Paris: IDEF, 1987).

Marks, Lara V., *Sexual Chemistry: A History of the Contraceptive Pill* (New Haven: Yale University Press, 2001).

McLellan, Josie, *Love in the Time of Communism: Intimacy and Sexuality in the GDR* (Cambridge: Cambridge University Press, 2011).

Natanson, Jacques, 'Education sexuelle et maturité sociale', *Revue française de pédagogie*, 9 (1969), pp. 14–18, doi:10.3406/rfp.1969.1778.

Neveu, Érik, 'Les sciences sociales doivent-elles accumuler les capitaux? À propos de Catherine Hakim, Erotic Capital, et de quelques marcottages intempestifs de la notion de capital', *Revue française de sciences politiques*, 63, 2 (2013), pp. 337–358, http://www.jstor.org/stable/43124237.

Odin, Roger, *Le Film de famille: Usage privé, usage public* (Paris: Méridiens Klincksieck, 1995).

Paci, Viva, 'Entre promesse et menace: Le cinéma regarde la télé', in *Télévision: Le moment expérimental*, ed. by Gilles Delavaud and Denis Maréchal (Rennes: Apogée, 2011), pp. 525–532.

Pavard, Bibia, 'Contraception et avortement dans Marie-Claire (1955–1975): De la méthode des températures à la méthode Karman', *Le Temps des medias*, 12, 1 (2009), pp. 100–113, doi:10.3917/tdm.012.0100.

Poels, Géraldine, *Les trente glorieuses du teléspectateur: Une histoire de la réception télévisuelle des années 1950 aux années 1980* (Bry-sur-Marne: INA, 2015).

Reagan, Leslie J., Nancy Tomes, and Paula A. Treichler, *Medicine's Moving Pictures: Medicine, Health, and Bodies in American Film and Television* (Rochester: University of Rochester Press, 2007).

Sauerteig, Lutz D. H., and Roger Davidson, eds., *Shaping Sexual Knowledge: A Cultural History of Sex Education in Twentieth Century Europe* (London: Routledge, 2009).

Sauvage, Monique, and Isabelle Veyrat-Masson, *Histoire de la télévision française: De 1935à nos jours* (Paris: Nouveau Monde, 2012).

Schaefer, Eric, *Bold! Daring! Shocking! True! A History of Exploitation Films, 1919–1959* (Durham, NC: Duke University Press, 1999).

Schwarz, Uta, 'Helga (1967): West German Sex Education and the Cinema in the 1960s', in *Shaping Sexual Knowledge: A Cultural History of Sex Education in Twentieth Century Europe*, ed. by Lutz D. H. Sauerteig and Roger Davidson (London: Routledge, 2009), pp. 197–213.

Schwarz, Uta, 'Vom Jahrmarktspektakel zum Aufklärungsinstrument: Gesundheitsfilme in Deutschland und der historische Filmbestand des Deutschen Hygiene-Museums Dresden', in *Kamera! Licht! Aktion! Filme über Körper und Gesundheit 1915 bis 1990*, ed. by Susanne Roeßiger and Uta Schwarz (Dresden: Sandstein, 2011), pp. 12–49.

Winkler, Anita, 'Biology, Morality and Gender: East and West German Sex Education in Films, 1945–70' (PhD diss., Duke University, Durham, 2014).

Verheyen, Nina, 'Der ausdiskutierte Orgasmus: Beziehungsgespräche als kommunikative Praxis in der Geschichte des Intimen seit den 1960er Jahren', in *Sexuelle Revolution? Zur Geschichte der Sexualität im deutschsprachigen Raum seit den 1960er Jahren*, ed. by Peter-Paul Bänziger, Magdalena Beljan, Franz X. Eder, and Pascal Eitler (Bielefeld: Transcript 2015), pp. 181–197.

Verheyen, Nina, 'Eifrige Diskutanten: Die Stilisierung des "freien" Meinungsaustauschs zu einer demokratischen Kulturtechnik in der westdeutschen Gesellschaft der fünfziger Jahre', in *Demokratie im Schatten der Gewalt: Geschichten des Privaten im deutschen Nachkrieg*, ed. by Daniel Fulda, Dagmar Herzog, Stefan-Ludwig Hoffmann, and Till van Rahden (Göttingen: Wallstein, 2010), pp. 99–121.

Zimmermann, Patricia R., *Reel Families: A Social History of Amateur Film* (Bloomington: Indiana University Press, 1995).

About the Author

Christian Bonah, MD, PhD, is professor for the history of medical and health sciences at the University Strasbourg, member of its Institute of Advanced Studies and principal investigator of the ERC Advanced grant BodyCapital. He works on comparative, social, and material history of health, health products and services and bodies especially in connection with media and law.
Contact details: bonah@unistra.fr

4. Measuring Subjectification: The Reception of Health Education Campaigns and the Evaluation Conundrum

Luc Berlivet

Abstract
The purpose of this chapter is to analyse how, from the 1970s onwards, the organization in charge of planning and implementing health education in France was led to reflect on the true effect on the public of the films, radio messages, posters, etc. it produced. After detailing how a tiny group of 'modernizers' aimed to harness the apparently pervasive power of advertising for the benefit of public health, I explore the difficulties they encountered in their attempt to evaluate their mass media campaigns. Interestingly, the conception of human behaviour and risk taking that underlay the evaluative method which they devised for that purpose strongly echoes some of Michel Foucault's most famous analyses on what he termed 'problematization' and 'subjectification' processes.

Keywords: health education; mass media; films; evaluation; effectiveness; risk; behaviour; problematization; subjectification

> An American study has shown that $1 invested
> in prevention can save up to $25 in medical expenses.
> – Annick Morel[1]

1 '*Une enquête américaine a montré qu'un dollar investi dans la prévention peut économiser 25 dollars en dépense de soin.*' Morel, *L'information*, p. 3. (Excerpted from a report by the head of IGAS, the general inspectorate for health and social affairs at the Minister of Welfare and Public Health.) All translations by the author unless otherwise stated.

Bonah, C. and A. Laukötter (eds.), *Body, Capital, and Screens: Visual Media and the Healthy Self in the 20th Century*. Taylor & Francis Group, 2020
DOI 10.5117/9789462988293_CH04

> We are working out social images, thus contributing to crafting little by little a new culture of health. This is how we will be able to contribute to the irreversible transformation of health behaviours.
>
> – Jean-Martin Cohen-Solal[2]

The atmosphere in the film is warm and relaxed. The two main characters, a woman and man, both equally young and good-looking, are enjoying a meal together. They might be on a date, who knows? What is sure is that they are at the restaurant: a nice, cosy eatery somewhere in the countryside, as attested by the leafy walls outside and the checked red-and-white tablecloth inside. The man picks up the bottle of wine on the table and is about to refill his companion's glass, but she stops him at the very last moment by putting her hand over the glass. She explains the meaning of this gesture by commenting, in a half-serious half-playful tone: '*un verre, ça va, trois verres ... bonjour les dégâts!*'[3]

The 21-second long film was aired as a commercial on 1 February 1984 in a public-health campaign designed to curb 'excessive drinking' in the general population. One in a series of eight films, it was produced by one of the most successful French advertising agencies of the time for the Comité Français d'Éducation pour la Santé (CFES, French Committee for Health Education). All the films, set in different social contexts (a bar, a cocktail party, etc.), picture a character (male or a female) anxious to avoid drinking too much for their liking, without looking like a ghastly bore, unable to relax and socialize (see, for example, Figure 4.1). In each film, this character finds the perfect way out of their dilemma by making the gesture described above, punctuated by the same words: the signature slogan, crafted as a pseudo-proverb. In the life of the CFES, the 'mass media campaign' proved to be a highlight, one of their most successful campaigns ever. The results of a survey that the Committee commissioned in the wake of the campaign showed that 82 per cent of the public had 'heard' the slogan, while 74 per cent of them

2 Cohen-Solal, 'Intervention'.

3 The slogan was penned by Daniel Robert, a famous French copywriter, to sound like a proverb. A tentative rendering would be: 'One single drink is all right! three drinks ... and you're asking for trouble.' The semiotic impact of the extremely colloquial '*bonjour les dégâts*' was very strong: It allowed for various layers of interpretation by referring both to 'a mess' and some 'harm'. The pseudo-dictum originally proposed by Robert: '*Un verre c'est bon, trois verres c'est con!*', was so colloquial ('One drink feels good, three drinks ... that's crap!') that CFES' senior staff worried about the reactions to a government-funded communication campaign that used rude words and unashamedly claimed that 'one drink is good'; Berlivet, 'Une santé à risqué'.

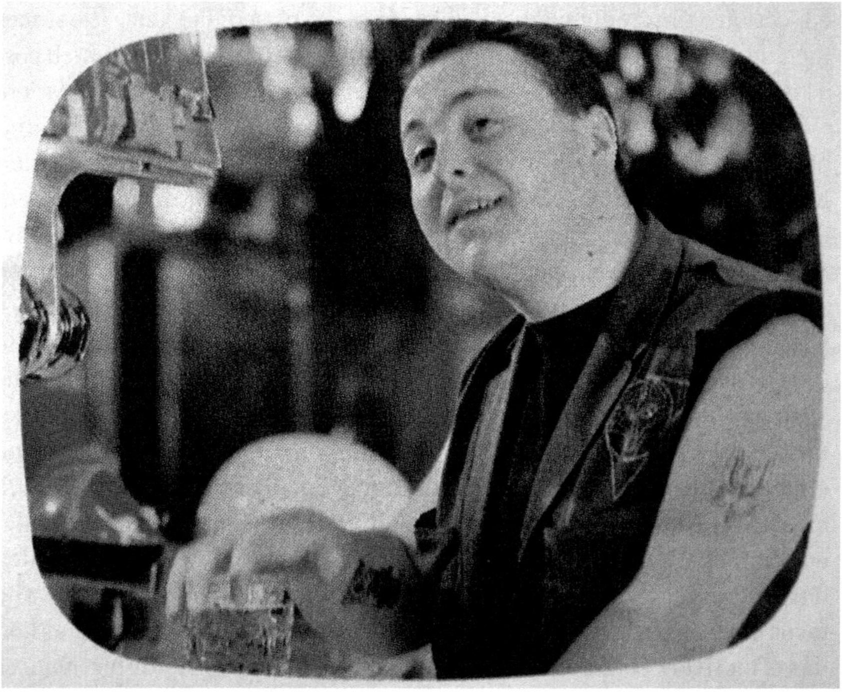

4.1. A tattooed French biker sitting at a bar drinking beer makes it clear to his friends that he does not want to be served again. Picture from the film *Le bistrot*, part of the 1984 CFES anti-alcoholism campaign *'Un verre ça va…'* (source: Santé Publique France).

could quote it (perfectly or approximately).[4] It has consistently ranked among the 'most successful' French public communication campaigns in surveys published by marketing experts since then.[5] The campaign also marked a key point in the development of a new approach to health education that aimed to break away from the previous communication strategy, which even French health education professionals deemed to be patronizing. The acceptability of health education in the eyes of the public, the policymakers who funded the CFES, and French health communication experts themselves, was at stake. The top-down approach that they had used since the mid 1970s to 'channel information' on health risks to the public was no longer acceptable; hence, the playful tone of the films and the cheerful punchline. Yet, the rationale behind this aggiornamento, as it was deemed internally, went beyond enhancing the social acceptability of health

4 See SOFRES, *Sondage d'impact de la campagne de prévention de la consommation excessive d'alcool*, May/June 1984, *CFES Archives*; Service Études et Recherches series, p. 15.

5 CSA, 'Les meilleurs slogans'; Saint-Michel, 'Les meilleurs slogans'.

education (admittedly, a crucial objective in its own right), since the stakes included the effectiveness of national, mass-media campaigns, which cost a lot and had required continuous increases in the CFES' budget allocation.

Is health education effective? What is the true impact, if any, of the kind of film mentioned above on the public's health? At a time when evaluation has become an obsession, these (admittedly) difficult questions seem inescapable. In the past decade or so, the rise of Evidence-Based Policy-Making (EBPM) in the wake of Evidence-Based Medicine, first in Europe and North America, and now as a key feature of Global Health programmes, has increased the pressure on public-health organizations to demonstrate the effectiveness, if not the cost-effectiveness, of their interventions. This is no easy task when it comes to health education, where 'Randomized Field Experiments', the so-called 'gold standard' of EBPM for evaluating effectiveness, are not always feasible, nor deemed desirable.[6] So much ink has been spilled discussing the 'evaluability' (or lack thereof) of public-health policies that the issue is now framed in an objectivist way, which has overshadowed many important questions. First and foremost, the focus on the methods and metrics of evaluation in the ongoing discussion has effectively eclipsed any critical examination of what effectiveness actually means to those in charge of implementing and, in many cases, also evaluating, health education programmes around the world, in profoundly different social and political contexts. To what extent did their conceptions of effectiveness, evidence, evaluation, etc. vary from context to context, and how did they evolve over time? And when, in the first place, did the various kinds of professionals who invented 'health propaganda' (as it was initially widely called) start bothering about the true impact of their interventions? Take the example of Lucien Viborel, arguably France's most prominent 'health propagandist', who he entered the field at the end of the First World War and remained active almost until his death in 1959.[7] It is striking how little attention was paid to this question in the many books and numerous articles he wrote and edited.[8] When, then, did preventive healthcare experts start to feel compelled to provide evidence of the impact of their own interventions, and how did that work out in the context in which they worked?

6 For a comprehensive overview of the methodology and a discussion of its strengths and limitations, see Gerber and Green, 'Field Experiments'.

7 For an outline of his approach to cinema as a health propaganda medium, cf. Viborel, 'Introduction'. See also Bonah, 'Health Crusades'; Vignaux, 'L'éducation sanitaire'.

8 See, for example, Viborel, *La technique modern*; Viborel, *L'éducation sanitaire.*

The main aim of this chapter is to further reflect on the public impact of health education as a means to preserve (human) body capital. It unfolds as a 'case' study of the transformation of the French approach, from the late 1970s to the 1990s. This reflection stemmed from the need to move beyond the mere analysis of moving images and their corresponding sounds, and even beyond studying the 'communication strategies' implemented by health education agencies, to taking into account the way these agencies themselves have tried to assess the reception and impact of their films, sounds, pictures, etc., on the targeted audience. I start by explaining how the tiny group of officials (a dozen at the most) who had been charged with 'modernizing' health education through the intensive (and almost exclusive) use of mass media, back in the mid 1970s, came to be obsessed with the effectuality of their interventions. I then detail the difficulties they encountered in their attempt to produce a meaningful evaluation of something as elusive as the reception of films, radio broadcasts, posters, and health messages. The toolkit they eventually devised, or, more exactly, adapted in order to assess the impact of their 'nation-wide media campaign' (as they called it), has proved to be of great interest, as it provides a window into the style of reasoning on 'risk behaviour' favoured by French health education specialists over some 20 years. Unravelling the rationale underpinning the technicalities of the evaluation process they designed helps us to understand their partly explicit, and largely implicit, view on human behaviour and the best way to change it. A view that strongly echoes some of Michel Foucault's most famous analyses on what he termed the 'problematization' and 'subjectification' processes.

'Modernizing' Health Education: The Lure of Advertising

The first French health education campaign that attempted to harness the alleged informative power of the 'mass-media' (the umbrella term used at the time for television and, to a lesser extent, radio) was launched on 1 October 1976 as part of a broader anti-smoking policy.[9] The experience was deemed so successful that it opened the way to a long series of '*grandes campagnes nationales d'éducation pour la santé*' ('large-scale national health education campaigns'), as they came to be called. French policymakers all

9 The campaign was conceived as the second stage of a policy framework, which had started to be implemented three months earlier, with the enactment (on 9 July 1976) of a law banning smoking in most public places and a ban on tobacco advertising; see Berlivet, 'Une santé à risqué'; Padioleau, 'La lutte contre'.

agreed that this mix of short films and brief radio messages broadcast in commercial slots, as well as billboard posters, had proved to be the only real tool available to them to reduce the human and economic burden induced by a wide range of '*comportements à risques*' ('risk behaviour'), such as smoking, drinking in excess, unhealthy diet, lack of exercise, etc. This uncritical faith in the power of 'mass-media' was certainly neither specific to France nor limited to the domain of public health. From road safety to the prevention of energy waste, through health education, the 1970s saw the development, in Western industrialized countries, of media campaigns aimed to persuade the public to modify a wide range of 'behaviour'.[10] What *was* perhaps specific to France, however, was that, between 1976 and 2002, public-health media campaigns remained the province of a single organization, the Comité Français d'Éducation pour la Santé ('French Committee for Health Education').[11] The CFES had been established in 1945 as the 'French Committee of Sanitary Education', with the mission to take over and 'modernize' the 'propaganda work' that had been undertaken by the 'Office National d'hygiène sociale' ('National Bureau of Social Hygiene') since its inception in 1924.[12] However, it was marred by a long period of institutional instability and budgetary misery, which ended in the early 1970s only after a reorganization process that included the renaming of the Committee in 1971. The old-fashioned, bureaucratic-sounding 'sanitary education' was dropped, for the purportedly more appealing 'health education'. In any case, until the mid 1970s, health education in France amounted largely to the publication of a magazine: *La santé de l'homme* ('Human health');[13] the publication and dissemination of booklets, brochures, and posters; and the organization of lecture tours at primary and high schools across the country, which sometimes included

10 Although this new kind of public policy drew a lot of public attention and attracted significant amounts of public money, analyses of this development by historians and social scientists are still relatively scarce. On the French case, see: Ollivier-Yaniv, *L'état communicant*; Berlivet, 'Une biopolitique'.

11 The CFES lost its *de facto* monopoly on mass-media health education campaigns between 1989 and 1994, when a specific organization was established to implement Acquired Immune Deficiency Syndrome (AIDS) prevention campaigns. From 1976, The Committee launched a series of 'national media campaigns' on: smoking (1976); the risks of a sedentary lifestyle (1977); improving the social integration of the disabled (1977); dental health (1978); alcohol abuse, 1984); the risk factors for cardiovascular diseases (1984); the hazards of illegal drugs (1986); AIDS (1987); domestic accidents (1990); 'the appropriate uses of pharmaceuticals' (1991); and advocating Measles, Mumps, and Rubella (MMR) vaccination (1993) and hepatitis B vaccination (1995).

12 See Lévy, 'L'éducation'; CFESS, *Au service*.

13 On the history of this health education journal established in 1942 by a physician, Pierre Delore, which became the CFES' home journal in the 1950s, see: von Bueltzingsloewen, 'Retour sur les origines'.

the screening of brief 'educational' films.[14] Experiments in the use of 'audio-visual means of communication' were carried out with the cooperation of the Office de radiodiffusion television française (ORTF, the then state radio and television monopoly), although questions were raised regarding the impact, if any, of such brief 'information programmes' aired on the only available television channel, that staged ritualistic conversations between a journalist and a medical doctor (often from the CFES) on various health problems.[15] A plan to use puppets as a means to reach and communicate health messages to children was made public in 1973, although it is difficult to assess the extent to which it was implemented, if at all.[16]

Planning and implementing the pioneer 1976 anti-smoking mass-media campaign was clearly not something on the same scale as touring two puppet masters across French primary schools. In order to facilitate the scaling up, Simone Veil hired Michel Le Net, deputy director of the road safety agency, at the time the only public organization in France with any experience in large-scale public communication.[17] Veil also secured massive increases in the CFES' budget: from 2.5 million francs in 1974 to 28.2 million five years later (a 1,028 per cent increase over the period), in order to cover the costs of audiovisual content (no one ever considered that the CFES could produce films or radio messages on their own) and advertising time/space. Together with his expertise in public communication, Le Net brought to health education his hyper-rationalist vision of human agency, not entirely uncommon in the *milieu* of the French state engineers who partially constituted the public-service elite to which he belonged.[18] As set

14 A physician by training, former Member of Parliament and former government minister, Aujoulat, headed both the CFES and the International Union for Health Education at the time; Aujoulat and Leclainche, 'La promotion'.

15 Entitled *'Je voudrais savoir …'* ('I would like to know …'), the 10-minute-long programme (funded by CNAM-TS, the main social security fund) was broadcast just after lunchtime on a weekday (usually on Tuesdays). The TV ratings were apparently very low. See Danzon, 'Le médecin', p. 154.

16 The announcement was made on France Inter, a public radio programme, in July 1973: http://www.ina.fr/audio/PHF08004709/inter-actualites-de-19h00-du-13-juillet-1973-audio.html, accessed 5 January 2018.

17 Le Net had been in charge of pioneering road safety media campaigns since 1973, the year when the inaugural campaign was launched to make it known to the public that a new law had made seat belts compulsory (in the front seats); Decreton, 'Les trois temps'.

18 Le Net, an 'Ingénieur des ponts et chaussées' (the state corps of civil engineers) by training, strongly believed that it was his 'scientific mind' that proved to be both the key to his success and what would later turn critics against him: 'The road safety world is an engineers' world […] there's a background of engineers, that is, scientists, that is, rational people. But medics did not think like that', 'Le milieu de la sécurité routière c'est un milieu d'ingénieurs […] la toile de

out in a preparatory report he drafted in the summer of 1976, the rational management of mass communication lay in a set of statistical indicators that were to be carefully reported on a single chart:

> The objective of this management chart [*tableau de bord*] is to monitor the evolution of the public's knowledge, ideas, and behaviour as regards smoking. It displays the shape of the mortality and morbidity curves which are linked to the use of tobacco products.[19]

In Le Net's rather simple, perhaps simplistic view, the difference between *prosper hoc* and *post hoc* values of the indicators would provide a precise measure of the impact of the campaign.

Unravelling the Social Fabric of Risk Behaviour: From Engineering Thinking to Social Psychology

The first of the two surveys (supposed to reveal baseline public opinion on smoking) was run in September 1976 by professional pollsters, on behalf of the CFES. The campaign proper was launched on 1 October and lasted until 30 November. During these 61 days, nine different films (20 seconds long each) were broadcast 87 times altogether on France's two existing TV channels (Télévision Française 1 and Antenne 2, both of which were part of the state-owned Office National de Radiodiffusion-Télévision Française). At the same time, 18 different oral messages (20 seconds long, on average) were aired 330 times overall on all the radio stations (either publicly or privately

fond était une toile d'ingénieurs, donc de scientifiques, donc de rationnels. Mais les médecins ne pensaient pas comme ça'; Berlivet, 'Une santé à risque'.

19 'Ce tableau de bord a pour objectif de suivre l'évolution des connaissances, des idées et du comportement du public dans le domaine du tabagisme. Il cherche à présenter les tendances des courbes de mortalité et de morbidité liées à la consommation des produits du tabac'; 'Tableau de bord anti-tabac', 28 July 1976, *CFES archives*; 'Service Études et Recherches' series, p. 1. Four kinds of data were deemed necessary to a proper monitoring of the intervention: i) an 'indicator of knowledge and opinion', based on surveys run before and after the campaign, and completed by an investigation in a maternity ward; ii) 'indicators of behaviour', based mainly on statistics regarding tobacco sales and smoking cessation counselling; iii) 'morbidity and mortality indicators' (in the end, only the latter was made available to the CFES); iv) 'indicators of action': claimed to measure the 'persuasion effort' exerted during the campaign period (said to be a function of the number of messages broadcast, the volume of edited pamphlet, etc.), 'indicateur de connaissance et d'opinion', 'indicateurs de comportement', 'indicateurs de morbidité et de mortalité', 'indicateurs d'action', 'l'effort de persuasion'.

owned).[20] Then, as early as January 1977, the results of a 'Recall test' (i.e. a post-campaign survey) provided the first hint at the public reception of all these health messages. Based on 450 face-to-face interviews (of which only 361 were actually used in the analysis),[21] the results of the market-research study were mixed: Whereas the 'memorization' of the films, the 'understanding of the message', and the memorization of the slogan were rated 'good' or 'very good' by advertising standards, 55 per cent of the respondents considered the campaign to be 'unconvincing', 57 per cent considered it to be 'ineffective', and 86 per cent of those who smoked said they would not quit.

These contrasting preliminary results fuelled doubts within the CFES about the self-styled 'scientific approach' advocated by Le Net.[22] Ironically, it was the young statisticians, social scientists, and preventive healthcare experts he had hired from outside or promoted from within the organization to implement his method, who first grew wary of his ultra-rationalistic take on human agency. This started after they learnt first-hand from the marketing experts and advertising executives hired for the campaign that changing human behaviour was more easily said than done. Internal dissension combined with external pressure as Simone Veil gradually became more critical of what she saw as Le Net's intellectual rigidity. Their clash ended in the early months of 1978, when Veil replaced him with Françoise Buhl, her public relations expert. Buhl immediately undertook to define a new, humbler approach to health communication.

What was already clear at that point to both the new generation of French health education professionals and their new director, was that the quest to improve the effectiveness of media campaigns would have to go hand in hand with a complete dissociation from the vision of prevention as 'normalization', which had been at the core of health education until then.[23] For various reasons, all of them believed unconditionally that breaking away

20 Cf. the 'Note documentaire n°125 de la Division de la presse et de l'information du Ministère de la santé', entitled: 'Premier Bilan d'Éducation sanitaire sur le tabagisme', undated but probably from December 1976 *CFES archives*; 'Centre de documentation' series, p. 2. In addition, 400,000 posters of various sizes were printed, and 1.5 million leaflets were distributed.

21 Centre d'Études et d'Opinion (CEO), 'Recall Test de la campagne sur le tabagisme', January 1977, *CFES archives*; 'Service Études et recherches' series. Despite the rather small number of interviewees, and the fact that they had not been randomly selected, but rather chosen through 'quota sampling' (see below), the market researchers presented the results as 'representative of the French population aged 15 and over'.

22 Le Net's two closest aides at the CFES confirmed that their relations with him had started to deteriorate during the implementation of the campaign; Berlivet, 'Une santé à risqué'.

23 For a comprehensive overview of this 'normalizing', 'accountability' approach to preventive healthcare, see Legrand, *Sur l'Éducation sanitaire*; Aujoulat, 'Communications et changements'.

from authoritarian, top-down approaches to health communication that tended too easily to 'blame the victim', was a precondition to any effective prevention. Whereas Françoise Buhl's main preoccupation was to shield the Ministry of Health from any accusation of attempting to manipulate public opinion on behalf of her former boss, there is clear evidence that her closest collaborators were receptive to the criticism of authoritarianism popularized by the countercultural movements of the time, and wary of the so-called 'medicalization' of society.[24] Their shared views were effectively summarized in a lecture by Buhl that was aired on the Bavarian state radio in 1980:

> Under no circumstances should one scare the audience or make them feel guilty. On the contrary, our intention is that everyone, conscious of the various risk factors that he or she is confronted with, takes his or her health in charge.[25]

And as is often the case in such situations, they turned towards the social sciences for guidance. The kind of applied social sciences they were looking for first materialized, in 1977, under the guise of so-called 'Motivation Research',[26] thanks to an encounter with Emeric Deutsch, a renowned social psychologist who doubled as a marketing guru. Deutsch, at the head of *SOFRES Communication* (the market-research branch of the French pioneer and still dominant polling firm), also held academic positions at the Institute of Psychology (Université Paris V) and Institut d'Études Politiques de Paris (Sciences Po, the Paris Insittute of Political Studies), where he introduced social psychology into the curriculum.[27] Attracted by both his academic and his professional reputation, CFES' Service Études et Recherches (research department) commissioned Deutsch to study the 'motivations' that led teenagers to take up smoking, despite their apparently unanimous, initial aversion to the taste of cigarettes. Based on 44 in-depth interviews with children and teenagers aged between eight and sixteen, his report detailed

24 Originally hired by Le Net, Claude Vilain and Marc Danzon were instrumental in the creation and growth of the CFES' research department. The former (a statistics and economics postgraduate who had also spent a sabbatical year 'on the road') was a keen reader of Ivan Illich and Thomas Szasz, whereas the latter (a medical doctor) had grown critical of 'modern western medicine' after discovering Canadian 'community health', in the mid 1970s; Berlivet, 'Une santé à risqué'.

25 Françoise Buhl, 'Intervention de Mme Buhl à la semaine internationale d'information sur l'éducation pour la santé par la radio et la télévision', Munich, 17–21 November 1980, *CFES archives*; 'Éducation pour la santé' series.

26 First introduced in France by Martineau, *Un guide*, although it did not become common practice until the mid 1970s; Lagneau, *La Sociologie*, p. 68.

27 Blondiaux, *La fabrique de l'opinion*, pp. 522–523.

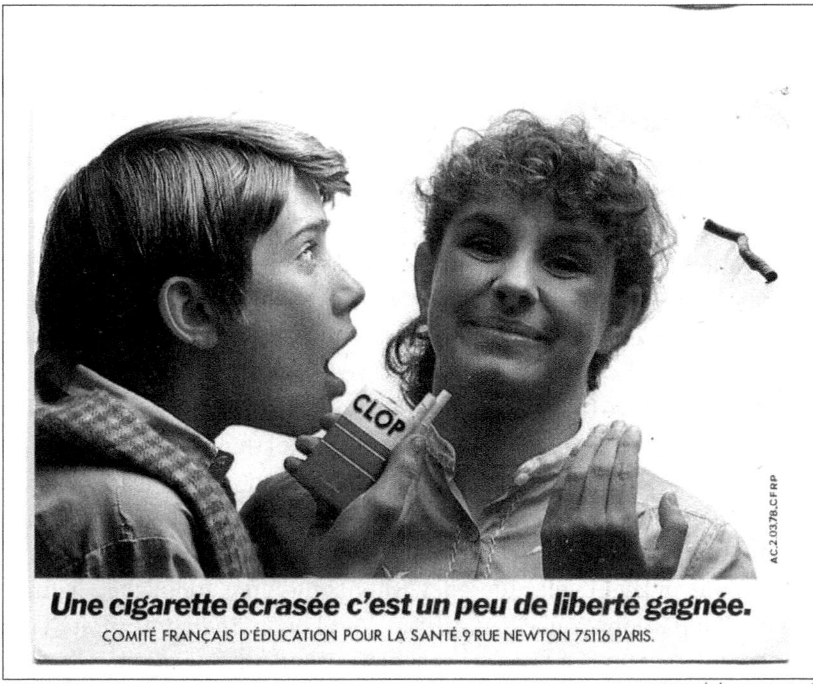

4.2. Picture from the 1978 CFES campaign on smoking *'Une cigarette écrasée ...'*.

the role played by peer pressure in this process, and ascribed the ultimate cause of smoking initiation to what he termed 'the social image of the cigarette', especially the 'smoker myth' (*'mythe du fumeur'*), which made teenagers want to emulate adults.[28] The reception of Deutsch's analysis within the CFES was enthusiastic to the point of entirely reframing their communication strategy on smoking around his argument. Since the 1978 campaign, which aimed to convince teenagers and young adults that the first step to 'win some freedom' was to 'stub a cigarette out', the explicit goal of French health education was always to undermine the positive 'social image' of cigarettes, and later (from the late 1980s onwards) to picture non-smokers as active, fun-loving, independent-minded people (Figure 4.2).[29]

28 'L'image sociale de la cigarette'; SOFRES-Communication, 'Les jeunes et le tabac: Étude psycho-sociologique', February 1978, *CFES archives*; 'Service Études et recherches' series), esp. pp. 37, 91–92.

29 The slogan of the 1978 campaign read: *'Une cigarette écrasée, c'est un peu de liberté gagnée!'* ('One crushed-out cigarette means a bit more freedom!'). For an analysis of the increasing use of social-psychological models at CFES, see Berlivet, 'Une santé à risqué', pp. 717–753; Berlivet, 'Une biopolitique'.

Deutsch's success also paved the way for an extensive use of social psychology in the planning of interventions on other health education topics. Nowhere was this as clear as in the case of the 1984 campaign 'on the prevention of excessive drinking', as it was euphemistically called, in which the films and slogan drew on in-depth preparatory research by yet another academic who doubled as a marketing expert: Eliséo Verón.[30] A semiotician and anthropologist of Argentinian origin, Verón undertook a qualitative investigation into what he termed 'the typology of drinking opportunities', which he divided into three different 'spheres': 'work related', 'with friends and acquaintances', and in the family.[31] In collaboration with a few research assistants, he analysed the social dynamic of drinking associated with each kind of sociability, to find out what sort of interactions led otherwise sensible adults to take in a much higher quantity of alcohol than they had originally planned, or even wanted to. They paid special attention to the ritual of the 'round' (*'la tournée'* in French), as interviewees were unambiguous about how engaging this generalized exchange of drinking was: 'One cannot turn down a drink', one of them volunteered, without worrying about the reactions of one's companions, since this refusal could be wrongly interpreted as a snub, an affirmation of exteriority which risked alienating the reluctant drinker from their peer group.[32] Building on their social-psychologic model of motivations for drinking, Verón and his colleagues suggested framing the communication in such a way that it provided those willing to avoid drinking in excess a pragmatic way to escape the 'round' without jeopardizing their social position. Following their intuition, the researchers started to explore the common knowledge on excessive drinking expressed in popular sayings: three full pages of the report were filled with dictums and aphorisms relating to drinking in excess.[33] The assumption was that such impersonal, apparently commonsensical, and still often ironic views could not be confused with

30 In his peripatetic career, Eliséo Verón held various academic positions in France, Argentina, and the United States. His book analysing the media coverage of the infamous Three Mile Island nuclear accident in the United States, had been published by one of the most highbrow French publishers a few years earlier; Véron, *Construire l'événement*.

31 'typologie des occasions de boire', 'sphères': 'la sphère du travail', 'des amis et des connaissances'; SORGEM, 'Stratégies de communication pour la prévention de l'excès de consommation de boissons alcoolisées', 7 October 1983, *CFES archives*; 'Service Études et recherches' series, p. 31. Here again, the research was based on unstructured interviews.

32 'on ne peut pas refuser de boure un coup'; SORGEM, 'Stratégies de communication pour la prévention de l'excès de consommation de boissons alcoolisées', 7 October 1983, *CFES archives*; 'Service Études et recherches' series, pp. 19ff.

33 SORGEM, 'Stratégies de communication pour la prévention de l'excès de consommation de boissons alcoolisées', 7 October 1983, *CFES archives*; 'Service Études et recherches' series, p. 19ff.

traditional medical (and pseudo-medical) advice on alcoholism that was seen as patronizing. Ingrained in popular sociability, proverbial sayings differed in form, if not in content, from these recommendations, and sounded more like a familiar 'voice of reason' that social drinkers could refer to without the fear of alienating anyone. The semiotician summarized his point in his report:

> The dictum calls on popular wisdom. The one who enunciates it does not pose as a specific moral authority [...]. The enunciator of a dictum is not therefore personally committed [in what he or she says] but increases his or her standing as he or she finds the right time to 'put it in'.[34]

The idea appealed very much to the CFES, and the copywriters hired for the occasion were asked to work along these lines. They ended up with a series of eight films framed around the narrative already described in the introduction to this paper: individuals belonging to various social classes and age groups, and portrayed in different settings (at work, at a restaurant, at a party, etc.) starting to drink together, until one of them makes it clear that they have had enough, by tapping their glass and saying, half jokingly: '*Un verre ça va, trois verres: bonjour les dégâts!*' Each film then ends with the campaign slogan: 'For our health, let's opt for moderation!' (See Figures 4.3 and 4.4)

The campaign proved to be a great success, at least by social communication standards. The results of a survey undertaken in 1984 on behalf of the committee showed that 70 per cent of the interviewees spontaneously remembered and quoted the famous '*Un verre ça va* ...' slogan, and remembered that it referred to an initiative on excessive drinking.[35] Moreover, 25 per cent of the interviewees who had watched the campaign on television or listened to it on the radio had discussed the films and the messages with their relatives or friends. The latter result was perceived as 'especially

34 'Le dicton fait appel à la sagesse populaire. Celui qui l'énonce ne se construit pas en tant qu'autorité morale particularisée [...]. L'énonciateur d'un dicton n'est donc pas engagé personnellement, mais il se valorise en trouvant le bon moment pour le 'placer'.' SORGEM, 'Stratégies de communication pour la prévention de l'excès de consommation de boissons alcoolisées', 7 October 1983, *CFES archives*; 'Service Études et recherches' series, p. 14.

35 SOFRES Médical, 'Sondage d'impact sur la campagne alcool', May/June 1984, *CFES archives*. Another overview assessment proudly claims that: 'The memorization of, and adherence to [the campaign] show the highest scores recorded so far in the field of social communication, even though the topic was especially difficult.' Cf. 'Un verre ça va, trois verres [...] bonjour les résultats !', 4 October 1984, *CFES Archives*; 'Service Études et recherches' series, p. 3.

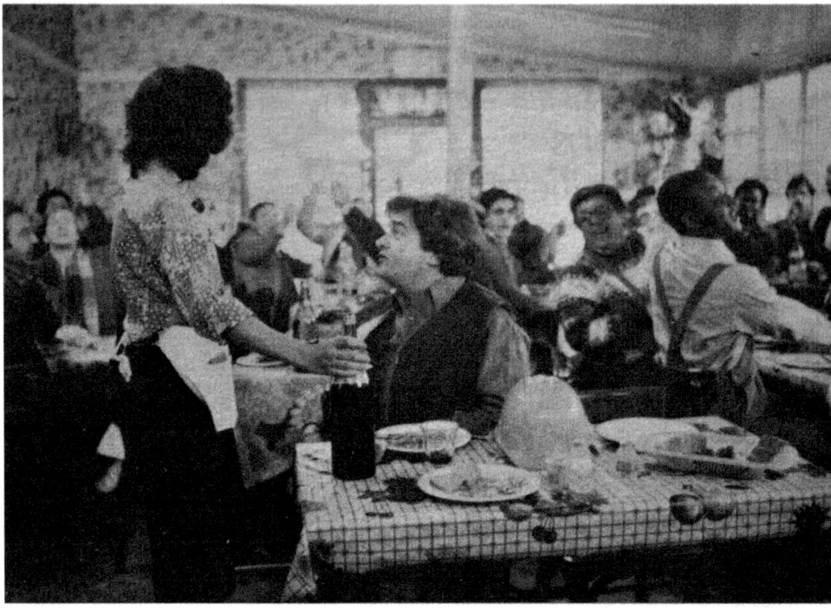

4.3. Lunch at a road restaurant where wine is included in the menu. Picture from the film *Le routier*, part of the 1984 CFES anti-alcoholism campaign *'Un verre ça va …'*, as reproduced in a magazine (source: Santé Publique France).

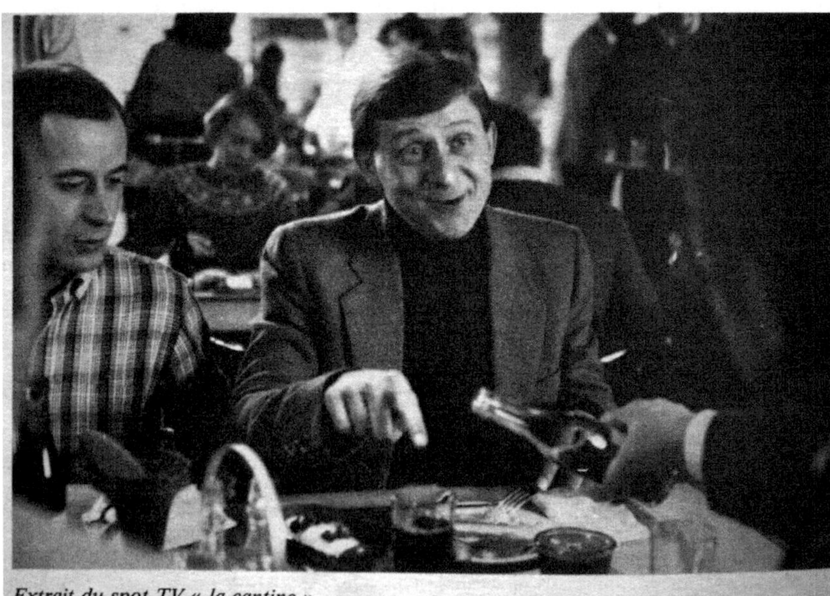

4.4. Lunch at a canteen comes with a glass of wine … but no more than that. Picture from the film *La cantine*, part of the 1984 CFES anti-alcoholism campaign *'Un verre ça va …'*, as reproduced in a magazine (source: Santé Publique France).

interesting, as it is an indicator of the penetration of the action within the social fabric [“*le tissu social*”]’.[36]

This was deemed to be especially significant by CFES’ research department, as problematization and subjectification were gradually becoming the twin objectives of health education.

The Evaluation Conundrum

In the new regime of French health education, reduced more or less to mass-media communication, the effectiveness of health advertising could no longer be taken for granted. However, what I found striking when going through the countless reports, articles, international conference presentations, and so on written by CFES officials from the late 1970s to the 1990s, is how defensive they sounded when it came to assessing the precise impact of their campaigns. Providing evidence of their effectiveness had become an utmost priority for two complementary reasons. On the one hand, the multiplication of mass-media interventions—aimed at an ever-increasing number of ‘health risks’—had attracted a lot of public attention, and the Ministry of Health faced growing pressure to demonstrate the effectiveness of their innovative policy. On the other hand, within the Committee itself, the ‘young Turks’, who had just revamped health education campaigns, were eager to prove that their approach was not only more respectful of individual self-determination, but also more effectual than Le Net’s. What made things all the more complicated, though, was that French health education had put itself in an ‘evaluation trap’.

The constant favouring of national, large-scale media campaigns over local, face-to-face intervention (‘*le travail de terrain*’ in CFES parlance), meant that it had become practically impossible to set up any ‘case-control evaluation’ of their interventions. What kind of population could act as a ‘control group’ at a time when virtually everyone was listening to the radio or watching television, and when billboards around the country were periodically covered with CFES posters? This was especially unfortunate as, in the late 1970s and early 1980s, the efforts of French biostatisticians and epidemiologists to promote ‘scientific evaluation’ of public-health intervention in the guise of randomized intervention trials had finally gained traction among the administrative and political elite. Daniel Schwartz, by far the most prominent medical

36 ‘particulièrement intéressant dans la mesure où il est un indicateur de la pénétration de l’action dans le tissue social’; ‘Action nationale “Un verre ça va … trois verres bonjour les dégâts”: Évaluation à court terme’, 7 August 1984, *CFES Archives*, ‘Service Études et recherches’ series.

statistician at the time—he had set up both the first French case-control study, in 1954, and the first French Randomized Controlled Trial (RCT), in 1961—kept warning against lapses in scientific vigilance, and advocated randomization over 'natural experiments' and 'quasi-experiments'.[37] In 1981, a brave team of epidemiologists who specialized in the assessment of social interventions had incurred Schwartz's wrath by publishing an evaluation of French road safety policy based on an ecological analysis of time series data.[38] Their statistical examination of trends in road accidents since the introduction of media campaigns established the effectiveness, albeit limited, of the approach. The CFES never found their own 'scientific' evaluators, as their repeated offers to collaborate with epidemiologists and social scientists, from the late 1970s to the late 1980s, were invariably turned down. Only in 1989 did they finally succeed in co-organizing, together with the Institut national de la santé et de la recherche médicale (INSERM, the national biomedical research institute), a conference on the 'effectiveness of anti-smoking prevention'. The invited speakers, however, had little to say about the impact of media campaigns, and the only case-control experiment discussed during the event (a 'field intervention' in the prevention of tobacco smoking among high school students in the Lyon area, which was not properly randomized) had been undertaken by a local volunteer organization with no link whatsoever to the CFES.[39] In fact, the only instance of randomized field intervention organized with the financial support of the Committee around that time was undertaken at the behest of the Ministry of Health by a team of epidemiologists belonging to an INSERM research unit (U. 292), with the goal to assess the effectiveness of interpersonal, face-to-face counselling in the prevention of sexually transmitted disease, *before* the launch of the first national media campaign on AIDS prevention, in 1987.[40]

Shunned by public-health scholars, the CFES research department turned to market-research experts for guidance, just like they had done a few years earlier when they embarked on an exploration of 'risk behaviour'. At first glance, what those experts had to offer looked rather disappointing to them: Marketing companies had long relied on a (more or less) standard toolkit to assess the impact of advertisements of all sorts, but the information provided by these 'post-tests', as they were called, seemed both rudimentary and

37 'expérimentations naturelles', 'quasi-expérimentations'; Schwartz, 'L'évaluation en santé', p. 103.

38 Hatton et al., 'L'effet'.

39 Sasco and Pobel, 'Une action éducative'.

40 Meyer et al., 'Prevention'.

poorly adapted to social communication. On closer observation, however, they started to figure out a way to make use of the evidence provided by these surveys to indirectly assess the impact of their interventions.

Post-tests are small-scale surveys routinely implemented after the end of an advertising campaign to 'measure' its impact on the audience. As most commercial surveys of any kind, they are based on 'quota sampling', as opposed to random sampling.[41] For all their claims of originality when it comes to measuring the impact of advertising campaigns, the post-tests devised by the different market-research firms that worked for the CFES from the 1970s to the 1990s all consisted of four series of questions that constituted as many separate but complementary 'tests'.[42] The 'impact measurement process' always started with a set of queries designed to assess the extent to which the sampled population remembered the media campaign. This 'recall test' or 'recognition test', as it is sometimes called, is by far the oldest component of modern post-tests, having initially been introduced in market research in the 1920s by Daniel Starch, one of the first in a long line of social scientists to work for advertising agencies.[43] Over the years, researchers explored in great detail the use of visual and verbal 'prompts' to stimulate the respondents' memory. The second series of questions in 'post-test surveys' aims to evaluate the level of 'memorability' of the campaign advertisements by the targeted population. Respondents were asked to summarize the 'plot' of the advertisements that they had seen on television and/or heard on the radio, to describe the posters, and, importantly, to quote the campaign slogan. Here again, prompts could be used if needed. A third series of questions aims to assess the so-called 'level of likeability' of the whole campaign. 'Likeability' has long become a complex, highly interesting notion in market research; it is is claimed to depend chiefly on the extent to which the audience has found the situation depicted in the advertisements to be 'believable', 'convincing', and 'true to life'. It is therefore considered to be a prerequisite to 'stimulate

41 Larsen, 'Quota Sampling'.

42 A late 1990s report by the CFES Research Department on the changes in their uses of 'post-campaign evaluations' over the previous 20 years provides insight on the differences and similarities between the set questionnaires used by the different French market-research firms at that time. See CFES, 'Les post-tests', *CFES Archives*, the 'Service Études et recherches' series (although undated, it was probably written in the last months of 1996).

43 The concept and the practicalities of the test itself were first outlined in the second, expanded edition of his (already classic) textbook: Starch, *Principles of Advertising* (1910). Starch taught the psychology of advertising at the University of Wisconsin and, later, at Harvard Business School. In 1924, he became the director of research at the American Association of Advertising Agencies, before establishing his own business, two years later; Applegate, *Rise of Advertising*, p. 163.

the interest' of the targeted audience. Finally, the last series of questions included in each post-test was designed to assess the so-called 'implicative power' (*'pouvoir d'implication'*) of the visual and sonic signs that make up the advertisements. In their attempts to evaluate whether their targeted audience 'had felt concerned' by the situations depicted in the advertisements, and 'could picture themselves' in the stories told, market researchers paid special attention to the respondents' answers to the closing question of the survey, which asks whether they had 'talked about the campaign' with friends and/or relatives.

Problematizing Health Risks: The Way to the Subjectification of the Healthy Self

CFES staff was faced with the challenge of turning the results of basic, small-scale surveys devised to assess the impact of commercial advertising into a source of meaningful information on the reception of their health education interventions. In this sense, the (routine) question of whether the targeted audience of a specific campaign had 'talked about it' turned out to be a lifeline. Around this query, described as providing the best proxy assessment to date of the 'implicative power' of any media campaign, they gradually crafted a full-fledged theory of preventive healthcare, including a firm stance on the best way to evaluate its impact. It was a theory that resonated surprisingly strongly with the two concepts of 'problematization' and 'subjectification' set forth by Michel Foucault in the late 1970s and early 1980s, at the very same time that the French Committee was undergoing its aggiornamento.

In an interview shortly before his death, Foucault clarified what he intended by 'problematization':

> Problematization doesn't mean the representation of a pre-existent object, nor the creation through discourse of an object that doesn't exist. It's the set of discursive or non-discursive practices that makes something enter into the play of the true and false, and constitutes it as an object for thought (whether under the form of moral reflection, scientific knowledge, political analysis, etc.).[44]

Saying that the handful of statisticians, social scientists, and physicians who were charged with redefining health communication after the departure

44 Foucault, 'Le souci de la vérité', p. 670, as translated by Crampton, 'Key Term'.

of Michel Le Net from the CFES gradually came to see media campaigns as 'problematizing tools' in all but name, may sound banal. Clearly, preventive healthcare always starts with framing social practices (i.e. 'behaviours' such as smoking and drinking, noncompliance, etc.) as 'problematic', in one way or another. What is specific here, however, is that this team, and consequently the whole organization, gradually came to evaluate the success or failure of their media campaign by the degree to which the targeted audience had subscribed to the 'problematization' brought forward by their advertisements.[45] This postulation was, in turn, grounded on the contention that such an adhesion was necessary to prompt, or at least to reinforce, a 'subjectification' process by which smokers, 'excessive drinkers', and sedentary middle-aged French people would finally awake to their inner nature of 'risky selves'.

Foucault laid out the clearest and most comprehensive definition of what he meant by 'subjectivation' in a 1982 article:

> This form of power applies itself to immediate everyday life which categorizes the individual, marks him by his own individuality, attaches him to his own identity, imposes a law of truth on him which he must recognize and which others have to recognize in him. It is a form of power which makes individuals subjects. There are two meanings of the word 'subject': subject to someone else by control and dependence; and tied to his own identity by a conscience or self-knowledge. Both meanings suggest a form of power which subjugates and makes subject to.[46]

The reason why the closing question of each post-test—'Have you discussed the campaign with people around you?'—eventually came to be seen as a key indicator of the success (or failure) of the CFES campaigns is therefore twofold: First, because 'talking about' smoking, drinking, or any other 'health risks' in everyday conversation with peers and relatives had long been pictured by social psychologists as a major contribution to the problematization of such 'behaviours';[47] and, second, because, according to these psychologists, discuss-

45 The focus on whether the targeted audience had 'talked about the campaign' was acknowledged very clearly by Christine Dressen, the then head of CFES' Research department: 'We look at it very carefully. This is clearly important to figure out whether people have seen the campaign, whether they understood it [...] and if they liked it too, that also is important. But it's more [...] I would even that that's the more important. It's the equivalent of a snowball effect: when one starts to talk about it, it makes people talk about it, it becomes a conversation topic.' Berlivet, 'Une santé à risqué', p. 881.

46 Foucault, 'Subject and Power', p. 781.

47 On the psychology of the 'risky self', see Ogden, 'Psychosocial Theory'.

ing these issues in public provided an opportunity for smokers, excessive drinkers, and so on to subjectify themselves as 'individuals at risk'. Talking about oneself was deemed the first, crucial step in a subjectification process described by health education specialists as the only way to 'free' oneself from the alienating influence of both advertisements and peer pressure, in order to finally fulfil one's potential.[48] As we know, Foucault discussed the role of first-person speech in the framing of identity at great length in the first volume of his *History of Sexuality*, which came out in 1976, a time when support groups had already made it a defining feature of their modus operandi.[49]

Interestingly, in the mid 1990s this approach to media campaigns (and the best way to assess their impact), which had been devised by health education professionals themselves on the basis of partly academic, partly applied psychological expertise, and could have been easily criticized as a mere exercise in self-legitimation, started to receive some strong scientific backing from an unlikely ally: French academic epidemiologists. It all started when researchers from one of the most prominent INSERM research units, specialized in public health (U. 292, again), was brought in to assess the impact of a health education programme that had just been launched by the Centre Régional d'Information et de Prévention du Sida (CRIPS, the Regional Centre for AIDS Prevention) of the Ile de France region. Starting in 1992 under the name *3,000 scenarii against a virus*, the programme called for teenagers under 18 years of age to write the screenplay for a short film (2 to 5 minutes long). A jury selected 31 of them, which were fully produced by CRIPS and their partners, and broadcast on all French TV channels in June and July 1994.[50] In order to evaluate the effectiveness of the campaign, the epidemiologists interviewed 1000 individuals aged between 15 and 49, who had watched and still remembered at least three of the 31 different films. Their conclusion strongly echoed the CFES' own take on what made a media campaign effective, perhaps partly due to the fact that one of the lead investigators had worked at the Committee's research department for a few years. The researchers detailed their views on the possible impact of educational films and related media in both their articles in a very telling way:

> The study here presented aimed therefore to assess whether these films induce any effect which we have every reason to think will help foster the

48 I elaborate further on this in Berlivet, 'Les ressorts'.

49 The introductory chapter to the first part of the book focusses on 'the incitement to discourse': Foucault, *La volonté de savoir*, pp. 25–49.

50 See Bajos et al., 'Evaluation'; Rudelic-Fernandez et al., 'Entre message didactique'.

> adoption of preventive health behaviours, namely a personal involvement accompanied by a questioning on one's own practices and/or discussions that can bring about change in existing social norms.[51]

And again:

> [E]ven if a communication campaign does not lead to immediate changes in health behaviour, as these models imply [suppose], one cannot conclude, for all that, that its effectiveness has been nil. [...] While the ultimate goal of public campaigns is to help encourage the adoption of [healthy] behaviours, they seem first of all to contribute to modifying social norms and to facilitating the questioning of individuals about their own practices. [...] This less direct impact of media campaigns requires the implementation of specific evaluation methods, based on intermediate indicators that measure factors known to promote the adoption of prevention behaviours.[52]

Despite the existing links between an INSERM researcher and CFES research department, the conclusions of the study were seen as a clear vindication of the approach to health education media campaigns developed by the latter, in the years between 1977/1978 and the mid 1990s.

Conclusion

To modern-day social scientists, exploring the historical trajectory of French health education can invoke a strong feeling of déjà-vu. The centrality of first-person speech in the problematization of 'risk behaviour', the role played by the subjectification of discourse in biopolitics and governmentality, even the (more Eliasian than Foucauldian) idea that increased self-control is the only way out of alienation and towards self-realization—this is well-known territory to us. What is more unexpected, perhaps even unprecedented, is

51 Bajos et al., 'Evaluation', p. 239.

52 '[m]ême si une champagne de communication n'aboutit pas à des changements de comportements immédiats, comme le supposent ces modèles, on ne peut pas pour autant en conclure que son efficacité est nulle. [...] si l'objectif ultime des campagnes publiques est de contribuer à favoriser l'adoption de comportements, celles-ci semblent d'abord contribuer à modifier les normes sociales et à faciliter le questionnement des individus sur leurs propre pratiques. [...] Cet impact plus indirect des campagnes médiatiques nécessite la mise en place de méthods d'évaluation spécifiques, basées sur des indicateurs intermédiaires qui mesurent des facteurs dont on sait qu'ils favorisent l'adoption des comportements de prévention.' Rudelic-Fernandez et al., 'Entre message didactique', p. 164.

that, back in the late 1970s and mid 1980s, a public organization was trying to build on social processes that had only started to be explored by social scientists and philosophers, in a reflexive way, in order to foster behavioural change, while doing its best to assess the definite and distinct impact of its own interventions. Equally interesting is the realization that the evaluation toolkit devised by the CFES' research department forced the institution to further clarify its views on behavioural change processes and, consequently, to refine its communication strategy.

The main question raised by these new insights is clearly whether the approach to evaluation that gradually emerged at CFES from the late 1970s onwards proved unique, or whether in other places, too, professionals, consultants, and/or scientists of different kinds also endeavoured (either contemporarily, later, or even sooner) to measure the 'subjectification effect' induced by mass-media campaigns. A comparative study of the role played by evaluation in organizations in charge of planning and implementing such campaigns, across countries, time, and policy fields (from public health, to road safety, to energy savings, etc.), could shed light on the differences in the problematization of effectiveness between national and thematic contexts. The differential importance assigned to the demonstration of effectiveness by private as well as public organizations, together with the great variety of answers over time and space to the question as to what constitutes a demonstration of effectiveness underlines the need for a contextual analysis of evaluation. Macro sociological explanations pointing to the rise of neoliberalism and the vogue of the New Public Management, although important, are insufficient here.

What we already know, however, is that evaluative methodologies aimed at measuring the subjectification effect of interventions whose efficacy could not possibly be assessed through experimental studies never became standard practice in public health at the international level. They are among a series of more or less (un)successful evaluative practices devised over the years, either to palliate the impossibility of randomized case-control studies or to circumvent a methodology that was being promoted by many as the 'golden standard' in evaluation studies, but was still criticized by some as unnecessarily arcane, not always as scientific as assumed, and ultimately unsatisfactory.[53] Further investigating these attempts, irrespective of their success or failure, would help complexifying the narrative of

53 Penissat, 'Quantifier', analyses the parallel attempt by statisticians at the French Department of Work to assess the 'specific effect' (*l'effet pur*) of active employment policies through the use of 'panel data' (or 'longitudinal data' as they are sometimes called).

'cost-effectiveness' by dispelling the erroneous perception that experimental studies are the 'natural' answer to all questions with regard to the evaluation of public policies and human interventions, more broadly.

That is not to say that CFES' approach and methodology to assessing the effect of its 'mass media campaigns' were entirely flawless. Being forced to settle for a proxy measure of the effect induced by their interventions, French health education specialists had no way to tell the Ministry of Health and their other backers how many smokers had quit 'because of' their campaigns. What their evaluation toolkit had to offer was nothing but a way to rank the different campaigns according to their (alleged) ability to induce first-person speech in the targeted audience on specific 'health risks', without ever knowing what those viewers-turned-speakers actually said about the campaigns, let alone whether their behaviour changed afterwards. This, however, did not stop the CFES from furthering their idiosyncratic approach to health education, increasingly building on humorous and subversive films in a way that was sometimes *risqué*. In 1993/1994, an anti-smoking campaign consisting of three advertisement films was launched. One of them pictured

> a *dignified, retired bourgeois* couple vainly trying to read in their living room while the sounds of a squeaking mattress of a young couple making love in the apartment above them grow louder. Resignedly, the wife comments, 'I liked it better when the kids upstairs used to smoke. They didn't go on for so long' ('*Les jeunes du dessus, je préférais quand ils fumaient. Ça durait moins longtemps*'). The last shot is a medium close-up of the offending couple's noisy box-springs, with the campaign's title superposed, 'Energy isn't meant to go up in smoke'.[54]

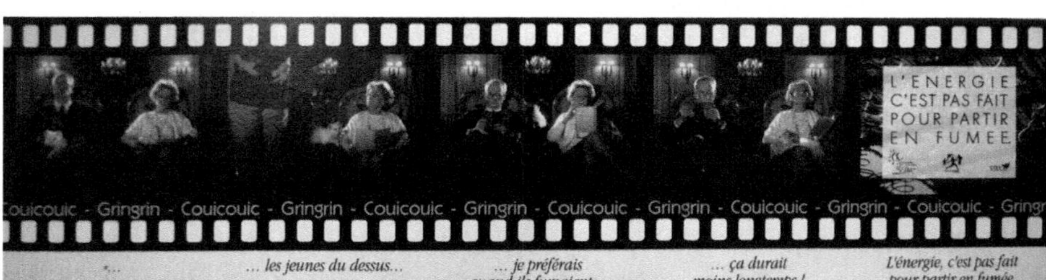

4.5. Pictures from one of the films of the 1993 CFES anti-smoking media campaign *'L'énergie c'est pas fait pour partir en fumée!'* (source: Santé Publique France).

54 Reid, *Globalizing Tobacco Control*, p. 176, emphasis added. The film is accessible at http://www.unairneuf.org/2012/06/culture-pub-cfes-fumee-tabac.html, accessed 12 June 2018.

Works Cited

Films, Television Programmes, and Recordings

'Je voudrais savoir …' funded by CNAM-TS, 1974–1984.
Le bistrot, commercial, CFES, 1984.
La cantine, commercial, CFES, 1984.
Le routier, commercial, CFES, 1984.

Books and Articles

Applegate, Edd, *The Rise of Advertising in the United States: A History of Innovation to 1960* (Lanham: Scarecrow, 2012).

Aujoulat, Louis-Paul, '"Communications et changements": Discours d'ouverture de la VIIème conférence mondiale sur l'éducation sanitaire et sociale, Buenos Aires, 7–12 septembre 1969', *La santé de l'homme*, 165 (November 1969), pp. 7–11.

Aujouat, Louis-Paul, and Xavier Leclainche, 'La promotion de la santé par l'information et l'éducation: Communication à l'Académie de médecine, séance du 5 mai 1970', *La santé de l'homme*, 169 (1970), pp. 2–7.

Bajos, Nathalie, Béatrice Ducot, Dana Rudelic-Fernandez, France Lert, and Alfred Spira, 'Evaluation d'un nouveau modèle de communication et de prévention du Sida: Analyse des réactions suscitées par la campagne "3000 scénarios contre un virus"', *Revue d'Épidémiologie et de Santé Publique*, 44 (1996), pp. 237–247.

Berlivet, Luc, 'Une biopolitique de l'éducation pour la santé: La fabrique des campagnes de prévention', in *Le gouvernement des corps*, ed. by Didier Fassin and Dominique Memmi (Paris: Éditions de l'École des hautes études en sciences sociales, 2004), pp. 37–75.

Berlivet, Luc, 'Une santé à risqué: L'action publique de lute contre l'alcoolisme et le tabagisme en France (1954–1999)' (PhD diss., University of Rennes 1, 2000).

Berlivet, Luc, 'Les ressorts de la "biopolitique": "Dispositifs de sécurité" et processus de "subjectivation" au prisme de l'histoire de la santé', *Revue d'histoire moderne & contemporaine*, 60, 4/4bis (2013), pp. 97–121, doi:10.3917/rhmc.604.0097.

Blondiaux, Loïc, *La fabrique de l'opinion: Une histoire sociale des sondages* (Paris: Seuil, 1998).

Bonah, Christian, '"Health Crusades": Environmental Approaches as Public Health Strategies against Infections in Sanitary Propaganda Films, 1930–60', in *Environment, Health and History*, ed. by Virginia Berridge and Martin Gorsky (Basingstoke: Palgrave Macmillan, 2011), pp. 154–177.

CFESS, *Au service de la santé publique, le Comité français d'éducation sanitaire et sociale, une organisation nationale dont l'objectif est de promouvoir la santé par l'éducation* (Paris: COFEP, 1967).

Cohen-Solal, Jean-Martin, 'Intervention du Dr Jean-Martin Cohen-Solal, Délégué général du Comité Français d'Éducation pour la santé', in *Actes de la XII'me conférence mondiale d'éducation pour la santé* (Dublin: n.p., 1985), p. 10.

Crampton, Jeremy W., 'Key Term: Problematization?, *Foucault Blog*, 26 April 2007, https://foucaultblog.wordpress.com/2007/04/26/key-term-problematization, accessed 15 February 2018.

CSA, 'Les meilleurs slogans des campagnes gouvermentales depuis trente ans: Sondage de l' Institut CSA', *Bleu Blanc Pub*, 0801249E, October 2008, http://www.lefigaro.fr/assets/pdf/Les%20meilleurs%20slogans%20des%20communications%20gouvernementales.pdf, accessed 8 February 2018.

Danzon, Marc, 'Le médecin et l'éducation sanitaire moderne' (Medical thesis, Université de Toulouse Jean Jaurès, 1972).

Decreton, Séverine, 'Les trois temps de la communication de sécurité routière', *Quaderni: La revue de la communication*, 33 (1997), pp. 85–98, doi:10.3406/quad.1997.1207.

Foucault, Michel, 'Le souci de la vérité', in *Dits et écrits, 1954–1988*, vol. 4, *1980–1988* (Paris: Gallimard, 1994), pp. 670–680.

Foucault, Michel, *Histoire de la sexualité*, vol. 1, *La volonté de savoir* (Paris: Gallimard, 1976).

Foucault, Michel, 'The Subject and Power', *Critical Inquiry*, 8, 4 (1982), pp. 777–795, http://www.jstor.org/stable/1343197.

Gerber, Alan S., and Donald P. Green, 'Field Experiments and Natural Experiments', in *The Oxford Handbook of Political Methodology*, ed. by Janet M. Box-Steffensmeier, Henry E. Brady, and David Collier (Oxford: Oxford University Press, 2008), pp. 357–381.

Hatton, Françoise, Marie-Hélène Bouvier, and Léone Maujol, 'L'effet des mesures de sécurité routière', *Revue d'Épidémiologie et de Santé Publique*, 29, 3 (1981), pp. 341–353.

Lagneau, Gérard, *La Sociologie de la publicité*, 2nd ed. (Paris: Presses universitaires de France, 1983).

Larsen, Michael D. 'Quota Sampling', in *Encyclopedia of Measurement and Statistics*, vol. 1, ed. by Neil J. Salkind (Thousand Oaks: Sage, 2007), pp. 812–814.

Legrand, Albert, *Sur l'Éducation sanitaire et sociale, Comité central d'enquête sur le coût et le rendement des services publics* (Paris: Services du Prime minister, 1972).

Lévy, Émile, 'L'éducation pour la santé: Avis adopté par le conseil économique et social au cours de sa séance du 23 juin 1982 sur le rapport de Monsieur Emile Levy', *Journal Officiel* (7 Octobre 1982), pp. 857–913.

Martineau, Pierre, *Un guide de la stratégie publicitaire: Motivation et publicité* (Neuilly-sur-Seine: Éditions Hommes et Techniques, 1959).
Meyer, Laurence, Nadine Job-Spira, Jean Bouyer, Elizabeth Bouvet, and Alfred Spira, 'Prevention of Sexually Transmitted Diseases: A Randomised Community Trial', *Journal of Epidemiology and Community Health*, 45, 2 (1991), pp. 152–158, http://www.jstor.org/stable/25567160.
Morel, Annick, *L'information et l'éducation sanitaires dans le système de santé français: État des lieux et propositions* (Vanves: CFES, 1995).
Ollivier-Yaniv, Caroline, ed., *L'état communicant, des formes de la communication gouvernementale*, special issue of *Quaderni*, 33 (Paris: Panthéon-Sorbonne-CREDAP, 1997).
Ogden, Jane, 'Psychosocial Theory and the Creation of the Risky Self', *Social Science & Medicine*, 40, 3 (1995), pp. 409–415, doi:10.1016/0277-9536(94)00150-R.
Padioleau, Jean G., 'La lutte contre le tabagisme: Action politique et régulation de la vie quotidienne', *Revue Française de Science Politique*, 27, 6 (1977), pp. 932–959, doi:10.3406/rfsp.1977.393754.
Penissat, Étienne, 'Quantifier l'effet "pur" de l'action publique: entre luttes scientifiques et redéfinition des politiques d'emploi en France', *Sociologies et Sociétés*, 43, 2 (2011), pp. 223–247, doi:10.7202/1008245ar.
Reid, Roddey, *Globalizing Tobacco Control: Anti-smoking Campaigns in California, France, and Japan* (Bloomington: Indiana University Press, 2005).
Rudelic-Fernandez, Dana, Nathalie Bajos, and France Lert, 'Entre message didactique et stratégie publicitaire: Usage de la fiction dans la communication préventive', *Ruptures: Revue transdisciplinaire en santé*, 4, 1 (1997), pp. 163–180.
Saint-Michel, Serge-Henri, 'Les meilleurs slogans des campagnes gouvernementales depuis trente ans', *Marketing-professional.fr*, 12 November 2008, http://www.marketing-professionnel.fr/breve-wp/les-meilleurs-slogans-des-campagnes-gouvernementales-depuis-trente-ans.html, accessed 5 February 2018.
Sasco, Annie, and Dominique Pobel, 'Une action éducative en milieu scolaire', in *La lutte contre le tabagisme est-elle efficace? Évaluation et perspectives*, ed. by Karen Slama, Serge Karsenty, and Albert Hirsch (Paris: INSERM, 1992), pp. 45–55.
Schwartz, Daniel, 'L'évaluation en santé', in *L'évaluation des politiques publiques*, ed. by Jean-Pierre Nioche and Robert Poinsard (Paris: Économica, 1984), pp. 93–105.
Starch, Daniel, *Principles of Advertising* (Chicago: Shaw, 1923).
Véron, Eliseo, *Construire l'événement: Les médias et l'accident de Three Mile Island* (Paris: Minuit, 1981).
Viborel, Lucien, 'Introduction: Le cinéma, créateur d'impressions distrayantes est, avant tout, un prodigieux agent d'éducation', in *Catalogue de la cinémathèque du ministère du Travail, de l'Hygiène, de l'Assistance et de la Prévention sociales,*

de l'Office National d'Hygiène Social et du Comité National de Défense contre la Tuberculose [Paris: n.p., undated].
Viborel, Lucien, *La technique moderne de la propagande d'hygiène sociale* (Paris: La Vie saine, 1930).
Viborel, Lucien, *L'éducation sanitaire: Science d'action* (Tours: Arrault, 1944).
Vignaux, Valérie, 'L'éducation sanitaire par le cinéma dans l'entre-deux-guerres en France', *Sociétés & Représentations*, 28, 2 (2009), pp. 67–85.
von Bueltzingsloewen, Isabelle, 'Retour sur les origines de La Santé de l'homme', *La santé de l'homme*, 420 (September 2012), pp. 17–18.

About the Author

Luc Berlivet is Chargé de recherche at the French National Centre for Scientific Research (CNRS), and lecturer at the School for Advanced Studies in Social Sciences (EHESS), in Paris. He has published extensively on the history of epidemiology, the various uses of statistics in public health, and the politics of health education.
Contact details: luc.berlivet@cnrs.fr

5. Swimming the Crawl to Educate the Modern Body: Visual Material and the Expanding Market for Participatory Sports in the USA, 1890s–1930s

Olaf Stieglitz

Abstract

This essay outlines how sports photography and film from the early twentieth century have been used to introduce US-Americans to a scientific understanding of human bodies and their motions. It asks how certain groups tried to make sure that this modern perspective became not only ubiquitous but also a marketable commodity. The essay focuses on crawl swimming because its motions became increasingly related to discussing modernity and modern bodies. Furthermore, crawl swimming was densely charged along racial and gendered lines: The modernity of the sporting body and its visual appeal rested significantly on ideas of racial hierarchies and a changing as well as problematic perception of women's roles in public. In that sense, swimming was doing gender as well as doing race.

Keywords: crawl swimming; *Crystal Champions*; sports photography; sports film; sports marketing; modernity; gender; race; whiteness; technology.

During the summer and fall of 1929, film audiences in the United States as well as in Europe could watch amazing, even spectacular scenes on the silver screen while waiting for the main picture. A popular short film of that season, *Crystal Champions*, took cinemagoers under water: Shot at a lakeside in Silver Springs, Florida, and using the newest photo technology (such as a high-speed underwater handheld camera) and an integrated soundtrack like those becoming more and popular in Hollywood productions, the

Bonah, C. and A. Laukötter (eds.), *Body, Capital, and Screens: Visual Media and the Healthy Self in the 20th Century*. Taylor & Francis Group, 2020
DOI 10.5117/9789462988293_CH05

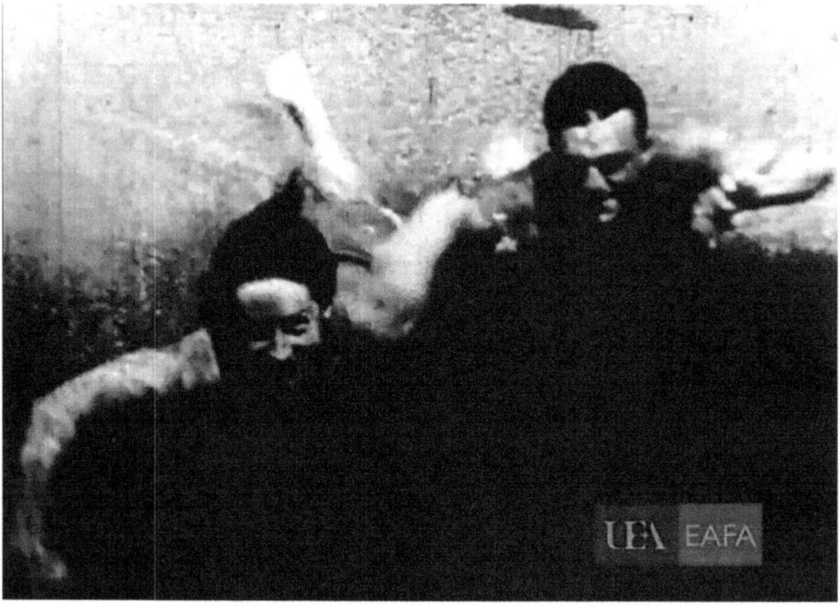

5.1. Still from *Crystal Champions* (USA, 1929), showing high-divers Helen Meany and Pete Desjardins. Permission by East Anglia Film Archive.

eleven-minute-long film depicted water sports from mostly previously unseen perspectives. With the help of this cutting-edge photo equipment, the film's opening sequence follows a group of teenage boys and girls on a diving treasure hunt to the bottom of the lake, showing underwater motions that had been impossible to depict before. Fascination then shifts to the expertly executed swimming styles of two world-record-holding champions, Martha Norelius and Johnny Weissmuller, who are shown demonstrating their skills in astonishingly detailed close-up shots from a variety of angles. While this part of the film celebrates underwater efficiency and elegance, the following sequence returns to the fun of water sports and tells the story of Newton Perry, who makes a living by diving for turtles—an occupation truly suitable for introducing new photo technology to a broader public. In its final minutes, *Crystal Champions* takes its audience airborne: Starring the two well-known high divers Helen Meany and Pete Desjardins, the film uses slow motion as well as shots from both above and below the divers to present close depictions of jumps from platforms located some 60 feet above the water (Figure 5.1).[1]

1 *Crystal Champions: A Grantland Rice Sound Sportlight for Van Beuren-Pathé*, 1 reel (11 min.), directed by Jack Eaton; performances by Pete Desjardins, Helen Meany, Martha Norelius, Newton

While contemporary reviews highlighted the amazing images of *Crystal Champions*, the fact that it was a sound short received even more praise.[2] Produced by Grantland Rice, the famous sports columnist also served as the film's narrator, and, given the novelty of sound film as a signature development of the film industry, it is no wonder that the synchronized words and orchestral music aroused a special curiosity. All in all, the release of *Crystal Champions* served several interrelated interests: First, the film was a valuable advertisement for Florida's tourism business; it depicted one of the state's main vacation spots and underscored its natural beauties as well as its recreational opportunities to an all-American and even international audience of potential visitors. In this regard, the film operated clearly within economic reasoning. Second, the film featured technological progress and linked it to creativity, success, achievement, and personal pleasure, using the world of sports as a well-established reference for that relationship. In doing so, it emphasized a certain understanding of American modernity that strongly rested on the idea of success and self-fulfilment through progress and ingenuity.[3] Since the First World War, American sports had increasingly been understood within this worldview, assuming that winning athletes were the result of technological superiority and intellectual reason, resulting in scientifically guided training. *Crystal Champions*, a fitness expert stated, served as a perfect example, because it 'helps intermediate and advanced swimmer[s] in improving skill'.[4] Third, *Crystal Champions* celebrated the potential of the human body, its capabilities and beauty, and charged it as a reservoir for achievement as well as pleasure. The film achieved this by building on the persuasiveness of visuality—narration and music were undoubtedly very important for the attractiveness of the film, but it nevertheless drew its overall appeal from its images of bodies in motion in, under, and above the water's surface. That this fascination with the human body rested on unmarked gendered and racialized assumptions establishes a core starting point for the analyses I am going to unfold on the following pages. Finally, as a fourth aspect, *Crystal Champions* pointed towards swimming as an activity that linked white, middle-class family life to a growing leisure time and vacation industry. Swimming here emerged as

Perry, and Johnny Weissmuller; released in May 1929. For another Grantland Rice water sports film production, *Aquatic House Party*, cinematographer Ernest Corts and director Jack Eaton received an Academy Award for best short film (1949).

2 Bradley, *First Hollywood*. Reviews of *Crystal Champions* were published in *Motion Picture News*, 27 April 1929, p. 1410 and *Variety*, 16 October 1929, p. 17.

3 Susman, *Culture as History*, esp. chapter 7.

4 Schutz, 'Motion Picture', p. 376.

a social action, a multigenerational lifestyle of consumption that expressed a gendered and racialized class identity.

In this essay, I will outline how sports images from the early decades of the 20th century, and especially photography and film, have been used to introduce Americans to a scientific understanding of human bodies and their motions, and how certain groups tried to make sure that this modern perspective became not only ubiquitous but also an attractive, sexualized, marketable commodity. The actual example I am going to focus on will be swimming, mostly because the motions of swimming became increasingly related to discussing modernity and modern bodies in the United States, an aspect that, moreover, addresses the capabilities of photography and film as modern media technologies in particular ways. Furthermore, swimming has been, and, in some regards, still is today, densely charged along racial and gendered lines: The modernity of the sporting body and its visual appeal, I argue, rested significantly on ideas of racial hierarchies and a changing as well as problematic perception of women's roles in public. In that sense, swimming was *doing gender* as well as *doing race*.

I will develop my argument in two steps: First, I am going to focus on popular advice literature published in the United States during the early 20th century, arguing that printing photos of bodies in motion significantly aided in establishing an understanding of what a modern body should look like and how it should function efficiently in a changing social and cultural setting. A combination of technological developments, a changing media environment, economic interests, and social trends all addressed the body as some sort of interface between individual and society, as a personal project to incorporate changing social values—or relate to them in a less affirmative fashion. In the second part of this essay, I underscore the rising importance of film after the First World War, with an emphasis on developments that accentuate the relevance of gender as a lens for understanding modern perspectives on American bodies.

The Science of Swimming: From Advice Literature to Moving Images

In the silent film comedy *College* (USA, 1927), starring Buster Keaton, we see the freshman protagonist, Ronald, arriving at his new school fully prepared to become a popular athlete. Ronald brings along all the necessary equipment needed to make the college's baseball, football, and track teams. Moreover, his suitcase contains copies of several advice booklets, all published in Spalding's

Athletic Library.[5] Since the late 1880s, more than 300 separate publications on sports and physical activities had been published by that company, which was part of the A.G. Spalding and Brothers' sports goods emporium, a Chicago-based but, at that point in time, nationally and internationally operating corporation that dominated the sale and marketing of sports apparel and equipment. These advice manuals were not peripheral to the company's activities, but were, instead, produced to create 'the greatest educational series on athletic and physical training subjects that has ever been compiled'.[6] Titles ranged from the simple *How to Play Baseball* to the more specialized *How to Play Shortstop*, from *Home Exercising* to *How to Live 100 Years* to *Ten Minutes' Exercises for the Busy Men*. Priced from 10 to 25 cents, many of these pamphlets saw multiple editions over the years, sold several hundreds of thousands of copies, and made their way into numerous school and public libraries. When freshman Ronald came to college in 1927, almost two generations of Americans had grown up reading sporting advice from Spalding's Athletic Library.

In offering a complete line of sports equipment, the mother corporation Spalding and Brothers' was an almost ideal example of a large-scale, ever expanding, vertically integrated, diversified, expertly managed, modern corporation. The large majority of its Athletic Library manuals fitted perfectly into that design: They were usually written by well-known expert authors such as former athletes, coaches, journalists, or other pundits; they claimed to contain state-of-the-art and practically tested knowledge; they almost always included advice pointing to embedding very specific corporeal practices into a much larger concept of taking care of one's body by observing questions of nutrition, hygiene, or sexuality; and they offered information relevant to different kinds of readers, from school kids and adult beginners to advanced athletes, to those seeking health and relaxation in physical activities, as well as to those wanting to push their personal records, to men and—increasingly important, especially after the First World War—women. Yet despite its wide appeal and distribution, one should keep in mind that those publications were almost completely marketed towards a white American middle class; references to racialized groups within society remained rare even during the 1920s and 1930s, when the world of sports started to acknowledge non-white athletes, at least sometimes.[7]

While the Spalding booklets dominated the market, many other publishing houses held important shares in it as well. Taken together, one comes

5 Stieglitz, 'Die Komödie als Bewegungsstudie'.
6 Levine, *A. G. Spalding*, p. 102.
7 Welky, *Everything Was Better*; Wolcott, *Race*.

across a financially lucrative segment of advice literature, which aims to place sports and physical activity within a dense discourse that linked health, nutrition, hygiene, and fitness to an active understanding of what a modern, white, urban American citizen should look like and should do.[8] A variety of magazines further broadened this objective, spanning from middle-class lifestyle publications such as *Vanity Fair* or *Collier's* to less expensive and less fashion-oriented outlets like *Physical Culture* (published by the both popular and controversial fitness advocate Bernarr Macfadden) to the many different special interest sports magazines.[9] And, in their aim to charge the moving body as modern, all these publications greatly relied on advanced printing technology and especially on photography. Drawings and engravings had been established features in advice manuals for a long time, but photography promised not only a more realistic but also a more detailed perspective on bodies in motion. And a focus on detail, on separating individual, specific elements of motions from one another, analysing complexity in synchronic and diachronic movements, became a core epistemological concern for the developing sports science after 1900.[10] Photographic and later filmic time-motion studies carried an enormous argumentative weight in expert discourses, and advice manuals for the ordinary sportsperson, plus magazine articles, were immensely influential in transmitting that notion to a larger American public.[11]

A perspective on swimming helps demonstrate that aspect. In some regards, this sport/fitness practice is a very suitable example because swimming boomed in the US during the early decades of the 20th century.[12] What made swimming especially appealing to many white, middle-class Americans was its twofold character that made the practice a serious sport or fitness pursuit as well as a leisure activity done for socialization—its popularity rested on the fact that one could spent a day at the beach but still claim to go swimming. A widely circulating safety discourse linked the two practices of swimming and bathing together, strongly demanding that, in order to enjoy the latter, one has to master the former. Although still heavily segregated along lines of race, gender, and class, the overall number of facilities and opportunities to swim increased greatly, and many commentators underscored the value of swimming for what they considered

8 Green, *Fit for America*; Mackert, 'I want to be'; Martschukat, 'Pursuit of Fitness'.

9 Stieglitz, 'Ikonen einer neuen Freiheit'.

10 Hoberman, *Mortal Engines*; Massengale and Swanson, *History of Exercise*; Carter, *Medicine*.

11 Braun, *Picturing Time*; Prodger, *Time Stands Still*.

12 Wiltse, *Contested Waters*.

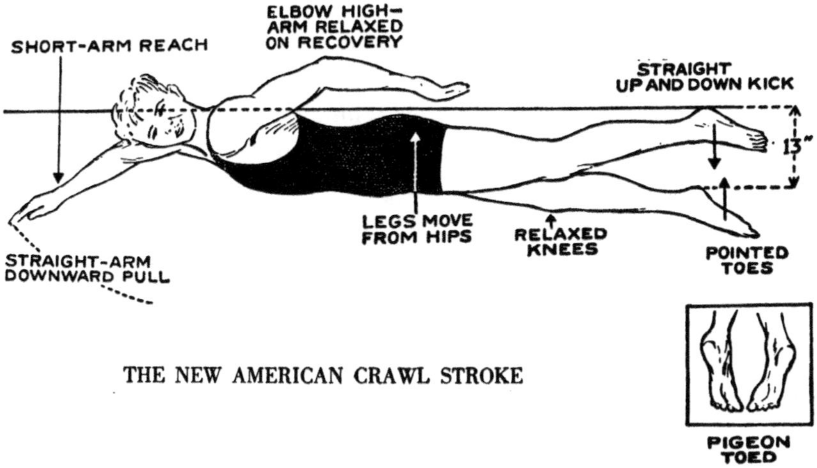

5.2. Sullivan, *Science of Swimming*, p. 32.

an all-round, well-balanced, healthy body development. The introduction and popularization of the new crawl style during these years resulted in a small swimming craze, and the motions of the crawl were regularly related to ultimate modern ideas of speed, efficiency, and streamlining.[13]

In other regards, though, swimming presents an unlikely and rather complicated example for my point. The technical possibilities for visualizing in- and underwater motions remained difficult until well into the 1920s. Photographic and filmic technology capable of depicting what usually remained invisible parts of swimming motions were usually too expensive and too much part of laboratory studies to find their way into commercial publications, but authors and publishers were very creative in dealing with that problem. The speed of some swimming styles, plus the necessity to protect the valuable camera equipment from getting wet, added to the difficulties—undesired sprays of water became a constant issue in depicting swimming in several advice manuals.

The process of modernizing what had formerly been called the 'ancient art of swimming' relied on the language and imagery of workplace studies and scientific management. A drawing taken from a 1934 publication (Figure 5.2) illustrates the constantly growing urge to split up the motions of swimming

13 A small sample of swimming manuals popular in this time period includes: Dalton, *Swimming Scientifically Taught*; Sterrett, *How to Swim*; Brown, *Modern Swimming*; Bachrach, *Outline of Swimming*; Sheffield and Sheffield, *Swimming Simplified*; Handley, *Swimming and Watermanship*; Handley, *Swimming for Women*; Sullivan, *Science of Swimming*.

in general and the crawl in particular into several individual analytical units. The language used the vocabulary of scientific management:

> [The crawl stroke] must enable [the swimmers] to so reduce the effort that they can develop greater speed and endurance than was possible [before] on the same output of energy. It would be illogical to believe [...] that methods which allow the contestant to travel faster and farther without increasing the strain, will not render equal service to the man or woman who swims for pleasure, exercise or necessity.[14]

Many advice texts actively established a close relationship between both the textual descriptions and the visual material they deployed, on the one hand, and the actual training practice of athletes and coaches on the other, a relationship based on a carefully guided cooperation between the human eye and camera lenses. In many sports, and swimming is no exception, coaches often remained reluctant to trust camera-produced images, arguing that their experienced expert eyes were able to detect more details and nuance than any technical device could. Confronted with this opinion, manual authors argued in favour of a reasonable compromise, and so, when author Gerald Barnes appealed to his reader to 'get someone to watch you', he pointed towards an all-round visual arrangement of analytical gazes that included instructive images, coaches' perspectives, and the self-observation of swimmers.[15]

Nevertheless, depicting in- and underwater motions in photographs remained problematic (Figures 5.3 and 5.4). Well into the 1920s, most manuals relied on two strategies to deal with that technological inadequacy. The first made use of a long-established practice of swim training, the on-land, so-called dry drill. From the perspective of authors and publishers, it served a valuable purpose, because it allowed for a combined illustration of three important aspects: Photos like these could be produced without the confusing effects of water; they could be staged by prominent, role-model swimmers; and they underlined the analytics by focussing on the detail arrangement of watching oneself and others. With the second strategy, manuals tried to combine studio photography with the explanatory opportunities offered by drawings. The artificially superimposed waterline, separating above- and underwater movements, indicated, at the same time, the limits of photography and the strong desire to use all visual means available to depict a scientific understanding of the sport.

14 Handley, *Swimming and Watermanship*, p. 20.
15 Barnes, *Swimming and Diving*, p. 5.

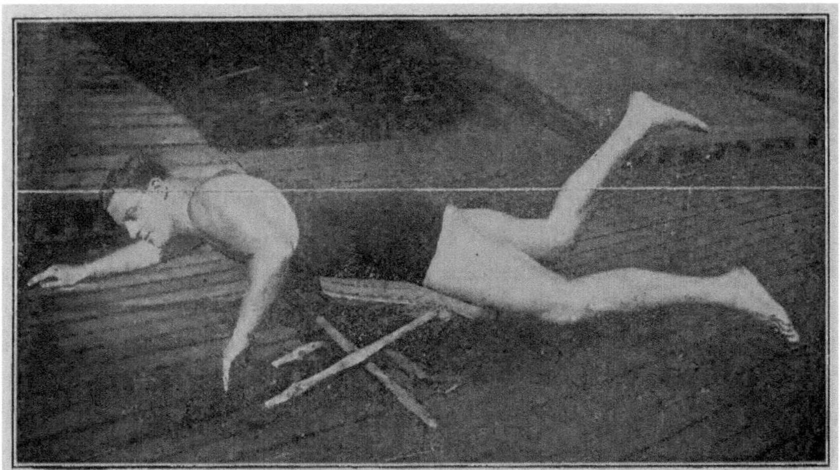

CRAWL–SECOND POSITION.

5.3. Daniels, *Speed Swimming* p. 30.

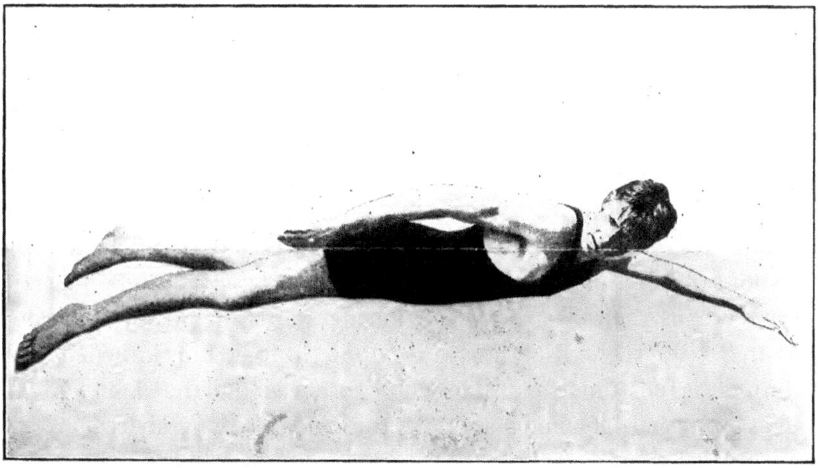

HERBERT VOLLMER, N. Y. A. C., SWIMMING THE TRUDGE-CRAWL.

5.4. Sterrett, *How to Swim*, between pp. 16–17.

Visualizing the Gendered Modernity of Swimming through Photography and Film

But the visual arrangement of how-to-swim manuals extended beyond images for instruction and self-instruction, and, with the advance of photo technology after the Great War, the depictions started to actively combine an analytical gaze on movements with notions related to physical appeal and thus to what were considered modern and very much gendered understandings of beauty and personality. The increasing importance of women's swimming was one influential part of that process.[16] A growing number of magazine articles and book chapters conveyed the message that learning to swim was the thing to do for young, white, middle-class women, often indicating that the newly gained political and social rights for women were well represented in the swimming boom.[17] Manuals now regularly included individual chapters on women's swimming, and many were indicative of the ambivalences that came with integrating women 'into citizenship in the sporting republic', to quote a phrase by historian Mark Dyreson: 'As women's sports boomed during the 1920s, American culture transformed female athletes into icons of liberty. At the same time, American culture also transformed female athletes into objects of desire.'[18] Photos of successful female swimmers and divers served as often-recurring examples of the 'modern athletic woman'.

'One of the weirdest of the many phenomena attendant upon the American sport scene is the worship [...] accorded to lady swimmers', wondered sports columnist Paul Gallico, observing that they 'have been photographed, biographed, feted, pursued by millionaires, popped into the movies, lionized, and [...] glorified, beyond all bounds of sanity and reason'.[19] Especially after the mid-1920s, these images became more sexually suggestive in character, presenting young sports-women in their swim-suits that indicated both athleticism and eroticism. A dense visual arrangement thus linked women's swimming to fashion, beauty, and physical attractiveness. Moreover, many advice texts and magazine articles underscored a close relationship to questions of conscious nutrition and dieting. A *Physical Culture* magazine essay serves as a suitable example: If 'Business Girls Should Swim for Better Posture', to quote its title, they were supposed to do it as knowledgeable swimmers, as costumers of fashionable sportswear and the 'right food', and thus as promising dates and potential future brides.[20] Many advice books also manoeuvred along that thin line separating empowering women through teaching a new, exciting, even liberating bodily practice on the one hand, and asking them to adjust to the new sexualized demands of the post-war years, on the other. Handbooks used photography for the twin purposes of teaching technique and displaying sex appeal at the same time. This combination

16 Bier, *Fighting the Current*.
17 Corsan, 'Learning to Swim'; Ford, 'Swimming for Ladies'.
18 Dyreson, 'Icons of Liberty', pp. 435, 438.
19 Gallico, 'Babes in the Drink', p. 49.
20 Macfadden, 'Business Girls'.

was regularly used, for example, by Spalding's sports booklets. In a volume authored by Louis Handley, one finds photos inspired by time-motion studies next to several pages of advertisement for Spalding swimsuits, all visually emphasizing the erotic appeal of an athletic body wearing this outfit.[21] This visual strategy became influential even in magazines such as *Vanity Fair* or *Physical Culture*; outside the realm of textbooks and without the necessity to claim the images' instructiveness, the staging of female swimmers in bathing costumes increasingly lost its reference to the actual practice of swimming. Although labelled as the result of an active, 'healthy' lifestyle in and around a pool or a beach, the mise en scène of many such images meant that the sport itself became an empty signifier.

Nevertheless, eroticizing the body in motion was not limited to women. One person in particular lifted the visual representation of crawl swimming and of the capable white modern athletic body on another level. Without any doubt, Johnny Weissmuller was *the* embodiment of American swimming during the 1920s, and, in addition to Hollywood actor Douglas Fairbanks, he constituted the most visual example of a modern, white masculinity.[22] His fame as a five-time Olympic champion was just the basis for his body being highly visible in magazines, advertisements, and newsreels during the 'Golden Age of Sports' era that produced and consumed (white) sport stars in unprecedented ways. Weissmuller's underwear and swimwear advertisements had almost pin-up quality; and when he became an actor and started to portray Edgar Rice Buroughs' Tarzan in twelve motion pictures from 1932 onwards, the public visibility of a crawl swimmer within US popular culture peaked in the most modern media available.[23]

In 1930, Weissmuller published his bestselling half textbook, half autobiography *Swimming the American Crawl*. Compared to its precursors, Weissmuller's manual broke new ground in actively bridging the gap between three media; it took photographs explicitly extracted from motion pictures and used them as illustrations in a book. These filmstrips demonstrated the publisher's desire to characterize Weissmuller as the ultimate product of scientific training methods supported by the newest technology, the true climax of swimming's 'modern' development, the fastest swimmer of the world using the fastest style photographed by the fastest cameras available. For that purpose, text and images corresponded closely with each other, as did autobiography and educational passages.

21 Handley, *Swimming for Women*. See also Wright, 'Spectacular Bodies'.

22 Pendergast, *Creating the Modern Man*.

23 Kirkham and Thumim, *You Tarzan*.

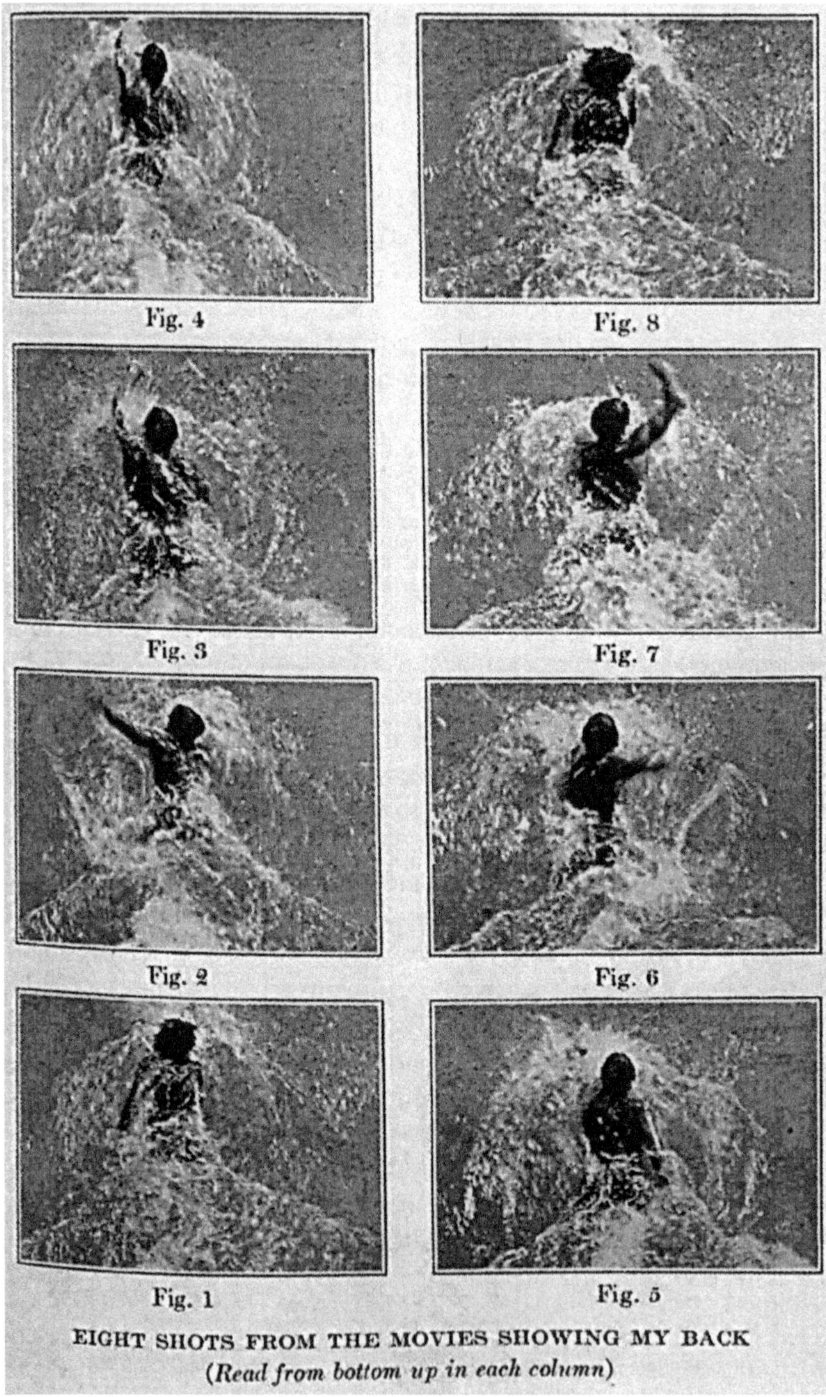

5.5. Weissmuller, *American Crawl*, p. 18.

Swimming the American Crawl contained several image series representing state-of-the-art photo technology, images of swimming that most Americans had rarely seen before (Figure 5.5). Shot by high-speed film cameras designed for depicting fast action under difficult circumstances, these illustrations made readers believe they could actually watch one of the educational films that the Olympic champion had earlier produced. The time gap between individual pictures within one series was significantly reduced compared to prior attempts, and together with a much more sensitive and stronger telephoto lens, the water spray now was no longer a handicap in visualization but an asset that added speed and authenticity to the focus on breathing technique. Moreover, Weissmuller used long paragraphs of text to comment on these images. He did that not only in a mode of explanation, for a detailed description of what readers could detect in and learn from them, but also to elaborate on the limits of representation: 'This clean recovery is not always apparent in the movies I have reproduced, as there is a lot of spray flying around, and the action is sometimes too swift for the camera.'[24]

Within the star persona of Johnny Weissmuller, several elements of the visual arrangement of modern bodies in motion merged. As scholarship on sports marketing during the 1920s and 1930s shows, his ubiquitous media presence made his body a marketable international icon of white Americanism.[25] With Johnny Weissmuller and his Tarzan films of the 1930s, the processes of Americanizing the crawl and labelling it as specifically 'modern' came almost full circle. Showing the masculine physique and actions of Tarzan in Hollywood films, starring the most famous swimmer of his times literally crawling through the African jungle, underscores the entangled genealogy of crawl swimming and its close relation to discourses of modernity, or, more precisely, to the multilayered contemporary debates involved in negotiating what that term was supposed to signify. Swimmers and coaches adopted the motion from a supposedly 'native' body movement, made it available to a larger portion of the American population, analysed it scientifically with advancing techniques of visualization, and ultimately refined it by American expertise into a motion perfectly suited for both speed and endurance.[26] It became the stroke of its time—fast, efficient, successful, streamlined. In the 1930s, Hollywood, with its worldwide appeal

24 Weissmuller, *American Crawl*, p. 17.

25 Dyreson, 'Marketing Weissmuller'.

26 Historians Gary Osmond and Murray Phillips documented the early history of the crawl in Australia around 1900 and underscored the importance of studying and adopting what were considered 'natural' motions of natives born in the Pacific islands. As Osmond and Phillips show, that process of appropriation was structured along notions of racial hierarchies. See Osmond and Phillips, 'Look'.

and commercial power, depicted the myth of the crawl, a myth of a white stroke with roots in nature that was capable of progressing 'Western' civilization into areas not yet touched by American spirit—and money.

Not only Hollywood but film in general added important new layers to that discourse. Before the First World War, depicting swimming was only marginal among the already immensely growing field of sports film that catered to the audience's desire to watch bodies moving on-screen.[27] The reason for this was mainly technical—because cameras could not be brought close enough to the water, and lenses were not advanced and fast enough to catch the ongoing action precisely. Moreover, much of the relevant motion happened below the water's surface and thus remained beyond the reach of the standard camera's view. This changed dramatically during the 1920s and the 1930s. Successful college coaches like Robert Kiphuth from Yale University or David Armbruster from the University of Iowa started to use visual techniques to optimize their training sessions, and textbooks began to include photographs used explicitly for visualizing motion occurring too fast to be grasped without it.[28] At the same time, a market for tutorial films developed in the field of physical education, including productions used for swimming classes in high schools as well as colleges.[29] Still, despite an increase in productions and the growth of distributive channels, educational films in the realm of sports and physical education only reached a limited audience of aspiring young athletes enrolled in sports programmes. Commercial films produced for release in cinemas all over the United States proved to be more influential: Over the course of the 1920s, ever more newsreels included sports in their programmes regularly, and, after short films became a common part of the overall moviegoing experience in the later years of that decade, sports-related examples became popular.[30]

During the summer of 1926, the increasing significance of newsreels for the popularization of swimming became especially evident. In August of that year, the 20-year-old Gertrude Ederle from New York succeeded in her quest to be the first woman to swim the English Channel, and she did so faster than any man before her.[31] To promote and finance the event, Ederle and her management relied upon cooperating with powerful media agents, making sure that the American public was not only constantly aware about

27 Streible, *Fight Pictures*.
28 Hughes and Stimson, 'Motion Pictures'.
29 Dear et al., *Motion Pictures in Sports*, pp. 29–30. Orgeron et al., *Learning*.
30 Bradley, *First Hollywood*.
31 Vertinsky and Job, 'Breaking Traditions'; Dahlberg et al., *America's Girl*.

what went on in Europe but was also able to get new visual impressions of the athlete's efforts. Newspapers and magazines covered the story closely, and when Americans watched the newsreels of her accomplishment, they could see how much preparation went into it: The film shows a young woman who is adjusting her body to the task by wearing special glasses and covering herself entirely with protective grease. The swim itself is depicted as complicated by waves but nevertheless easy—while it lasted, she crawled without much visible discomfort alongside the boats that transported her aids. This impression might, of course, be the effect of the brevity of the newsreel and the long-distance shots of the cameras.[32] Still, Ederle became a star, and swimming for women reached its peak in popularity.

Compared to those often rather franticly produced newsreels, professional short film productions had huge advantages for selling corporeal practices to moviegoers. Depicting swimming in such productions was not exactly a novelty in the 1920s, the Australian-born swimmer Annette Kellerman already performed successfully in front of film cameras before the Great War, becoming a star in feature films and semi-documentaries with titles such as *The Mermaid* (1911), *Neptune's Daughter* (1914), or *A Daughter of the Gods* (1916).[33] But, while these films certainly aroused (erotic) interest in female bodies performing ballet in the water, their actual imagery remained very suboptimal, leaving more to fantasy than to clear vision. Productions from a later period allowed for improved representations, and *Crystal Champions*, shot only three years after Ederle's channel crossing, is a suitable case in point. A well-financed collaboration between a prominent sports journalist, a gifted cinematographer using cutting-edge technology, an experienced director, the chamber of commerce of a popular vacation resort, and a handful of both successful and good-looking athletes, *Crystal Champions* made use of twin developments within American culture. It related a changing cinema experience that incorporated the short film as a valued part of an evening's entertainment, and a new emphasis on actively combining the biopolitical obligation on fitness and health to notions of pleasure and self-fulfilment.[34] Nevertheless, the collaboration at that particular moment is also a strong reminder of how much remained excluded from the circulating images. At a time when Silver Springs, Florida, was still a strictly segregated vacation spot that allowed non-white Americans only as

32 The newsreels are available among the Universal Newsreels on the Associated Press Archive website, http://www.aparchive.com. Moreover, Universal also features a channel containing their material on https://www.youtube.com.

33 Catapano, 'Perfect Woman'; Stieglitz, 'Ikonen einer neuen Freiheit'.

34 Mrozek, 'Sport in American Life'.

servants in their hotels, when journalists such as Grantland Rice still served as gatekeepers making sure that African-American athletes held marginal roles at best in what they described as 'America's Golden Age of Sports', and when Hollywood and other players in the film industry clearly separated between a 'white' and a 'black' cinema, *Crystal Champions* was indicative of the contemporary whiteness of bodies in motion.

To generalize, it becomes evident that the practice of swimming and its representations in visual media became intrinsically linked. The popularity of swimming, as both a sport and a leisure or vacation activity, rested on constant and high-quality visibility, and the inherent difficulties in depicting in- and underwater action stimulated crucial technological developments in photo and film technology. Its close affinity to the realms of fashion, nutrition, and fitness allowed images of swimming to become omnipresent elements within these areas of white middle-class identity politics.

Conclusion: The Athletic Body as Future's Project

Visual representations of fit, white, middle-class families grew increasingly prominent after the First World War (Figure 5.6).

The modern, athletic body became a project for the immediate generational future, and many sports and physical-culture publications and films pointed at the necessity for developing an active, healthy lifestyle from early on—the first few sequences of *Crystal Champions* depicting youngsters swimming and diving are strong reminders of that. Parents were supposed to take responsibility and educate their children in matters of health-related physical culture. Again, swimming played an important role for that development, for several reasons. The number of public and private pools was increasing and learning the crawl was continuously described as accessible and easy, so parents could teach their children themselves. Moreover, learning to swim was, by now, strongly linked to urbanization and suburbanization, and the ever-recurring hint at life-saving techniques added a notion of safety to living in a changed, modern environment. Most of all, though, swimming fitted nicely into established illustrations of eugenic appeal in interwar popular culture.[35] Already strongly associated with notions of purity, hygiene, and a 'balanced' ideal of the body, swimming American children signified a true promise for good citizenship: '[T]he best ideals may be inculcated' by swimming, one manual stated, 'such as courage, self-confidence, leadership,

35 Currell and Cogdell, *Popular Eugenics*.

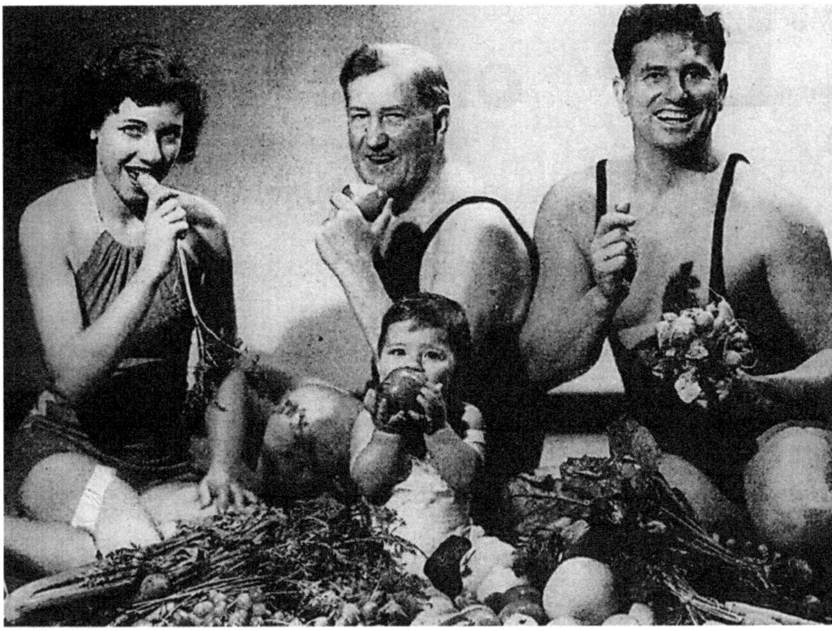

5.6. From *Physical Culture* (July 1937), p. 4.

a democratic spirit, good sportsmanship, self-sacrifice and heroic service'.[36] At a time when the promises of modernity became increasingly uncertain for white, middle-class Americans, a fit, beautiful body in motion was reassuring; at times when 'weakness was a crime', to paraphrase the motto of fitness entrepreneur Bernarr Macfaddens, swimming seemed to keep that promise, and, in closely interacting with texts, visual culture underscored this concern immensely.[37] Photos and film were considered superior educational instruments in circulating notions of 'modern' bodies in notion, and, as this essay shows, this sort of modernity rested on an unmarked whiteness. Not only did the visual representations exclude non-whites to a large degree, but, even more importantly, they helped normalize the idea of white bodies as endowed with certain abilities and a certain beauty. Moreover, the motions of swimming and its representations were also and more clearly coded along lines of gender. Swimming in the US not only mirrored gender relations, it took an active part in negotiating and developing notions of masculinity and femininity within an intersectional social structure that related aspects of race, ethnicity, age, and capability to these categories.

36 Sheffield and Sheffield, *Swimming Simplified*, p. xii.

37 Ernst, *Weakness is a Crime*; Adams, *Mr. America*; Stieglitz, 'Man of Your Years'.

Works Cited

Films, Television Programmes, and Recordings

Aquatic House Party, directed by Jack Eaton, Paramount Pictures, released on 31 March 1950.

College, directed by James W. Horne and Buster Keaton; performances by Buster Keaton, Anne Cornwall, and Harold Goodwin; United Artist, released 27 September 1927.

Crystal Champions: A Grantland Rice Sound Sportlight for Van Beuren-Pathé, 1 reel, directed by Jack Eaton; performances by Pete Desjardins, Helen Meany, Martha Norelius, Newton Perry, and Johnny Weissmuller; Universal, released in May 1929.

A Daughter of the Gods, directed by Herbert Brenon; performances by Annette Kellermann, William E. Shay, and Hal De Forest; Fox Film Co., released 17 October 1916.

The Mermaid, performance by Annette Kellermann, released in 1911.

Neptune's Daughter, directed by Herbert Brenon, performance by Annette Kellermann, Universal, released 25 April 1914.

Books and Articles

Adams, Mark, *Mr. America: How Muscular Millionaire Bernarr Macfadden Transformed the Nation through Sex, Salad, and the Ultimate Starvation Diet* (New York: Harper Collins, 2010).

Bachrach, William, *The Outline of Swimming: An Encyclopedia of the Sport* (Chicago: J. B. Bradwell, 1924).

Barnes, Gerald, *Swimming and Diving* (New York: Charles Scribner's Sons, 1922).

Bier, Lisa, *Fighting the Current: The Rise of American Women's Swimming, 1870–1926* (Jefferson, NC: McFarland, 2011).

Bradley, Edwin M., *The First Hollywood Sound Shorts, 1926–1931* (Jefferson, NC: McFarland, 2005).

Braun, Marta, *Picturing Time: The Work of Etienne-Jules Marey (1830–1904)* (Chicago: University of Chicago Press, 1992).

Brown, J[oseph] H[enry] P[atrick], *Modern Swimming: An Illustrated Manual* (Boston: Small, Maynard & Co., 1916).

Catapano, Peter, '"The Perfect Woman": Annette Kellerman and the Spectacle of the Female Form', *Proteus: A Journal of Ideas*, 25, 2 (2008), pp. 23–27.

Carter, Neil, *Medicine, Sport and the Body: A Historical Perspective* (Basingstoke: Bloomsbury, 2012).

Corsan, G[eorge] H., 'Learning to Swim is Easy', *Physical Culture*, 40, 2 (August 1918), pp. 21–24 and 75.
Currell, Susan, and Christina Cogdell, eds., *Popular Eugenics: National Efficiency and American Mass Culture in the 1930s* (Athens: Ohio University Press, 2006).
Dahlberg, Tim, Mary Ederle Ward, and Brenda Green, *America's Girl: The Incredible Story of How Swimmer Gertrude Ederle Changed the Nation* (New York: St. Martin's Press, 2009).
Dalton, Frank Eugen, *Swimming Scientifically Taught: A Practical Manual for Young and Old* (New York: Funk & Wagnalls, 1912).
Daniels, C[harles] M[eldrum], *Speed Swimming* (New York:American Publishing Co., 1922).
Dear, Elaine M., Louise S. Kjellstrom, and Jenny E. Turnbull, *Motion Pictures in Sports: A Bibliography and Film List, Presented by the Motion Picture Committee of the National Section of Women's Athletics of the American Association for Health, Physical Education, and Recreation* (Washington, DC: American Association for Health, Physical Education, and Recreation, 1939).
Dyreson, Mark, 'Icons of Liberty or Objects of Desire? American Women Olympians and the Politics of Consumption', *Journal of Contemporary History*, 38, 3 (2003), pp. 435–460, https://www.jstor.org/stable/3180646.
Dyreson, Mark, 'Marketing Weissmuller to the World: Hollywood's Olympics and Federal Schemes for Americanization through Sport', *International Journal of the History of Sport*, 25, 2 (2008), pp. 284–306, doi:10.1080/09523360701740398.
Ernst, Robert, *Weakness is a Crime: The Life of Bernarr Macfadden* (Syracuse, NY: Syracuse University Press, 1991).
Ford, Corey, 'Swimming for Ladies', *Vanity Fair* (May 1927), pp. 49 and 94.
Gallico, Paul, 'Babes in the Drink', *Vanity Fair* (January 1936), pp. 49 and 58.
Green, Harvey, *Fit for America: Health, Fitness, Sport and American Society* (New York: Pantheon, 1986).
Handley, L[ouis] de B[reda], *Swimming and Watermanship* (New York: Macmillan, 1927).
Handley, L[ouis] de B[reda], *Swimming for Women: Preliminary and Advanced Instruction in Competitive Swimming, Fancy Diving and Life Saving* (New York: American Sports Publishing Co., 1928).
Hoberman, John M., *Mortal Engines: The Science of Performance and the Dehumanization of Sport* (New York: Free Press, 1992).
Hughes, William L., and Pauline E. Stimson, 'Motion Pictures in Health and Physical Education: Sources, Films, Descriptions, and Prices', *Research Quarterly*, 9, 1 (1938), pp. 104–153, doi:10.1080/23267429.1938.11802422.
Kirkham, Pat, and Janet Thumim, eds., *You Tarzan: Masculinity, Movies and Men* (London: Lawrence & Wishart, 1993).

Levine, Peter, *A. G. Spalding and the Rise of Baseball: The Promise of American Sport* (New York: Oxford University Press, 1985).

Macfadden, Helen, 'Business Girls Should Swim for Better Posture', *Physical Culture* (July 1937), pp. 46–47.

Mackert, Nina, '"I want to be a fat man / and with the fat men stand": US-Amerikanische Fat Men's Clubs und die Bedeutungen von Körperfett in den Dekaden um 1900', *Body Politics*, 2, 3 (2014), pp. 215–243, http://bodypolitics.de/de/wp-content/uploads/2015/07/Heft_3_10_mackert_fat_End.pdf, accessed 27 July 2018.

Martschukat, Jürgen, 'The Pursuit of Fitness: Von Freiheit und Leistungsfähigkeit in der Geschichte der USA', *Geschichte und Gesellschaft*, 42, 3 (2016), pp. 409–440, https://www.jstor.org/stable/24891243.

Massengale, John D., and Richard A. Swanson, eds., *The History of Exercise and Sport Science* (Champagne, IL: Human Kinetics Publishers, 1997).

Mrozek, Donald J., 'Sport in American Life: From National Health to Personal Fulfillment, 1890–1940', in *Fitness in American Culture: Images of Health, Sport, and the Body, 1830–1940*, ed. by Kathryn Grover (Amherst: University of Massachusetts Press, 1989), pp. 18–46.

Orgeron, Devin, Marsha Orgeron, and Dan Streible, eds., *Learning with the Lights Off: Educational Film in the United States* (New York: Oxford University Press, 2012).

Osmond, Gary, and Murray G. Phillips, '"Look at that Kid Crawling": Race, Myth and the "Crawl" Stroke', *Australian Historical Studies*, 37, 127 (2006), pp. 43–62, doi:10.1080/10314610608601203.

Pendergast, Tom, *Creating the Modern Man: American Magazines and Consumer Culture 1900–1950* (Columbia, MO: University of Missouri Press, 2000).

Prodger, Phillip, *Time Stands Still: Muybridge and the Instantaneous Photography Movement* (New York: Oxford University Press, 2003).

Schutz, Louise, 'Motion Picture Sports for Women', *Journal of Health and Physical Education*, 8, 6 (1937), pp. 376–392, doi:10.1080/23267240.1937.10619792.

Sheffield, Lyba, and Nita Sheffield, *Swimming Simplified* (New York: A. S. Barnes and Company, 1927).

Sterrett, James H., *How to Swim: A Practical Manual of Swimming by a Practical Swimmer and a Guide to the Novice as well as the Expert* (New York: American Sports Publishing, 1917).

Stieglitz, Olaf, 'Ikonen einer neuen Freiheit? Das Frauenschwimmen und die Ambivalenzen seiner Sichtbarmachung in den USA zwischen den Weltkriegen', in *Anerkennung und Sichtbarkeit: Perspektiven für eine kritische Medienkulturforschung*, ed. By Tanja Thomas, Lina Brink, Elke Grittmann, and Kaya de Wolff (Bielefeld: Transcript, 2018), pp. 69–85.

Stieglitz, Olaf, 'Die Komödie als Bewegungsstudie: Spielfilme und ihr Platz in der visuellen Welt des Sports in den 1920er Jahren', in *Arbeit am Bild: Visual*

History als Praxis, ed. by Jürgen Danyel, Gerhard Paul, and Annette Vowinckel (Göttingen: Wallstein, 2017), pp. 217–235.

Stieglitz, Olaf, '"A Man of Your Years Shouldn't Expect to Be Able to Do Those Things"—Älter werden in Bernarr Macfaddens Physical Culture-Welt', in *Körperführung: Historische Perspektiven auf das Verhältnis von Biopolitik und Sport*, ed. by Stefan Scholl (Frankfurt am Main: Campus, 2018), pp. 99–130.

Streible, Dan, *Fight Pictures: A History of Boxing and Early Cinema* (Berkeley: University of California Press, 2008).

Sullivan, Frank J., *The Science of Swimming* (New York: American Sports Publishing Co., 1934).

Susman, Warren I. *Culture as History: The Transformation of American Society in the Twentieth Century* (New York: Pantheon Books, 1984).

Vertinsky, Patricia, and Christiane Job, 'Breaking Traditions, and Swimming Out of Place: Getrude Ederle and "The Greatest Sports Story in the World"', *Stadion: Internationale Zeitschrift für Geschichte des Sports*, 31, 1 (2005), pp. 111–134.

Weissmuller, Johnny, *Swimming the American Crawl* (Boston: Houghton Mifflin, 1930).

Welky, David, *Everything Was Better in America: Print Culture in the Great Depression* (Urbana: University of Illinois Press, 2008).

Wiltse, Jeff, *Contested Waters: A Social History of Swimming Pools in America* (Chapel Hill: University of North Carolina Press, 2007).

Wolcott, Victoria W., *Race, Riots, and Roller Coasters: The Struggle over Segregated Recreation in America* (Philadelphia: University of Pennsylvania Press, 2012).

Wright, Ellen, 'Spectacular Bodies: The Swimsuit, Sexuality and Hollywood', *Sport in History*, 35, 3 (2015), pp. 441–463, doi:10.1080/17460263.2015.1072578.

About the Author

PD Dr. **Olaf Stieglitz** teaches North American History at the University of Cologne (Dept. of History / Institute of North American History). His main areas of research and teaching are U.S. Social and Cultural History; Gender History & History of the Body; Sports History as Cultural History, Visual Studies. He is currently finishing a book project entitled 'Modernity in Motion – Visualizing Athletic Bodies, 1890s-1940s'.
Contact details: olaf.stieglitz1@uni-koeln.de

6. *Inside Magoo* (1960): Comedic Commentary on 1950s America and Cancer

David Cantor

Abstract

This chapter traces the role of humour in *Inside Magoo* (1960), an educational film released by United Productions of America (UPA) for the American Cancer Society (ACS). Humour, I suggest, provided 1) a response to ACS's concerns that public fears of cancer led people to avoid appropriate medical help, and 2) a commentary on 1950s America from the perspective of someone – Mr. Magoo – who rejected the post-war world of white, male, middle-class, consumerist suburbia. This film was thus not only about cancer. It wrapped the ACS message within humorous observations on life in the 1950s to charm audiences into adopting ACS approaches to the disease; a technique, I suggest, that was common to other UPA cancer educationals of the 1950s.

Keywords: Mr. Magoo; educational film; United Productions of America (UPA); American Cancer Society (ACS); *The Lonely Crowd* (Riesman)

In 1959, Stephen Bosustow appeared on television to discuss the role of the arts and entertainment in cancer control. Bosustow was the head of United Productions of America (UPA), the film company that had, in 1949, created the nearsighted character, Mr. Magoo, one of the most popular animated figures in the cinema of the 1950s. Bosustow was asked how he would try to persuade a man who was ignorant of the warning signs of cancer and who likely wouldn't act on them anyway. 'There are several ways we can do this', he answered, using the example of an educational film storyboard with Mr. Magoo. 'One, we can scare the daylights out of him—and in this case all he

Bonah, C. and A. Laukötter (eds.), *Body, Capital, and Screens: Visual Media and the Healthy Self in the 20th Century*. Taylor & Francis Group, 2020
DOI 10.5117/9789462988293_CH06

has to do is turn the dial to avoid the experience. Second, we can *charm* him into accepting the information and leave it up to him as to what happens afterwards.'[1] The following year, Bosustow turned the storyboard into a cancer education film, first called *Magoo's Check-up*, later *Inside Magoo.*[2]

There are two forms of charm to consider here. One is that Magoo himself lives a charmed, almost magical life. His poor eyesight means that he constantly mistakes what is going on around him, which takes him on an improbable, comedic route to the doctor and a check-up. The details of this journey will come later in this chapter. Suffice to say here that the film revolves around Magoo's frantic efforts to avoid the cancer message of the film's sponsor, the American Cancer Society (ACS), and that the message only gets through to him because of his misinterpretation of a series of accidents as warning signs of cancer. A further series of lucky events and misinterpretations then delivers him to the doctor's office and his salvation. This form of charm is wholly within the world of the film, and results in relief and joy for Magoo at the news that he does not have cancer. This is not only a story about how to control cancer, but also about how physicians could control anxiety about the disease.

The second form of charm—the one to which Bosustow refers—concerns the relationship of the film to its audience. The figure of Mr. Magoo, his quasi-magical life, the improbable course of events, the humour of his misconceptions, and the film's comic commentary on life in the 1950s were all intended to charm an audience, and to engage its loyalty to Mr. Magoo, to UPA, and to the educational message of its sponsor, the ACS. Charm in this form in *Inside Magoo* was a type of cultural capital that could be converted into other forms of capital: income and audience loyalty for UPA, support for the ACS' view of cancer control, and (the promise of) health and well-being for audiences. This is a film that used the animated body of a seemingly nearsighted, old, bald, small, and portly man to ensure that UPA flourished commercially and to approach a disease that, in the early 1960s, could lead, in the world outside the cartoon, to death, debility, financial ruin, broken families, and social stigma. No small wonder then that Bosustow and the ACS wanted to avoid scaring the daylights out of the viewer.

1 Quoted in Corwin, 'Tactic', p. 10, emphasis added.

2 For the storyboard, see 'Inside Magoo' (*Cancer News*); 'ACS Re-signs UPA'. The film was distributed by Columbia Pictures and was available free from the ACS; 'Magoo Cancer Cartoon'. There are few archival records on this film; see the sparse documentation in the Technicolor and the Abe and Charlotte Levitow collections held in Special Collections at the Margaret Herrick Library.

This chapter has two main goals. First, it explores how UPA deployed Mr. Magoo to address the problem of fear. The American Cancer Society had long had an ambivalent attitude towards fear. On the one hand, the Society argued, a healthy fear of the disease could drive people to the doctor and ensure timely medical intervention, early in the natural life of this group of diseases or some precursor. The disease, the ACS explained, began as a small circumscribed anomaly, and intervention was best undertaken early, ideally before it turned malignant, grew too large, or spread to other parts of the body. On the other hand, however, the ACS also argued that fear of the disease or its treatment could also dissuade people from this course of action, with the result that they delayed seeking appropriate medical help and arrived in the doctor's office with untreatable cancers. So, the question was how to promote the healthy fear of the disease without encouraging the unhealthy sort that resulted in delay. UPA's solution was to make audiences laugh at their own fears, as expressed by cartoon figures such as Mr. Magoo. The actor Jim Backus (the voice of Magoo) captured the point when, in the live-action section of *Inside Magoo,* he tells his viewers that 'by being funny I hope I can make you watch and think about something you maybe don't want to think about'.

A second goal of this chapter is to explore the film's commentary on 1950s America. This will be done by comparing *Inside Magoo* with two earlier films UPA made for the ACS—*Man Alive!* (1952) and *Sappy Homiens* (1956)—both of which, like *Inside Magoo,* were animated health education cartoon comedies targeted at men. However, whereas the two earlier films were comic parodies of middle-class suburbia, *Inside Magoo* approached its subject from a very different perspective. Whereas the protagonists of *Man Alive!* and *Sappy Homiens* were harassed men trying to navigate their way through middle-class life (and the fear of cancer), Mr. Magoo, with his homburg and fur-lined coat, came from a higher social and economic class, his nearsightedness a metaphor for a personality type that did not easily fit into post-war white, middle-class suburbia. These films were thus much more than films about cancer. They sought to persuade men to seek early detection and treatment for this group of diseases by embedding their fears of cancer within humorous observations on life in the 1950s. It was such comedic commentaries that UPA hoped would charm an audience into thinking about cancer.

UPA and the ACS

Founded in 1943, the company that came to be known as UPA got its start creating commissioned films (industrials, political campaign films, and educational and training films for the United States government) and, later, theatrical shorts and, still later, in the 1950s, television programmes. It quickly gained a reputation for pioneering new approaches to animation. With a smaller staff than larger established rivals such as Disney, UPA adopted a method of cel animation, eventually labelled limited animation, which lessened the work of producing cartoons. In part, this meant that UPA reduced or limited the number of frames it used to construct movement within a film, but it also, compared to Disney, limited movement within the film itself in at least two ways. First, in Disney films such as *Snow White* (1937), *Pinocchio* (1940), or *Fantasia* (1940), a character's face might be drawn and redrawn to accompany the movement of its eye or nose; UPA cut much of this movement, limiting it, at times, to a single body part, the rest of the body frozen in place. Second, compared to the distinctive, individuated complex of movements that made up a Disney animated character, UPA's characters often had a much more limited repertoire of movements (produced by the repeated used of a series of cels, at least more repeatedly than in Disney productions). In such ways, UPA hoped to reduce the workforce needed for artwork, speed up the production time, and cut costs.[3]

Man Alive! was the first film the ACS commissioned from UPA and it marked a transformation in cancer education film-making.[4] It was the first to pair limited animation with humour in the United States. Some earlier films had had humorous moments, but, in general, cancer educationals were not known for comedy. *Man Alive!* was the first to use humour throughout and was followed by *Sappy Homiens* and *Inside Magoo*, both, like *Man Alive!*, targeted at men. Comedy cartoon animation was not aimed at women in this period, except for some advertising spots. Their cancer education films tended to be melodramas and how-to films such as *Breast Self-Examination* (1950).

All three films followed the UPA house style of limited animation with minimal detail, quick edits, abrupt scene transitions, a borrowing from a wide range of artistic influences, and an imaginative flexibility towards size, shape, colour, timing, and visual perspective. Some of the humour was slapstick, the central characters undergoing humiliation and embarrassment before being saved by medicine. Ed Parmalee (the star of *Man Alive!*) and Sappy, for example, are Everyman figures whose pride and fear lead to discomforting mistakes before they are restored to dignity, emotional equilibrium, and health by medical advice. (Two of UPA's founders, John

3 Abraham, *When Magoo Flew*; Barrier, *Hollywood Cartoons*.

4 Cantor, *Man Alive*; Cantor, 'Uncertain Enthusiasm'. On health education films more generally, see, Bonah et al., *Health Education Films*.

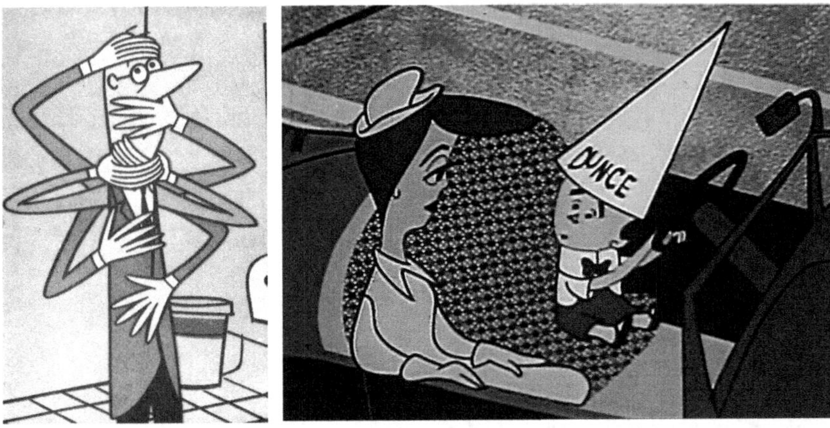

6.1. a (left): 'Sappy Examines himself', *ACS Bulletin*, 5, 9 (5 March 1956), p. 2, reprinted with permission of the American Cancer Society, Inc. All rights reserved. b (right): Screenshot of Ed Parmalee's transformation into a child dunce.

Hubley and Zachary Schwartz, had argued that the nature of animation demanded a return to symbols such as Everyman.)[5] Magoo, by contrast, never seems to be aware of his humiliation, despite his pessimism when he fears he may have cancer. The humour resides in the audience seeing what he cannot see, his misinterpretations of what is going on around him, and his improbable passage to the doctor.

There is also humour in the bodies of the main protagonists. Ed and Sappy both have malleable bodies: They physically shrink with fear, expand with (over)confidence, joyfully leap impossible heights, gain some extra arms (Figure 6.1a) and legs, change into other figures (a child dunce [Figure 6.1b], devil, Eskimo, or caveman), among other transformations. Magoo does not transform to the extent of Ed and Sappy: His eyeballs occasionally expand, but gross transformations are often in his imagination, such as when he sees his distorted self in a fairground mirror, which he mistakes for a real change in his body. Such transformations and exaggerations help create the antic humour of the films, as do other visual tricks and sleights of hand. In *Man Alive!*, Ed does not dress himself—his clothes fly off the valet stand and apply themselves to his body. Sappy's wife does not remove his coat—it magically appears in her hands. Magoo does not crash blindly through a fence on-screen, but the jarring sound effects, the hole in the fence, and the tire marks on the ground indicate what has happened.

None of the protagonists know their bodies or what, if anything, might be wrong with them; part of the humour is Ed's, Sappy's, and Magoo's misguided,

5 Hubley and Schwartz, 'Animation Learns', p. 363.

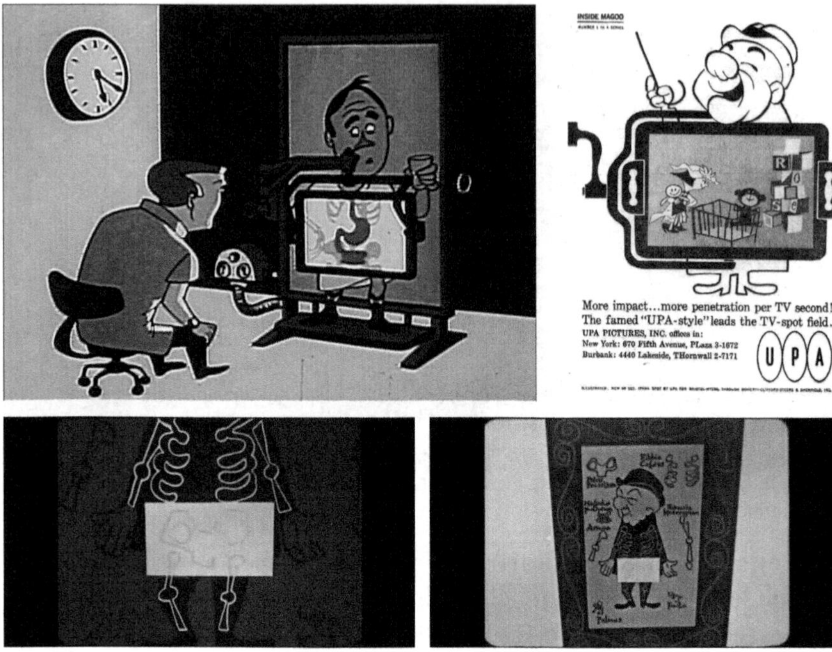

6.2. From fluoroscope to highlighter: a (top left): Screenshot from *Man Alive!*; b (top right): *Billboard*, 67, 51 (17 December 1955), p. 32; c–d (bottom left/right): Screenshots from *Inside Magoo*, reprinted with permission of the American Cancer Society, Inc. All rights reserved.

anxious efforts to understand their conditions. Occasionally, the films take us inside the body to show us what cancer is, such as illustrations of how cancer is formed and spreads at the cellular level in *Man Alive!* (8 mins. 34 secs.), *Sappy Homiens* (4 mins. 42 secs.), and *Inside Magoo* (1 min. 48 secs.), the last of which is lifted from *Man Alive!* But none of the three protagonists can see cellular changes without the aid of technology; their knowledge is limited to gross symptoms (or their absence) that might or might not denote cancer. The technology in *Inside Magoo* is that of film production: The narrator describes how animation can take the viewer places where live action could never go. But, in general, it is not the technology of the educational film that does this, but that of medicine. Ed's stomach problems, for example, are examined through a fluoroscope (Figure 6.2a), an image that was later taken up playfully by UPA (Figure 6.2b) in a 1955 print advertisement (coincidentally, also called *Inside Magoo*), and then in stylized form (Figures 6.2c–6.2d) in the film *Inside Magoo* as a coy means of highlighting where in the body cancer often affects men. Ironically, the narrator never speaks the name of that part, and the fluoroscope-cum-highlighter does not show much besides some bones.

Physically, Ed and Sappy are the opposite of Magoo. Ed and Sappy are white and middle-class, of working age and in good health, although stressed; Ed is more heavily built than Sappy. Magoo, by contrast, is stout, wealthy, elderly, retired, and bald—commonly compared to the American actor and comedian W. C. Fields.[6] They also differ graphically in other ways. Ed and Magoo are closer to what Robert Cannon, the director of one of UPA's most successful modernist theatrical cartoons, *Gerald McBoing-Boing* (1950), describes as three-dimensional characters set in the illusion of a three-dimensional, scaled setting (the house, the car, the doctor's office). Howard Rieder notes that, in Magoo, this is 'a halfway point between the extreme literalism of Disney and the stylized animation of the more off-beat UPA films'.[7] The same can also be said about Ed. Sappy is a different sort of graphical character, closer to Cannon's description of Gerald. Sappy shares a flat nearly two-dimensional shape with Gerald, with minimal detail. He is also sometimes, like Gerald, part of the overall design of the frame, his movements within the frame what Cannon called 'design in motion'.[8] Thus, when Sappy comes home, he does not change his distracted leaning-forward, looking-down posture, so his wife, son, and daughter all must adapt to him as they kiss him welcome. As with Gerald, Sappy's background is sparse: His lounge, for example, is little more than a television, side table, and chair set against a single flat block of colour, just as Gerald's rooms are denoted by the presence of a stylized sofa and lamp with hardly any other detail.

I write of these as tendencies, for all the films shade into one another. The background in *Sappy Homiens*—as in the bathroom scene (Figure 6.1a)—sometimes edged more towards the three-dimensional, as does, sometimes, the figure of Sappy himself. Similarly, the three-dimensional illusion of the background for Ed and Magoo sometimes disappears. Ed's anger is illustrated when the background detail disappears and is replaced with a block of red; his icy distain by a block of blue. Both also draw on German expressionism: Both Gerald and Ed are dwarfed by a railway crossing sign that signals the dangers of the outside world for Gerald and the danger signals of cancer for Ed. *Inside Magoo* also makes a 'vivid use of color', suggesting graphically, as Cannon puts it, 'that there is a great deal in the world to see, but Magoo walks blindly through it'.[9]

6 Rieder, 'Memories of Mr. Magoo', pp. 19–22.

7 Rieder, 'Memories of Mr. Magoo', p. 19. See also Rieder, 'Development of the Satire', p. 86. More generally on UPA's influence on post war modernist aesthetics see Bashara, *Cartoon Vision*.

8 Quoted in Rieder, 'Memories of Mr. Magoo', p. 19.

9 Rieder, 'Development of the Satire', p. 87. For the use of perspective in Magoo cartoons, see Bashara, *Cartoon Vision*, pp. 32, 35.

The Paths to the Doctor and *Inside Magoo*

The narratives of all three films trace the reluctance of their protagonists to go to the doctor, the circuitous, sometimes improbable paths by which they get there, the reasons why they delay (often fear), and the comforting results of their decision to seek medical help. Neither Ed nor Magoo have cancer, despite the fears which prompt them to delay seeking help. Indeed, *Man Alive!* and *Inside Magoo* end with their relief and joy at not having cancer and, learning from this experience, their determination to go for regular check-ups. Such reassuring messages—that most warning signs do not turn out to be cancer—were a common theme of ACS cancer education programmes, seeking to counter the fears that prompted people to delay seeking help.[10] For example, Oliver Dancer—the star of a 1956 UPA-like spot—comes to a similar conclusion. Despite his belief that a diagnosis of cancer is a death sentence, the lump that Oliver finds while shaving turns out not to be cancer.[11]

Ed's path to joy and relief begins inauspiciously. He dreads he may have cancer and avoids going to the doctor for fear of the diagnosis, just as he fears going to a reputable mechanic when his car's engine makes a strange noise. In the case of the car, the result is disastrous: Clyde, a crooked car mechanic, destroys the engine. Ed narrowly avoids a similar disaster with his body, when he is dissuaded from going to a quack (Clyde's identical twin) and seeks medical attention from a regular physician. As the narrator explains to him, his body is like a car engine—a metaphor never deployed in cancer education films aimed at women at this time—in that it gives warning signs of impending trouble.[12] The good news for Ed is that he does not have cancer, and his relief melts away all the fears that led him to delay. According to the ACS, '[h]umor is mixed with its grim significance as a Mr. Everyman avoids having his car properly serviced, or going to a doctor for checking of a symptom that may mean cancer. Both car and disease give their warnings'.[13] The film, the ACS claimed, was 'easier to take than many of the purportedly educational films that produce only boredom instead of knowledge'.[14]

Man Alive! was a major hit for the ACS.[15] Most cancer educationals were shown in informal settings: workplaces, clubs, clinics, classrooms, tents,

10 For other examples of relief, see Cantor, 'Uncertain Enthusiasm', pp. 67–68.

11 'Strange Case'.

12 Reagan, 'Engendering', pp. 1782–1783.

13 'Coast Reviewers', p. 4.

14 'Coast Reviewers', p. 4.

15 Cantor, *Man Alive*.

fundraisers. They were rarely shown in the cinema, unless it was hired for a special event. *Man Alive!*, by contrast, was one of a select few cancer educational films that was regularly shown in theatres as part of the regular film schedule, as a short subject that accompanied the feature. Demand was so great that the ACS found itself rushing to produce more copies. The film thus attracted attention far beyond the world of cancer education. It was the subject of a four-page spread in *Life Magazine*, with around 13 million readers, and was nominated for an Oscar in 1952.[16]

The success of *Man Alive!* prompted the ACS to partner again with UPA to release *Sappy Homiens* in 1956. As with Ed Parmalee, Sappy's journey to the doctor begins unpromisingly. Sappy, like Ed, avoids a visit to his doctor by hiding in the bathroom, secretly examining himself, and finding no danger signals of the disease. Sappy changes his view, however, when he watches television. Every channel has the same programme, with Sappy-like figures talking and singing to him, even when he turns the TV off. Eventually, he is pulled into the set, where he joins his other selves. There, he learns to save his life by going for a regular medical check-up since, as he is informed, it is quite possible to have cancer without realizing it. 'The cartoon moves briskly and brightly through the trials and tribulations of Sappy Homiens and his all-too human fears', noted the ACS, '[t]he film provides humour, but with an important lesson that can save lives'.[17] Part of the briskness was provided by a special jazz composition for the film, composed by the West Coast jazzman, Shorty Roberts, who had composed scores for other UPA films.[18]

There were several different versions of the film: some black-and-white, some colour, some longer, and some shorter. One film was 14 minutes long, with live action in which the UPA writer, Leo Salkin, contemplates how to do the task set up by the ACS (called *Sappy Homiens—The Story of an Animated Cartoon*); a shorter version of this film (under a shorter title) runs for 7 minutes and comprises the cartoon alone.[19] Some of these films were destined for television, as well as for the usual informal places where ACS films were shown.[20] Moreover, with the success of *Man Alive!* in mind, in 1958, the ACS began putting prints of *Sappy Homiens*—along with *Man Alive!* and a live-action educational, *The Other City* (1957)— into the hands of commercial

16 'Grim but Funny'.
17 'This Is Your Life'.
18 Feather, *Encyclopedia*, pp. 19, 142.
19 'This Is Your Life'. For a storyboard, see Salkin, *Story-Telling Home Movies*, pp. 88–91.
20 See ACS advertisement in *Broadcasting: Telecasting* (19 March 1956), p. 101.

film distributors for screening in cinemas as part of the regular schedule.[21] The film was honoured at the 1956 Edinburgh International Film Festival.[22] However, despite this, and Sappy's 'irresistible but hard-hitting humor', it did not gain the same recognition and distribution as *Man Alive!*[23] The smaller budget and the cruder animation perhaps worked against the film.

Sappy Homiens was followed by *Inside Magoo* in 1960. Magoo, like Ed and Sappy before him, avoids going to the doctor. We first meet him when he bursts out of his house, not by the front door, but through the glass window beside it. His cheerful obliviousness and myopia are established, as he mistakes a sprinkler for rain, and the sudden stop of his car by crashing into a water hydrant as a sign of good brakes. Although he has already tried to avoid the warnings about cancer on the car radio, he is pursued by an advertising billboard mounted on a truck that warns of the early warning signs of cancer, and to go to a physician the moment one is spotted. Magoo escapes the truck: 'Magoos never get cancer', he claims.

Then follows a series of mishaps. Magoo visits a funfair, mistaking it for a cinema. He sees his misshapen self in a distorting mirror and remembers the warning about sudden growths being a warning sign of cancer. He knocks a painter on his ladder and mistakes the red paint that falls on his head for blood coming from somewhere unexpected, another warning sign. He is hit by a hammer and a lump forms; the unexplained pain is yet another warning. Finally, some candy floss flies into his face and he starts coughing, another warning sign—a persistent cough. The viewer knows that Magoo is not exhibiting any of these symptoms, but Magoo does not and he begins to worry. He has many warning signs of cancer.

Magoo now goes to the doctor, but via an unlikely route. Mistaking a removal van for a doctor's office, Magoo climbs in and seats himself, his pessimism growing as he watches what seems to be a corpse under some sheeting: It is nothing of the sort. Then, removal men carry Magoo into a doctor's waiting room, where Magoo cheers up thinking that a table lamp is an attractive female nurse. He enters the doctor's office fearful of his fate—'the last of the Magoos', he mourns. The hands of a clock move a couple of hours and then Magoo exits the office elated. He does not have cancer—he leaps in the air and dances with the table lamp/nurse. (There are echoes here of Ed Parmalee's joyful leap when he gets the same news.)

21 Ross, 'Motion Pictures', p. 29.

22 '29 American Films', p. 28.

23 US Public Health Service, *Cancer Film Guide*, p. 22.

Then Magoo turns to his audience facing the camera and tells us all to get a check-up.

As with *Sappy Homiens*, there are several different versions of *Inside Magoo*. One was a 6-minute version for motion-picture theatres, which comprised only the cartoon. There were also two 15-minute versions for television, clubs, organizations, and Crusade training sessions. Both the longer films included additional live-action sequences. The first dramatized the Society's April Cancer Crusade, explaining the importance of public contributions to the ACS.[24] The second bookended the cartoon with two live-action sequences directed by John F. Becker, a two-time Peabody winner, and head of the ACS' motion-picture production, who had joined the ACS in 1954. The sequence at the start of the film provides a short history of the motion picture, culminating in the development of animation and the cancer cell scenes described earlier. The sequence that follows the animation echoes themes in the cartoon: A lamp turns into a nurse (played by Joi Lansing), Jim Backus is suddenly undressed for a medical examination, and Bosustow disappears to make way for a doctor (Jim Corey). Corey's examination of Backus is lightened by the latter's comedic reactions, before Magoo himself returns, entering the live action.

1950s America

If UPA film-makers hoped to charm male audiences through humour and visual style, they also sought to charm them through commentaries, sometimes parodies, of 1950s America. *Man Alive!*, for example, sought to entice its male audiences by wrapping its cancer-control message in a story about the dangers of the city, the psychology of fear, and the pleasures and pains of affluent white suburbia, car ownership, and companionate marriage.[25] It portrayed a world in which men had to identify and confront their inner fears, listen to the wisdom of their wives, and turn to reputable professionals when necessary, be they car mechanics or physicians.

Wives, in particular, were important to this film. The ACS argued that many men were not only fearful of the disease but regarded an interest in their own health as a sign of weakness. Someone had to persuade them otherwise, and, as an ACS slogan put it, 'a nagging wife can save your life'.[26] *Man Alive!* thus turned the stereotype of the nagging wife (and the henpecked

24 I have not found a copy of this version.

25 Cantor, *Man Alive*.

26 Ross, 'Motion Pictures', p. 31.

husband) around to make a comedic virtue of them both, just as it turned male humour about women drivers on its head. Ed is shown to be a stubborn figure who ignores the warning signs of his car (and body) going wrong as well as the wise advice of his wife Marion that he go to a reputable mechanic (and doctor). His claims to knowledge are shown to be bogus by know-nothings and charlatans who only make things worse. Yet, paradoxically, it is not his wife who eventually persuades him to go to the doctor, but the male narrator. A woman might nag, the suggestion is, but it takes the calm reasoning of a male narrator (or a comic film) to get a man to the doctor.[27]

Sappy Homiens also sought to wrap its cancer message in a comic commentary on 1950s America. The film begins with a careworn Sappy returning home (likely from the office), his wife and kids welcoming him home with a kiss, before (after the panic of his self-examination) he sits down in front of the TV. He is portrayed as a good father, a good husband (doing the washing up in a woman's frilly apron, a mixed symbol signifying both emasculation and a good helpmate), and as a hard worker (in an office with a teetering pile of paper in his in tray and a mess of documents around an overflowing bin) trying to pay off the mortgage (to a sinister banker in a top hat), keep the wolf from the door, and retire at 65. But all this is endangered by his foolishness, as a Sappy-like figure within the TV tells him: his unwillingness to take time off for a check-up. Thus, unlike with Ed, it is not the film's narrator who urges him to go to the doctor, but his television alter egos, who show him how self-diagnosis can be misleading. Cancer, they tell him, can happen without any symptoms, and only a doctor can spot its presence. Thus, this surreal, fantastical story also playfully gestures towards contemporary faith in the unique ability of the new medium of television to transform beliefs and behaviour.[28] After all, it is the Sappy-like figures within the television who persuade Sappy himself to change his attitude and behaviour towards cancer.

Man Alive! and *Sappy Homiens* thus do much more than present anxieties about cancer. They evoke both the promise of post-war affluence— spacious modern houses, television, automobiles, freeways peppered with advertising billboards, the suburbs—and also the many anxieties that went with this world: broken cars, costly repairs, financial ruin, con men, and grasping financiers.[29] Ed, more than Sappy, captures another issue—what it meant

27 Cantor, *Man Alive*.

28 Seed, *Brainwashing*.

29 Cantor, *Man Alive*. On efforts to redefine masculinity more generally, see Gilbert, *Men in the Middle*.

to be a man within the context of a companionate marriage. He fails to see the reality of his wife's greater wisdom and is unwilling to compromise with her because of his fears, screaming his anger at her, until he is told by the narrator to go to a professional and to listen to his wife. More generally, Ed is a man who constantly represses his anxieties, as does Sappy, and their films suggest that it is only by understanding the psychology of fear and how it clouds a man's judgements that they will be able to adapt to this post-war suburban world, seek professional help, and listen to the advice of organizations like the Cancer Society and (in Ed's case) their wives.[30] Here, cancer is both a metaphor for the anxieties of living in post-war suburbia and a real cause of such anxieties: Contemporary reports suggested that the high cost of cancer care often resulted in immiseration, and that the disease disrupted families and 1950s gender roles, with men taking over care from their sick wives and wives having to go out to work.[31]

Inside Magoo also provides a commentary on the post-war world. However, where *Man Alive!* and *Sappy Homiens* are accounts of how men might live in white, consumer, suburban culture, *Inside Magoo* is, in part, a rejection of that world, or at least a failure to adapt to it. Ed and Sappy both live in modern houses—sparsely furnished and orderly—which they share with their wives and, in Sappy's case, children. Ed also drives a sports convertible (albeit one with some engine trouble). Magoo, by contrast, apparently lives alone in a Victorian house (cluttered with newspapers collecting on his roof) and drives an ancient jalopy, which meets its end in this film when it is wrecked on the fire hydrant.[32] Ed is anxious about his car problems. Magoo is blithely unaware of his.

Moreover, while Ed is prey to the temptations of the city from which white suburbanites were fleeing in the 1950s, Magoo, in this film, is not. Ed is an innocent in a world of urban predators: the dodgy car mechanic, the fraudulent quack, and the know-nothings who offer bad advice. He is always tempted by this dangerous world, where his claims to knowledge are revealed as phoney. Magoo is faced with shysters and con men in his other films, which, combined with his nearsightedness, inevitably carries him almost to his doom, which he improbably avoids. Here, he faces no such threats. Instead, he cheerfully wanders through this film, misinterpreting

30 UPA's educationals often explained the psychology of maladaptive behaviours such as bad driving, dangerous flying, not going to the doctor, or not listening to wives; Cantor, *Man Alive*, p. 6.

31 For further discussion of this, see Cantor, *Man Alive*, pp. 7–9.

32 In other 1950s films, Mr. Magoo shares his house with his nephew Waldo.

the world as he goes, until his unfounded pessimism prompts him to see a physician. The clutter and disorder of the city are threats to Ed and to his path to a recognized physician, unlike the clutter and mayhem around Magoo, which somehow delivers him to the doctor.

Inside Magoo thus presents a very different view of post-war America to those of *Man Alive!* and *Sappy Homiens*. Magoo lives in this world, but seems unaware of it, mistaking everything around him. As the historian of UPA, Adam Abraham, puts it, he 'perceives a world that everyone else—conformist, suburban-migrating, baby-booming consumers—fails to see'.[33] In *Inside Magoo*, such elements of consumer culture are represented by the newspaper headline on cancer Magoo fails to see; the advertising billboard that Magoo tries to ignore, but which follows him wherever he goes; the radio that Magoo cannot turn off no matter how he tries, until, paradoxically, the radio announcer tells him how; and the Playland fairground where the ACS' message finally gets through. It is there that Magoo mistakes paint for blood, a distorted mirror reflection for growths, a hammer blow for an unexplained pain, and a cough caused by cotton candy for another early warning sign of cancer. Even the doctor's office is a playful parody of modern medicine. There is a copy of *Live* magazine in the reception, a play on *Life*, the magazine that Ed Parmalee pretends to read while fearfully waiting for the doctor, and which Bert Hansen tells us was in every physician's waiting room at that time.[34]

Rejecting Consumer Culture?

There is an irony to Magoo's rejection of consumer culture, for, since 1956, he had increasingly turned his hand to marketing. Magoo had started life in theatrical shorts—short films shown before the feature film in commercial cinemas, or during a matinee show for children.[35] However, by the end of the 1950s, the market in theatrical shorts seemed to be drying up and UPA's own ventures into the new medium of television seemed to be stymied. So UPA turned Magoo into an advertiser and educator as the company sought to navigate the leaner years of the late 1950s—the very promotional activities Magoo so casually ignored in his films.

Bosustow first licenced Magoo for advertising purposes in 1956, when he was employed to sell Rheingold beer. The following year, the Radio Corporation

33 Abraham, *When Magoo Flew*, p. 161.

34 Hansen, *Picturing Medical Progress*, Chapter 9.

35 On UPA and advertising, see Abraham, *When Magoo Flew*, Chapter 8.

of America (RCA) put out a long-playing record, *Magoo in Hi-Fi*: a promotion of high-fidelity records and music equipment of which RCA was an innovator.[36] In 1958, he could be found promoting the Carling Brewing Company's Stag Beer. Then, in 1959, the film producer Henry G. Saperstein took out a licence on Mr. Magoo, and Bosustow sold him the entire company a year later.[37] Under Saperstein, Magoo became the focus of a complicated set of co-promotions all linked to Mr. Magoo's first feature film, *1001 Arabian Nights* (1959). The film was co-promoted with a General Electric campaign that used Magoo to sell their light bulbs,[38] and with another campaign to sell US Savings Bonds: 'Your magic carpet to the future—US Savings Bonds—Says Mister Magoo of "1001 Arabian Nights".'[39] A third co-promotion was with *Inside Magoo*.[40]

Magoo's efforts to ignore the world of marketing in *Inside Magoo* were thus a paradox.[41] He might have tried to ignore this world in the film, but he had been driven into it by changing consumer habits after the arrival of the television which had threatened UPA. Many animators had moved to better paid positions in television commercials, so that, when Bosustow sold UPA in 1960, only a few of the best remained. The company was a ghost of its earlier incarnation, but it had a strong film back catalogue and characters, such as Magoo, which Saperstein could licence or use in other formats, including television. Mr. Magoo followed the money, moving from theatrical shorts to the small screen (*Inside Magoo* itself was a regular feature on television well into the 1960s).

Inside Magoo was thus as much about the health of UPA as it was about promoting healthy bodies. It also came to be used to combat calls for greater film censorship, weakened during the 1950s by competition from television and antitrust legislation that opened the door to foreign films that did not follow to the Hays Production Code. Such developments, in turn, prompted demands for a return to stricter censorship. This is not the place to describe in full the industry's response to such demands. However, one of the ways they did so was to highlight the educational role of film. In this context, *Inside Magoo* was screened for this purpose by the film distributor, Robert W. Selig, to parent-teacher associations to illustrate family entertainment and educationals produced by the industry.[42]

36 Hollis, *Toons in Toyland*, pp. 171–172.
37 On Magoo as an advertising icon more generally, see 'Inside Magoo or What Makes'.
38 'Near-sighted Magoo was Far-sighted'; 'Myopic Magoo'.
39 'Treasury Department Tie-in'; 'Near-Sighted Magoo Helps'.
40 'Inside Magoo', p. 11.
41 On UPA and consumerism, see Klein, *Seven Minutes*, esp. Chapter 22.
42 'Selig Plan'.

Inner- or Other-Directed

Magoo, Ed, and Sappy are also commentaries on the 1950s in another way: They are light-hearted spoofs of the inner-directed and other-directed personalities found in David Riesman's influential book, *The Lonely Crowd: A Study of the Changing American Character* (1950).[43] In 1957, the psychologist Milton Rosenberg portrayed Magoo as a comic 'inner directed personality'.[44] 'Inner-directed' types were individualists, according to Riesman, who navigated social life by using moral codes internalized in childhood, instead of external codes imposed by sensitivity to the views of others. For Rosenberg, Magoo's values parody some of the features of the inner-directed personality. His character was made 'in equal parts of eccentric individuality, square shooting, get-up-and-go vigor, and classic persistence'.[45] Magoo, for Rosenberg, never questions the tenets of his existence, speaks his mind, and is unconcerned about what others think. Indeed, Rosenberg argues, 'this belief in himself, rooted in his internal loyalty to a moral view of existence, keeps him whole and secure in the face of dangers that, because of his *faith* rather than his myopia, are not visibly real'.[46] Magoo, he concludes, 'may have his greatest appeal in the eyes of lonely "inner-directed" persons caught up in an increasingly "other-directed" round of existence'.[47]

From such a perspective, Magoo's nearsightedness becomes a metaphor for his inner-directedness, allowing him to make sense of the crazy world around him. Indeed, at times, it is joined by another, more curmudgeonly, metaphor for inner-directedness, where Magoo is not so much someone who cannot see the world as it is, as someone who refuses to see that way. As the advertising executive, Art Bellaire, put it: 'He opens his eyes once in a while, but he doesn't always like what he sees, so he closes them again.[48] Bellaire's agency had surveyed Magoo's theatrical shorts while working on the advertising campaign that used Magoo to sell General Electric (GE)

43 Riesman, *Lonely Crowd*.

44 Rosenberg, 'Mr. Magoo as Public Dream'. Abrahams's discussion of this issue follows Rosenberg's suggestion (*When Magoo Flew*, p. 163). On inner-directed art house audiences and a preference for the Mr. Magoo type of cartoon, see Smythe et al., 'Portrait', p. 50. See also Lehman, *Colored Cartoon*, pp. 111–112. More generally, see Wells, *Animation and America*, Chapter 3.

45 Rosenberg, 'Mr. Magoo as Public Dream', p. 341.

46 Rosenberg, 'Mr. Magoo as Public Dream', p. 342, emphasis in original.

47 Rosenberg, 'Mr. Magoo as Public Dream', p. 342. Bashara refers to Magoo as having a pre-modern understanding of the modern world; *Cartoon Vision*, p. 63. In fact, Riesman associated inner-directed types not with the premodern world, but with nineteenth-century urban industrial modernity.

48 'Adapting a Cartoon Idol', p. 42.

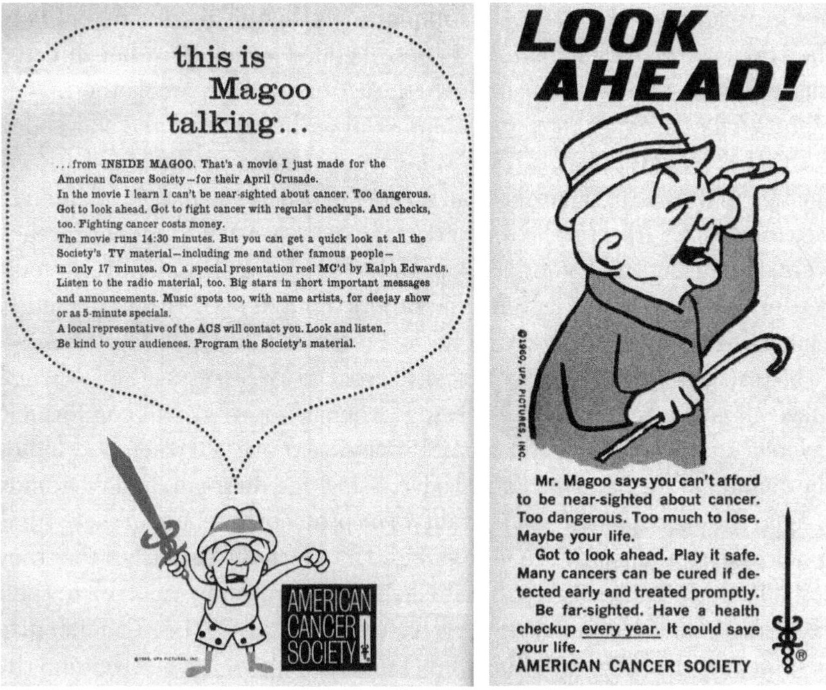
this is
Magoo
talking...
...from INSIDE MAGOO. That's a movie I just made for the
American Cancer Society—for their April Crusade.
In the movie I learn I can't be near-sighted about cancer. Too dangerous.
Got to look ahead. Got to fight cancer with regular checkups. And checks,
too. Fighting cancer costs money.
The movie runs 14:30 minutes. But you can get a quick look at all the
Society's TV material—including me and other famous people—
in only 17 minutes. On a special presentation reel MC'd by Ralph Edwards.
Listen to the radio material, too. Big stars in short important messages
and announcements. Music spots too, with name artists, for deejay show
or as 5-minute specials.
A local representative of the ACS will contact you. Look and listen.
Be kind to your audiences. Program the Society's material.
AMERICAN CANCER SOCIETY
LOOK AHEAD!
©1960, UPA PICTURES, INC.
Mr. Magoo says you can't afford to be near-sighted about cancer. Too dangerous. Too much to lose. Maybe your life.
Got to look ahead. Play it safe. Many cancers can be cured if detected early and treated promptly.
Be far-sighted. Have a health checkup every year. It could save your life.
AMERICAN CANCER SOCIETY

6.3. a (left): from *Broadcasting*, 58, 2 (23 May 1960), p. 112; b (right): from *Popular Mechanics*, 115, 1 (January 1961), p. 79.

lightbulbs (if he wants to see, he can with GE), and his observation also applies to *Inside Magoo*. Magoo does not want to listen to the radio (his eyes open briefly) that he cannot switch off, and he does not want to see (his eyes open briefly again, perhaps surprised) the advertising billboard that chases him. Paradoxically, it is only when he returns to his myopic, inner-directed world that the messages about the danger signals get through, his old certainty that Magoos never get cancer disappears, and he goes to the doctor. Thus, it is his myopia that metaphorically opens his eyes, and, after the good news that he does not have cancer, he urges the viewer to get a check-up. Posters produced as part of the advertising campaign echoed this point: 'Mr. Magoo says you can't afford to be nearsighted about cancer. Too dangerous. Too much to lose. Maybe your life. Got to look ahead.' (Figure 6.3b) Magoo, however, is still in his myopic state, looking ahead with closed eyes, playfully warning the viewer not to follow his lead or maybe to enter the myopic world that opened his eyes.

If Magoo represents a comic version of an inner-directed personality, Ed and Sappy seem to represent comic versions of other-directed personalities—younger men than Magoo, whose character type reflects the demands of a bureaucratized society. Riesman argued that, instead of listening to their own voices and following a set of embedded principles, other-directed men cultivated a special sensitivity to the actions and wishes of others. They monitored colleagues for signs of approval or disapproval and succeeded within bureaucratic structures by this constant management of self. In fact, such men, Riesman suggested, had no core of self. Instead, they adapted to circumstance with a series of superficial masks. Never confident that they were evaluating the situation accurately, they were chronically anxious, constantly trying to figure out what others thought of them and to modify their self-presentation accordingly.

Like Magoo, Ed and Sappy both seek to avoid the ACS' message. But, whereas Magoo is converted to the ACS message when he returns to his comfortable myopic, inner-directed world, Ed and Sappy are converted when they follow the dictates of the mass media and advertising that Riesman thought unduly shaped the other-directed personality. The problem as set out in these films is not that Ed and Sappy are manipulated by the mass media, but that they resist it. Both films suggest that it is when Ed and Sappy are true to their other-directed selves that they convert to the message of the ACS. They also suggest that the boundaries between Ed's and Sappy's inner selves and the world of the media are quite blurry. Thus, Ed is converted by the narrator of the film, who may also be his inner voice, or the voice of expert male authority. Sappy is converted, as I've mentioned, by his other selves, the ones he joins inside the television. As such, where Magoo's conversion comes about because of his nearsightedness (the metaphor for his inner-directedness), Sappy and Ed are converted by their other-directedness (metaphorically indicated by the narrator's voice for Ed and the television alter ego for Sappy). UPA has turned Riesman's critique of other-directed personalities on its head.

Yet, all these films also suggest that health and well-being come from setting limits on personality, whether inner- or outer-directed. In the case of Ed and Sappy, the films show how such limits could be set by recognized experts. Such experts would, the films suggest, allow them to reduce their anxiety about cancer and, indeed, of other aspects of contemporary life: broken cars, unpaid bills, nagging wives, shysters, and greedy bankers. Thus, experts teach Ed or Sappy how to listen to wives and the media, avoid tricksters and charlatans, seek sanctuary in the suburbs, cultivate self-understanding, and recognize the limits of their own knowledge and the psychological motivations behind their maladaptive behaviours. For example, Ed's anxieties about the health of his body are constantly exacerbated by the advice of con men and the ignorant. It is only when he turns to recognized experts that he can discount their suggestions, and, despite his continued fears of cancer, seek appropriate help. Experts, in short, are presented as a means by which other-directed personalities can anchor their beliefs and behaviours and adjust their sensitivity to the opinions of others in ways that promote healthy bodies and psychological well-being.

Something similar is also true for inner-directed personalities such as Magoo. Magoo's anxieties about cancer are not matched by anxieties about the contemporary world of the sort that afflict Ed and Sappy. Indeed, he seems cheerfully, perhaps wilfully, to ignore such anxieties, until the messages on the advertising billboard—representing consumer marketing—prompt him to briefly doubt his inner certainty that Magoos never get cancer. His world turned upside down by advertising is only returned to normal by a recognized expert—the off-stage doctor. Magoo now has perspective in which a regular check-up can prevent both cancer and the anxiety about it. Indeed, given that his eyes are closed, this new view seems to come from within his myopic, inner-directed world view. Magoo's myopic personality, out of tune with the 1950s, has changed slightly because of expert opinion and luck.

Conclusion

The three films under consideration in this chapter portray bodily and emotional health as things that could be converted into what Bourdieu describes as various forms of capital: social, economic, symbolic, and cultural. Thus, on the one hand, *Man Alive!* and *Sappy Homiens* both invoke the tropes of post-war suburban prosperity and status to which Ed and Sappy aspire, the anxieties that come with such a life, and how their fears of cancer hobble their enjoyment of such a life. Furthermore, in *Sappy Homiens*, in particular, cancer is also invoked as a threat to all that a man may work towards—a home, family, and retirement—and the loss of status that might follow. On the other hand, *Inside Magoo* is, in some ways, a comedic rejection of the post-war world that Ed and Sappy embrace. Magoo has none of the anxieties of Ed or Sappy, and he ambles through the film seemingly blind to what is happening around him. However, just as Ed and Sappy are troubled by the ACS' message, so, eventually, is Magoo. Magoo might have rejected the world of post-war consumer culture, but, like Ed and Sappy, his world is disturbed by symbols of modern advertising and marketing: advertising billboards, radio, television, and pamphlets.

All three men share one handicap—they are paralyzed by fear, and much of the comedy of the films focusses on how it makes them avoid going to the doctor. In this sense, Ed and Sappy are both like Magoo, unwilling or unable to see the world as it is. Indeed, Magoo's other handicap—his nearsightedness—can be seen as a comic metaphor for the fantasy worlds into which those fearful of cancer might retreat, and the ignorance which individuals (including Ed and Sappy) may have of what is going on in their bodies. The ACS argued that only a recognized physician could determine whether a patient had cancer. And it is such physicians—and experts and expert knowledge more generally—that are presented as a solution to the anxieties produced by consumer advertising, even that produced by the ACS. The films thus evoke broader cultural concerns about the ability of marketing to manipulate and mislead, and the roles of experts in countering such effects. The irony here is that Magoo himself turned to advertising in the 1950s, to sell beer, light bulbs, and UPA's feature films, and that *Inside Magoo* was a part of this turn.

But there is a further paradox here. The very solution that the films propose—going to the doctor at the first sign of the disease—itself raised the spectre of financial hardship, and the stigma of dependency and pauperism.[49] The National Cancer Institute (NCI), the Federal government's main anticancer agency, noted that the high cost of cancer treatment strained family finances, as did the unwillingness of employers to hire 'cured' patients because of the increased risk of compensable illness, to say nothing of the disablement and disfigurement that often followed surgery. Families lost status and self-respect, the NCI argued, and were forced to accept charity or other relief, as their dreams of sharing in post-war prosperity slipped away. UPA might have sought to project medical reassurance about cancer, but it could do little to solve the conundrum of such high costs. Had Ed, Sappy, or Magoo in fact been treated for or even cured of cancer, the forms of capital outlined by Bourdieu might have been much more difficult for them to obtain.

Works Cited

Films, Television Programmes, and Recordings

1001 Arabian Nights, directed by Jack Kinney, UPA, 1959.
Breast Self-Examination, directed by Alexander Gansell, ACS, 1950.
Fantasia, directed by Samuel Armstrong et al., Walt Disney Productions, 1940.

49 United States Congress, *Health Inquiry*, p. 102.

Gerald McBoing-Boing, directed by Robert Cannon, UPA, 1950.
Inside Magoo, directed by Abe Levitow and John F. Becker, UPA/ACS, 1960.
Magoo in Hi-fi: Mother Magoo Suite, RCA Victor, Camden, NJ, 1957.
Man Alive!, directed by William T. Hurtz, UPA/ACS, 1952.
The Other City, produced and directed by John F. Becker, ACS, 1957.
Pinocchio, directed by Ben Sharpsteen et al., Walt Disney Productions, 1940.
The Strange Case of Oliver Dancer, ACS, 1956.
Sappy Homiens, directed by Leo Salkin, UPA/ACS, 1956.
Sappy Homiens—The Story of an Animated Cartoon, directed by Leo Salkin, UPA/ACS, 1956.
Snow White and the Seven Dwarfs, directed by David Hand et al., Walt Disney Productions, 1937.

Books and Articles

'29 American Films Are Presented at Edinburgh, Venice Festivals', *Business Screen Magazine*, 17, 6 (1956), pp. 28 and 62.
'ACS Re-signs UPA', *Motion Picture Daily*, 86, 86 (2 November 1959), p. 4.
Abraham, Adam, *When Magoo Flew: The Rise and Fall of Animation Studio UPA* (Middletown, CT: Wesleyan University Press, 2012).
'Adapting a Cartoon Idol to Sales', *Printer's Ink*, 277 (24 November 1961), pp. 40–43.
Barrier, Michael, *Hollywood Cartoons: American Animation in Its Golden Age* (New York: Oxford University Press, 2003).
Bashara, Dan, *Cartoon Vision: UPA Animation and Postwar Aesthetics* (Oakland, CA: University of California Press, 2019).
Bonah, Christian, David Cantor, and Anja Laukötter, eds., *Health Education Films in the Twentieth Century* (Rochester, NY: University of Rochester Press, 2018).
Cantor, David, *Man Alive! (1952): Cartoon Fun with Cancer, Cars and Companionate Marriage in Suburban America* (Bethesda: National Library of Medicine, 2014), https://www.nlm.nih.gov/hmd/collections/films/medicalmoviesontheweb/pdf/manalive.pdf, accessed 6 August 2018.
Cantor, David, 'Uncertain Enthusiasm: The American Cancer Society, Public Education, and the Problems of the Movie, 1921–1960', *Bulletin of the History of Medicine*, 81, 1 (2007), pp. 39–69, http://www.jstor.org/stable/44451738.
'Coast Reviewers Praise ACS Film', *ACS Bulletin*, 2, 8 (12 January 1953), pp. 1 and 4.
Corwin, Emil, 'Tactic', *Cancer News*, 13, 3 (Summer 1959), pp. 9–12.
Feather, Leonard, *The Encyclopedia Yearbook of Jazz* (New York: Horizon Press, 1956).
Gilbert, James, *Men in the Middle: Searching for Masculinity in the 1950s* (Chicago: University of Chicago Press, 2005).
'Grim but Funny', *Life*, 32 (21 April 1952), pp. 99–100.

Hansen, Bert, *Picturing Medical Progress from Pasteur to Polio: A History of Mass Media Images and Popular Attitudes in America* (New Brunswick, NJ: Rutgers University Press, 2009).

Hollis, Tim, *Toons in Toyland: The Story of Cartoon Character Merchandise* (Jackson: University Press of Mississippi, 2015).

Hubley, John, and Zachary Schwartz, 'Animation Learns a New Language', *Hollywood Quarterly*, 1, 4 (July 1946), pp. 360–363, doi:10.2307/1209495.

'Inside Magoo', *Cancer News*, 14, 1 (Winter 1960), pp. 11–14.

'Inside Magoo Or What Makes a Top TV Sales Personality Tick', *Sponsor*, 18, 27 (6 July 1964), pp. 43–47.

Klein, Norman M., *Seven Minutes: The Life and Death of the American Animated Cartoon* (London: Verso, 1993).

Lehman, Christopher P., *The Colored Cartoon: Black Representation in American Animated Short Films, 1907–1954* (Amherst: University of Massachusetts Press, 2007).

'Magoo Cancer Cartoon Available to Exhibitors', *Motion Picture Daily*, 87, 30 (15 February 1960), p. 3.

'Myopic Magoo Eyes Beauty Tourneys as Col. Sets "Arabian Nights" Campaign Afloat', *Film Bulletin*, 27, 25 (7 December 1959), p. 22.

'Near-Sighted Magoo Helps Treasury Float Bond Issue', *Film Bulletin*, 27, 24 (23 November 1959), p. 18.

'Near-Sighted Magoo was Far-Sighted GE TV Buy', *Sponsor*, 18, 27 (6 July 1964), pp. 46–47.

Reagan, Leslie J., 'Engendering the Dread Disease: Women, Men, and Cancer', *American Journal of Public Health*, 87, 11 (1997), pp. 1779–1787.

Rieder, Howard [Edward], 'Memories of Mr. Magoo', *Cinema Journal*, 8, 2 (Spring 1969), pp. 17–24, doi:10.2307/1225373.

Rieder, Howard Edward, 'The Development of the Satire of Mr. Magoo' (MA thesis, University of Southern California, 1961), uscthesesreloadpub_Volume8/etd-rieder-527270.pdf, accessed 6 August 2018.

Riesman, David, *The Lonely Crowd: A Study of the Changing American Character* (New Haven: Yale University Press, 1950).

Rosenberg, Milton J., 'Mr. Magoo as Public Dream', *Quarterly of Film Radio and Television*, 11, 4 (Summer 1957), pp. 337–342, doi:10.2307/1209993.

Ross, Walter, 'Motion Pictures Worth 10,000 Lives', *Business Screen Magazine*, 20, 2 (1959), pp. 28–31.

Salkin, Leo, *Story-Telling Home Movies: How to Make Them* (New York: McGraw-Hill, 1958).

Seed, David, *Brainwashing: The Fictions of Mind Control: A Study of Novels and Films since World War II* (Kent: Kent State University Press, 2004).

'Selig Plan Answers Industry Criticism by Showing Family Films to Civic Units', *Motion Picture Daily*, 87, 42 (3 March 1960), pp. 1 and 3.

Smythe, Dallas W., Parker B. Lusk, and Charles A. Lewis, 'Portrait of an Art-Theater Audience', *Quarterly of Film Radio and Television*, 8, 1 (Autumn 1953), pp. 28–50, doi:10.2307/1209911.

'The Strange Case of Oliver Dancer', *Cancer News*, 10, 2 (Spring 1956), p. 23.

'"This Is Your Life": Sappy Learns A Lesson', *ACS Bulletin*, 5, 9 (5 March 1956), p. 2.

'Treasury Department Tie-in for "Arabian"', *Motion Picture Daily*, 86, 99 (20 November 1959), p. 2.

United States Congress, House Committee on Interstate and Foreign Commerce, *Health Inquiry: The Toll of Our Major Diseases: Their Causes, Prevention, and Control: Preliminary Report of the Committee on Interstate and Foreign Commerce* (Washington, DC: United States Government Printing Office, 1954), http://docs.newsbank.com/select/serialset/123255C7D 853E3D8.html, accessed 7 August 2018.

U. S. Public Health Service, *Cancer Film Guide*, rev. ed. (Washington, DC: U. S. Public Health Service, Cancer Control Branch, Public Health Service Publication no. 848, 1963).

Wells, Paul, *Animation and America* (New Brunswick, NJ: Rutgers University Press, 2002).

About the Author

David Cantor is a researcher (*investigador*) at the Instituto de Desarrollo Económico y Social (IDES), Buenos Aires, Argentina. His edited books are: *Reinventing Hippocrates* (2002); *Cancer in the Twentieth Century* (2008); with Christian Bonah and Matthias Dörries, *Meat, Medicine, and Human Health in the Twentieth Century* (2010); with Edmund Ramsden, *Stress, Shock, and Adaptation in the Twentieth Century* (2014); and, with Christian Bonah and Anja Laukötter, *Health Education Films in the Twentieth Century* (2018). He is series coeditor of *Social Histories of Medicine* (Manchester University Press). Contact details: djcantor@hotmail.com

7. 'One Feels so Much in These Times!' Emotional Education and the Construction of New Subjectivities: Sex Education Films in Early 1960s GDR

Anja Laukötter

Abstract

Shown in different formats—from cinema to television—in a variety of settings, this chapter outlines the role these films played in discourses on sex education in the GDR in the 1960s, which for their part were highly influenced by psychology and pedagogy. The article will argue that these films not only served the pedagogical function of teaching viewers about sexuality, but also aimed to (re-)produce the ideal of the 'new man' for a newly emerging socialist society that was to be founded on a new way of educating emotions. Since the education of youth was regarded a key issue for the construction of new selves, the medium of film with its special attractiveness for the young generation can be viewed as an instrument for forming new subjectivities.

Keywords: sex education; television; GDR; West Germany; emotion/feeling; sexuality; pedagogy; child; parents; teacher/educator; filmic techniques

Introduction

Anita runs home crying and throws herself onto the sofa. Her mother enters the room and asks 'What's the matter?', but Anita keeps crying. Her father chimes in: 'Every day it's the same drama.' The mother asks her husband: 'Do you understand all this?' Tracking shot through an empty classroom. 'Anita loves Peter' is written on the blackboard. Voice-over: 'Eleven- and twelve-year-old boys and girls sit in this classroom. Last month, three vulgar

Bonah, C. and A. Laukötter (eds.), *Body, Capital, and Screens: Visual Media and the Healthy Self in the 20th Century*. Taylor & Francis Group, 2020
DOI 10.5117/9789462988293_CH07

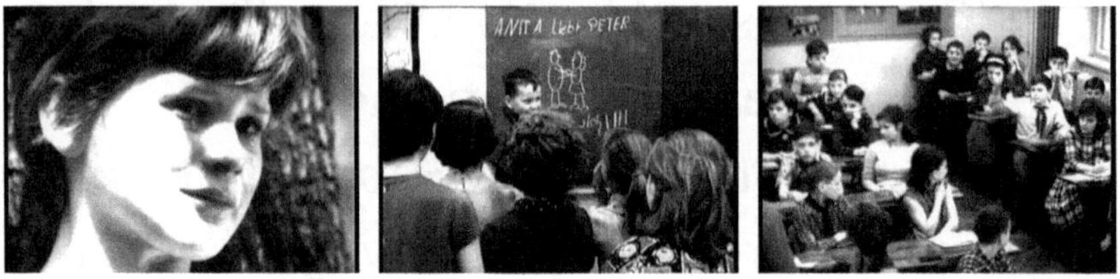

7.1. Three stills from *Sagst du's deinem Kinde?* ('Will you tell your child?'), 1963. © DEFA-Stiftung/ Günther Biedermann.

romance novels and multiple photos were exchanged among the pupils. Seventeen obscene drawings were drawn, nine love notes were written. What's behind all of this?' In the classroom, a teacher asks her class how many pupils have spoken about the topic of today's lesson with their parents. Voice-over: 'Studies conducted at various schools have shown that only 4 per cent of pupils aged twelve to thirteen have spoken with their parents about relations between man and woman and the difficulties that go along with them. Out of 1,000 pupils 40, out of 100 only 4, in this class only one.'[1] One boy raises his hand (Figure 7.1).

Voice-over: 'What do parents have to say about this?' In a parent-teacher association meeting, mothers discuss their experiences: insecurity on their part, reticence on the part of their children. It is not only the parents who are confronted with 'this problem', states one father, the school shares responsibility in the matter. Clearing his throat, he refers to biology lessons and examples from the animal kingdom. A discussion ensues. Anita's mother says: 'Yes, but the type of education we're talking about will make our children curious and then they'll just be on the lookout for indecent things everywhere they go.' A father counters: 'This sort of education can't be over and done with in a single talk. I mean, it's a process sort of thing. Education is always like that, from the very beginning.' He continues that he and his wife always answer their son's questions honestly and openly, qualifying: 'Nevertheless, I must be open and honest with you, too: That thing, it's still a bit difficult for me too.' Other mothers claim that their children still play and don't yet 'experience sexual urges', that the topic is a burden, and that

1 'Jeden Tag dasselbe Theater.', 'Verstehst Du das?', 'Anita liebt Peter', 'In diesem Klassenzimmer sitzen 11- bis 12-jährige Jungen und Mädchen. Im letzten Monat gingen hier drei vulgäre Liebesromane und mehrere Fotoserien von Hand zu Hand. Siebzehn obszöne Zeichnungen wurden angefertigt und neun sogenannte Liebeszettel geschrieben. Woran liegt das?', 'Untersuchungen an verschiedenen Schulen ergaben: nur 4 Prozent der Schüler des 12. und 13. Lebensjahres sind von ihren Eltern über die Beziehungen zwischen Mann und Frau den damit zusammenhängenden Problemen aufgeklärt worden. Von 1.000 Schülern 40, von 100 4, in dieser Klasse einer.'

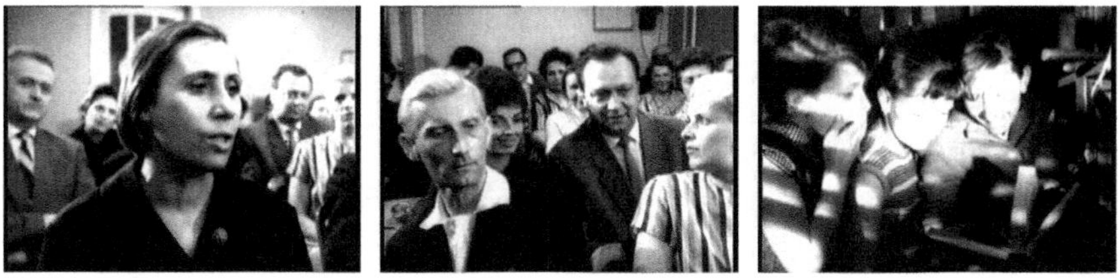

7.2. Three stills from *Sagst du's deinem Kinde?* ('Will you tell your child?'), 1963. © DEFA-Stiftung/ Günther Biedermann

it can wait, because there's still 'plenty of time'. Voice-over: 'Whoever still thinks in this way underestimates the development of their children and thus their own responsibilities as parents.'[2] (Figure 7.2) [...]

Voice-over: 'Educators must be conscious of children's enthusiastic search for role models, but they must also work discreetly to guide this search.' Shot on Peter, who is reading the book *Vom Leben erzogen* ('Brought up by life'). Voice-over: 'Above all, however, children should see their own mother and father as the role models most worthy of imitating. Even in the minutiae of everyday life.' The boy's mother brings dinner into the living room. The father warmly greets her and puts a coat on his wife's shoulders. The mother thanks him and gives him a kiss while the boy watches. Voice-over: 'Later on in life, such observations will help determine Peter's own behaviour.'[3] [...]

Peter puts a coat on Anita's shoulders as they stand on the lake shore during a field trip. Voice-over: 'For Peter, what his father does is a matter of course. But what Anita also perceives as a matter of course is not seen by her parents in the same way.' At home, Anita's father makes a patronizing comment about his daughter brushing her hair. Her mother says that 'it's not right' that Anita and Peter are always together. When checking his daughter's homework, Anita's father finds a letter from Peter. The father reads sections of the letter to his wife, saying to Anita: 'This is the most ridiculous thing I've ever seen. At your age, it's just plain silly.' Anita asks

2 'Was sagen die Eltern dazu?','Nun, wieso, Aufklärung, wie die hier verlangt wird, da werden die Kinder neugierig und sehen überall bloß was Unanständiges.', 'Diese Aufklärung, die ist doch nicht mit einem Gespräch beendet. Das ist doch ein, naja ich möchte sage, ein Prozess. Das ist Erziehungsarbeit von klein auf.', 'Allerdings muss ich auch offen und ehrlich sagen: Das letzte, naja, das fällt mir auch noch sehr schwer.', 'nicht geschlechtlich empfinde', 'Wer heute noch so denkt, unterschätzt den Reifegrad seiner Kinder, ebenso wie seine Erziehungsaufgaben.'

3 'Das ständige Suchen nach Vorbildern, das alle so begeisterungsfähig macht, muss von allen Erziehern bewusst, aber unaufdringlich gelenkt werden.', 'Das nachahmenswerteste Vorbild jedoch, sollten Vater und Mutter selbst sein. Auch in den alltäglichsten Kleinigkeiten.', 'Diese und ähnliche Beobachtungen werden später Peters eigenes Handeln bestimmen.'

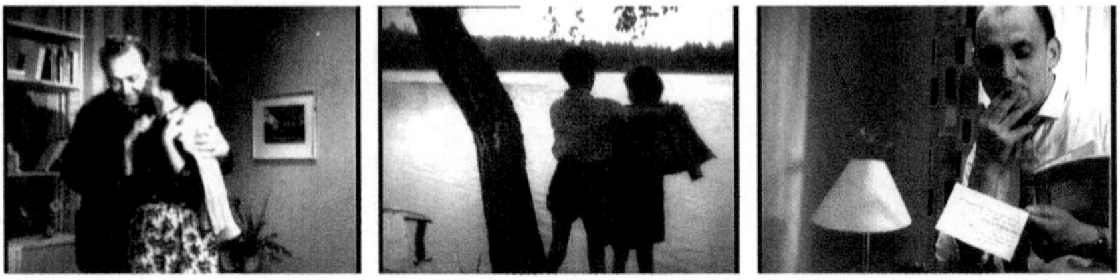

7.3. Three stills from *Sagst du's deinem Kinde?* ('Will you tell your child?'), 1963. © DEFA-Stiftung/ Günther Biedermann

to have the letter back. Her father answers: 'Of course, have it framed.' He tears up the letter and throws the pieces in the trash. Voice-over: 'Does Anita's father understand the way this bitter irony hurts her? He destroys the most important thing by being so bitterly ironic: Her trust.[4] Anita stares at him and leaves (Figure 7.3).

These scenes are taken from Götz Oelschlägel's film *Sagst du's deinem Kinde?* ('Will you tell your child?'), produced and screened in the German Democratic Republic (GDR) in 1963. The film is the first in a series of four films called *Beziehungen zwischen Jungen und Mädchen* ('Relations between boys and girls'), which deals with issues of sex education. Shortly thereafter, the second film, *Weil ich kein Kind mehr bin* ('Because I'm no longer a child'), was released; in 1964, the third, titled *Partner* was released; and, in 1965, the fourth with the title *Keine Scheu vor heiklen Fragen* ('Don't be shy with delicate questions') was released. In March 1965, Oelschlägel was awarded with the prestigious Art Prize of the GDR (*Kunstpreis*) for these films, and the first two in particular.[5]

These so-called 'popular science films', released by the Deutsche Film AG (DEFA) Production Studios, belong to the health education film genre developed in Europe and the United States beginning in the 1910s.[6] Over the run of their history, sex education was a central topic of these films, but it was not the only one. Usually commissioned by public-health organizations or ministries of health, the aim of these films was to inform and warn the public about health dangers and to train them to practise good health habits.

4 'Was sein Vater tut, ist auch für Peter so gut wie selbstverständlich. Doch was Anita als selbstverständlich erscheint, ist es keineswegs für ihre Eltern.', 'nicht gerne sieht [...] es sich nicht schickt', 'Alberner geht es wohl nicht mehr. In Deinem Alter, das ist doch geradezu lächerlich.', 'Selbstverständlich, lass ihn dir doch einrahmen.', 'Ob der Vater ahnt, was er mit dieser verletzenden Ironie in ihr zerstört? Das wichtigste. Ihr Vertrauen.'

5 Jahn, 'Partner'; 'Kunstpreisträger 1965'.

6 For the historical development of these films, see, for example, Bonah et al., *Health Education Films*; Bonah and Laukötter, 'Moving Pictures and Medicine'.

In the GDR, DEFA Studios and the Hygiene Museum in Dresden were the primary producers and distributors of such films.

Throughout the series *Beziehungen zwischen Jungen und Mädchen*, the director Oelschlägel defends an open approach to questions about sexuality and promotes a new way of discussing them. While the film *Partner* thematized issues of intimacy among adults, the other three films focussed on a younger age group. The first film (along with parts of the fourth) was a sex education film addressed to adolescents aged eleven to twelve, and the second film, *Weil ich kein Kind mehr bin*, targeted teens aged thirteen to sixteen. The films depict everyday scenes in the lives of adolescents, taking up a pedagogical approach to the issues of 'relations between boys and girls'. Thus, these films deal with questions of so-called puberty.

In the run of the 20th century, more and more significance was placed on this phase of development in the life of human beings. The establishment of paediatrics as a discipline turned the physical, mental, and emotional development of young people into an object of medical science and treatment. Interest in this phase of development was also spurred by the newly developing fields of pedagogy and psychology.[7] Although there were diverging developments and opinions on the topic throughout the 20th century, the claim can be made that, through the post-war period, pubescent youth were viewed as a cohort group who were all in a constant state of learning. This, combined with their limited life experience, made it imperative that they receive special guidance and be protected from harmful influence, a thesis confirmed by the scene from *Sagst du's deinem Kinde?* cited in the introduction.

Shown in different formats—from cinema to television—in a variety of settings, the chapter outlines the role these films played in discourses on sex education in the GDR, which, for their part, were highly influenced by psychology and pedagogy. The article will argue that these films not only served the pedagogical function of teaching viewers about sexuality, but also aimed to (re)produce the ideal of the 'new man' for a newly emerging socialist society that was to be founded on a new way of educating emotions. Since the education of youth was regarded as a key issue for the construction of new selves, the medium of film, with its special attractiveness for the younger generation, can be viewed as an instrument for forming new subjectivities.

In a close reading of the narrative strategies used in these films, and especially those of *Sagst du's deinem Kinde?*, this chapter will explain how they tried to help parents and educators navigate the difficulties of their

7 Hall, *Adolescence*. For a close reading of this relationship, see Laukötter, 'How Films Entered'.

child's or pupils' puberty. Based on an aesthetics designed by the director to help create a 'socialist consciousness', the film's pedagogical message puts the significance of feelings centre stage. In that sense, as the following analysis will show, the films target less the physical body as the topic to be discussed and the object to be worked on and changed. Thus, Oelschlägel did not construct the body as a form of capital to be bargained with (as those in the East thought was characteristic of the West). Instead, he focussed on the right management of emotions as the starting point and driving force for bringing new subjectivities into being. Viewed through the lens of Pierre Bourdieu's concept of different capitals, for Oelschlägel, feelings were the currency most adequate to describe the individual's position in a socialist society.

Moreover, this chapter will analyse the particular use of various film techniques to educate the emotions in this fashion. Framed in an educational and scientific setting, the films plead for parents to foster feelings such as trust, empathy, and love for one's child. Thus, the chapter will argue that the films go beyond showing parents the 'right way' to raise their child, by inviting the audience to mimic the film's emotional suggestions. In that sense, the film adopts a performative role, seeking not only to depict action, but also to effectuate it with the ultimate aim of producing socialist subjects.

Sex Education in East (and West) Germany

The history of sex education in the GDR is strongly related to its counterpart in West Germany. This is especially true for the 1950s and 1960s, when East German health educators treated developments in the West as examples of how not to do things. At the same time, in both East and West, ideas about sexuality and sex education underwent a number of diverse, sometimes contradictory changes. Historians have demonstrated that the move from a conservative view of sexuality in the early years of West Germany to a more liberal approach in the period around 1968 was more complex than this linear narrative might lead one to believe. Just as well, multiple case studies have been published that refute Dagmar Herzog's claim that, in the GDR—in contrast to West Germany—sexuality was not treated as an aspect of grappling with the legacy of Nazism.[8] From a broader perspective, one could argue that, despite their fundamental differences, both West Germany

8 Herzog, *Sex after Fascism*; Fenemore, 'Growing Pains'.

and the GDR oscillated between periods of reform and modernization, on the one hand, and periods of conservative regression, on the other.[9]

In the West, the shift towards a more progressive approach to sexuality found expression in various cultural phenomena: the success of Beate Uhse's sex shops; advice literature such as Oswalt Kolle's 1967 book *Dein Mann, das unbekannte Wesen* ('Your Husband, That Mysterious Being') and Günter Amendt's 1970 bestseller *Sexfront* ('Sexfront'); and in popular films like Kolle's 1968 blockbuster *Das Wunder der Liebe: Sexualität in der Ehe* ('The Miracle of Love: Sexuality in Wedlock'). Even the film series *Schulmädchen-Report* ('Schoolgirl Report') screened from 1970 to 1980—a mixture of sex education film and soft porn—enjoyed success.[10] These works tested the limits of speech about and depictions of sex in a new way.[11] They were popular, but also controversial, leading to protests such as the petition movement 'Clean Movie Screen' (*Saubere Leinwand*) as well as demonstrations in front of cinemas. Moreover, as Franz X. Eder has argued, the individual's sexual lust advanced to a duty for the individual self-management. In a capitalist environment, sexual issues developed into a separate area of life, in which not only the sexual appetite had to be fed but in which new consumerist desires were also created: It took up Fordist notions of more work and more (sexual) experience, in which the body was conceived of as a new form of capital.[12]

According to Mark Fenemore, the GDR underwent a shift in attitudes towards sexuality in the mid 1950s. This shift was partially due to the fact that Erich Honecker had withdrawn from youth politics, but was instead driven by Walter Ulbricht's speech at the Fifth Parliament of the Free German Youth (FDJ) on 26 May 1955.[13] In his speech, Ulbricht called upon the daily paper *Junge Welt* ('Young world') to publish articles addressing topics related to sexuality on the grounds that they were relevant for young people.[14] Alongside *Junge Welt*, many other papers followed Ulbricht's advice by publishing articles on sexuality with titles like: 'Vor einer ernsten Frage: Wer spricht mit wem über die Liebe?' ('A serious question: Who speaks with whom about love?')[15] or 'Eine ältere Frau heiraten?' ('Marrying an older woman?').[16]

9 See Laukötter, 'Politik im Kino'.
10 Miersch, *Schulmädchen-Report*.
11 Herzog, 'Das späte Menschenrecht'.
12 Eder, 'Das Sexuelle beschreiben', p. 116.
13 Fenemore, 'Growing Pains', p. 75. Cf. also Fenemore, *Sex, Thugs*, pp. 107–108.
14 Ulbricht, 'Antwort auf aktuelle Fragen'.
15 'Pelzer, 'Vor einer ernsten Frage'.
16 Bauer, 'Eine ältere Frau heiraten?'.

Junge Welt also published articles like 'Ein Buch über Liebe' ('A book about love'), which discussed Rudolf Neubert's book *Die Geschlechterfrage: Ein Buch für junge Menschen* ('The question of sex: A book for young people'); the paper also published articles by Neubert himself.[17] In 1952, Neubert, who held progressive positions on questions of sexuality, became Professor of Social Hygiene at the University of Jena.[18] His publications, such as *Was sage ich meinem Kinde? Einige Ratschläge für Eltern* ('What Should I Tell My Child? Some Advice for Parents') and the vision of a new society that they put forth were the complete opposite of the gynaecologist Wolfgang Bretschneider's conservative ideas.[19] In his books intended for a popular audience, among them *Sexuell aufklären, rechtzeitig und richtig* ('Sex Education Right and On Time'),[20] Bretschneider thematized parents' anxieties about discussing procreation with their children, argued against masturbation, and made a plea for abstinence.[21] The discourse of the 1950s and 1960s was not only concentrated on parents' role in a child's upbringing, especially in their function as bearers of knowledge, but also on the role of educators. Questions about the way sex education was administered in schools, its tasks, and its functions were hotly debated. Politicians and medical doctors, but also psychologists and pedagogues played an increasingly important part in these debates. The latter also undertook scientific surveys of pupils' knowledge on the subject. Education, including sex education, was part of a wider political programme with the aim to increase the birth rate.

The films of Götz Oelschlägel taken up here belong to this period of GDR history, a period whose end coincided with the release of the last film in the series, *Keine Scheu vor heiklen Fragen* (1965). They thus constitute an exemplary case study that offers an interesting perspective on what could be said and shown in this period.[22] The end of this phase is marked by the 1965 Eleventh Plenum of the Central Committee of the Socialist Unity Party of Germany (SED), which introduced a new approach to youth culture and cultural politics in general.[23] Alongside banning many books and plays, as

17 'Ein Buch über Liebe'; Neubert, *Die Geschlechterfrage*.

18 In the Weimar Republic, Neubert was a researcher and, occasionally, travelling salesman for the Hygiene Museum in Dresden, which he led for a short time after the war. He was forced to step down due to his membership in the NSDAP, but, shortly thereafter, was able to take up a position as a professor in Jena. See Fenemore, 'Growing Pains', pp. 74–75.

19 Neubert, *Was sage ich*.

20 Bretschneider, *Sexuell aufklären*.

21 Fenemore, 'Growing Pains', p. 79.

22 Niemeyer and Pfeil, *Der deutsche Film*.

23 Agde, *Kahlschlag*. See also Fenemore, 'Growing Pains', p. 84.

well as music seen as 'too Western', party officials at the congress demanded reforms in sex education.[24]

The Audience of the Films and their Different Media Formats

Oelschlägel's films do not only belong to this liberal period merely by virtue of their years of production. Their content directly grapples with the aforementioned debates. Thus, the films' message—that one should trustfully interact with adolescents and take their problems and questions seriously, including the 'touchy topics'—was addressed not to young people, but to parents and educators. These films were teaching tools for the generation in charge of guiding younger people. Oelschlägel explicitly discussed his intended audience in an interview: 'Parts 1 and 2 are clearly addressed to parents and educators. They warn against taboos, which are rooted in misunderstanding; the films are designed to help grown-ups foster trustworthy understanding for the problems of adolescents.'[25] *Partner* was the exception: its target audience was the 'young generation', which is to say young adults.

The films themselves make it clear that 'parents' and 'educators' are their addressees. The voice-over repeatedly emphasizes 'parents'' role in raising their children. Beyond that, 'parents' always figure prominently in the individual case studies. They have discussions with their children and debates with 'educators' at parent-teacher association meetings. In the film *Sagst du's deinem Kinde?*, grandparents are included among the 'parents'. The episode revolving around the young girl Sigrid thematizes the role grandparents can play in educating their grandchildren about sexuality and hygiene, while also indirectly addressing the conflict between generations: Because her grandmother was unwilling to discuss the 'touchy topics', Sigrid is surprised when she has her first period (Figure 7.4).

The group 'educators' is also treated from different perspectives. In most of the scenes involving 'educators', teachers feature as the main characters, either in their interactions with pupils or in their interactions with parents at parent-teacher association meetings. In some of the scenes, however, the 'educator' group is expanded to include counsellors, psychologists, and

24 See Regina Mönch's somewhat polemical article: Mönch, 'Kontrollverlust', p. 83. See also: Schwarz, 'Vom Jahrmarktspektakel', pp. 45–46.

25 'Teil 1 und 2 wenden sich in ihrer Aussage eindeutig an Eltern und Erzieher. Sie wollen vor falsch verstandenen Tabus warnen und bei den Erwachsenen vertrauensvolles Verständnis den Heranwachsenden und ihren Problemen gegenüber wecken und fördern.'; 'Ist Liebe ein romantischer Begriff'. All translations by the author unless otherwise stated.

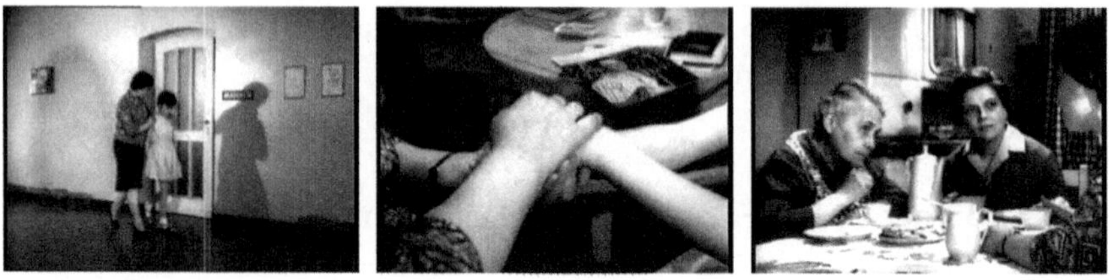

7.4. Three stills from *Sagst du's deinem Kinde?* ('Will you tell your child?'), 1963. © DEFA-Stiftung/ Günther Biedermann

others. For instance, the fourth film, *Keine Scheu vor heiklen Fragen*, depicts a psychologist teaching sex education.[26] And, in *Sagst du's deinem Kinde?*, the leader of the communist youth organization Freie Deutsche Jugend (FDJ) helps guide the young Sigrid through her sexual maturation. She not only educates Sigrid about 'natural things', but also advises Sigrid's mother and grandmother on how to cope with the difficulties they experience raising the young girl.

In contrast to the 'parents', the 'educators'' actions always go in the right direction: They speak openly with their pupils about all their questions and do not shy away from discussing 'natural things', namely, questions about procreation. One voice-over says:

> That the troop leader approaches [Sigrid] at precisely this moment is a matter of chance. But it is no matter of chance that the young girl trusts her. She earned this trust by being open in discussion and by consistently fulfilling her pedagogical duties. No good upbringing can do without such trust.[27]

While some parents still need to learn how to behave correctly, the educators as representational actors of the state not only know the best path of education, but are portrayed as examples worthy of imitation by the audience, inviting the parents watching the film to mimic the portrayed performance.

The audience Oelschlägel wanted to reach also determined the way the films were screened. In contrast to many health education films of the time, the films in Oelschlägel's series were not merely intended to be shown in cinemas as a part of the side show.[28] In the interview cited above,

26 Cf. also Jahn, 'Keine Scheu'.

27 'Dass die Pionierleiterin gerade in diesem Augenblick [zu Sigrid, AL] kommt, ist Zufall. Kein Zufall aber ist, dass sie das Vertrauen des jungen Mädels hat. Es ist durch Offenheit und pädagogische Konsequenz erworben. Es gibt keine gute Erziehung ohne dieses Vertrauen.'

28 Bonah and Laukötter, 'Moving Pictures and Medicine'.

Oelschlägel said: 'Like its predecessors, the film [*Partner*] will not be part of the official side show schedule. And I think that is right because these films are designed to promote an exchange of ideas. The most important part of their intended effect is a lively debate on the issues they address.'[29] Accordingly, the films (often the whole series) were shown at events for parents (parent-teacher association meetings) and pedagogues (teachers' committees, pedagogical institutes where teachers were trained, principals' conferences).[30] The films were supposed to be especially interesting for 'the parent-teacher associations [*Elternbeiräte*], in particular the committees for pedagogical propaganda'.[31] The press reported on screenings at special events like the 'Pedagogical Week' (*Pädagogische Woche*), an event for teachers' occupational training first held in February 1965 at the Teachers' House in Berlin. There, the first three films were screened for teachers and parent-teacher associations.[32] Films from Oelschlägel's series were also shown at events like the 'Seminar for Marriage Counselling', where doctors held talks on family laws, and 'Marriage Counselling from a Medical Perspective'.[33] A conference on 'Problems of Sex Education' featured a viewing of the first two films.[34]

The films were also shown at multiple film festivals, including at the Documentary and Short Film Festival of the GDR and at a special event at the Edinburgh Film Festival.[35] *Keine Scheu vor heiklen Fragen* was even shown at Cannes and at the Eighth Leipzig International Festival for Documentary and Short Films, where films from Canada, Iceland, Cyprus, and other 'capitalist countries' were also screened.[36] The participation in these film competitions, where Western countries competed, underlines the political value and importance of films for the GDR: They were regarded as strong currencies in the international contest on the superior form of society. The

29 'Der Film wird, wie auch seine beiden Vorgänger, nicht ins offizielle Beiprogramm gehen. Und ich finde das gut so. Denn unsere Filme sind so angelegt, daß sie zum Gedankenaustausch auffordern.'; 'Ist Liebe ein romantischer Begriff'.

30 Peschke, 'Drei Filme'; Jahn, 'Sagst Du's'. On the role of the various committees, see: Droit, *Vorwärts*, pp. 75–86.

31 'Elternbeiräte, speziell die Kommissionen für pädagogische Propaganda'; Peschke, 'Drei Filme'.

32 I.G. 'Erste "Pädagogische Woche"'; Erdmann, 'Lektion und Filmabend'.

33 'Seminar für Eheberatung', 'Eheberatung in medizinischer [...] Sicht'; Ena, 'Seminar für Eheberatung'.

34 'Probleme der sexuellen Aufklärung und Erziehung'; EB, 'Beratung für Eltern'.

35 'Filme für Millionen'; 'Festivale'; Z., 'Beiträge in Edinburgh'.

36 See the advertisement in *Berliner Zeitung*, 21, 334 (5 December 1965), p. 4; 'Erste Gäste eingetroffen'; 'Filme aus aller Welt'; Antosch, 'Farbenreiche Filmpalette'.

jury gave the film 'special praise'.[37] In an interview, Oelschlägel states that the first two films were sold 'in Holland, Sweden, Denmark, and of course in the other socialist countries'. He also stated: 'The West German distributor Walter Leckebusch, who acquired the rights to distribute them [the first two films], also signed a pre-contract for the distribution rights to *Partner* at the last Documentary and Short Films Festival in Leipzig without seeing it.'[38]

In 1968, a year in which the decisions of the Eleventh Plenum of the Central Committee of the SED had already begun to have their effects and the 'sexual revolution' in West Germany was being taken to the streets, *Keine Scheu vor heiklen Fragen* and at least two of the other films were screened on GDR television in response to the dominant forms of 'filthy education'.[39] Handwritten remarks on the official film board's protocols, which had to be completed before a film could receive permission to be screened, indicate that further screenings of the films were planned through the end of the 1970s and the beginning of the 1980s.[40]

Besides the fact that these films were put to multiple uses over a longer period of time, the different media in which they were shown is remarkable: These films were not only produced for the cinema screens in different settings (from festivals to schools), but also for television. The change in media, however, took place without any changes to the films themselves. The practice of presenting films in different formats was not limited to Oelschlägel's series, but was applied to other productions, too.[41] The obvious explanation is that this was a cost-saving measure. However, Oelschlägel's series was produced on expensive 35mm film material (while, in West Germany, comparable productions were produced on much cheaper 16mm film material): The use of superior film stock

37 Knietzsch, 'Festival mit Niveau'; advertisement in *Berliner Zeitung*, 21, 334 (5 December 1965), p. 4.

38 'nach Holland, Schweden, Dänemark und natürlich in die sozialistischen Länder', 'Der Westdeutsche Verleiher Walter Leckebusch, der sie ebenfalls ankaufte, hat z. B. auf dem letzten Dokumentar- und Kurzfilmfestival in Leipzig unbesehen einen Vorvertrag für die "Partner" abgeschlossen.'; 'Ist Liebe ein romantischer Begriff'.

39 'Keine Scheu vor heiklen Fragen'.

40 See BA Filmarchiv: DR 1-Z/4081a, Protocol No. 0308/63, 29 July 1963 (on *Sagst du's deinem Kinde?*); DR 1-Z/4647a, Protocol No. 0498/63, 4 December 1963 (on: *Weil ich kein Kind mehr bin*); 2248/2248c, Protocol No. 0519/64, 7 December 1964 (on *Beziehungen zwischen Jungen und Mädchen, III. Teil*); 2247c/2247, Protocol No. 0219/65, 27 August 1965 (on: *Keine Scheu vor heiklen Fragen*).

41 See, for example, the series *Wegweiser Gesundheit*, which was produced between 1974 and 1984; Schwarz, 'Vom Jahrmarktspektakel', pp. 31, 46. See also Hauptstaatsarchiv Dresden, 13658 Deutsches Hygiene-Museum Dresden, F V Bd. 2, pp. 21–46.

implies that the quality of these productions might have been seen as more important than their cost. In the end, though, screening the films in multiple formats might be better explained if one considers that cinema and television were not regarded as fundamentally different or even different at all. At the same time television evolved into a mass medium, it also developed in the GDR of the 1960s along 'ideological guidelines': TV formats, themes, and statements were under state control.[42] In terms of the topic of Oelschlägel's series, one might argue then that the specific message of the series—the education of the emotions—was not viewed as pertinent for parents and teachers only, but as something that had relevance for everyone in the GDR.

Film Techniques Used in the Series

The Discussion

When the films were screened to parents, the film's producers recommended that a 'discussion' be held afterwards, 'preferably accompanied by doctors',[43] a recommendation based on the assumption that parents would 'have a lot of questions'.[44] Sometimes, psychologists led the discussions. In the first half of the 20th century, screenings of health education films were commonly preceded by 'scientific' presentations held by doctors.[45] This technique of rhetorically reframing the film was supposed to lead the audience to receive the film in the intended way.[46] Most sources contain little information about the discussions held after screenings. We know that such discussions took place, but the insufficient source material makes it difficult to know exactly what was discussed and how the discussions (as a way of processing the viewed material) were organized. Thus, sources like Inge Gerlich's articles in the *Berliner Zeitung*, in which she reports on the discussions that followed screenings of films from Oelschlägel's series, are a boon for the historian. In one of her reports, Gerlich anonymizes the discussion participants, calling them 'a father' or 'a biology teacher' when 'quoting' their opinions.[47] In a report on a screening of *Partner*, however,

42 Steinmetz, 'Television History', p. 142; Gumbert, *Envisioning Socialism*, p. 59.
43 'am besten im Beisein von Ärzten'; Peschke, 'Drei Filme'.
44 'Fragen auf dem Herzen haben'; Jahn, 'Sagst Du's'.
45 Gerlich, 'Die Mär vom Klapperstorch'.
46 Laukötter, 'Listen and Watch'.
47 Gerlich, 'Die Mär vom Klapperstorch'.

she names the experts who participated when citing their contributions to the discussion: Elfried Göldner, High Court Judge; Dr. Lotte Winter, School Psychologist, Pankow; Dr. Linda Ansorg, Associate Professor for Civil and Family Law at the Humboldt University; Dr. Bernd Bittighöfer (named without his professional background).[48]

The discussion was a central aspect of the films themselves as well. Talks between doctor and patient are a technique of health education films well-known in the historiography. In the films of the first half of the 20th century in particular, the doctor plays the role of an adviser to the patient, dominating the 'discussion' as the real-life incarnation of knowledge itself. In contrast, Oelschlägel places both on equal footing, transforming the discussion into a dialectical dialogue of statement and objection. The frequent use of such dialogues distinguishes Oelschlägel's take on the discussion from earlier health education films. The different forms of dialogue used by Oelschlägel are also exceptional: Along with the one-on-one discussion, he also depicts 'debates' between educators and parents as well as roundtable discussions like the one in the parent-teacher association meeting in the film *Sagst du's deinem Kinde?*. Throughout the four films, discussions between child and parent/educator are depicted as the incarnation of trust and as a necessary precondition for finding a solution. Thus, Oelschlägel promoted a cooperative parent-child relationship based on trust and empathy, and the film emphasized solutions reached by consensus rather than by command.

The films themselves directly address the sociopolitical implications of these democratic interactions. Similarly, the documented discussions after the screenings reflect on them, too: A father states that there were no simple answers for the difficulties parents experienced when trying to talk to their kids about sex. Instead, he thinks it must be left to parents to find the right words: 'The truth alone decides. But unfortunately, parents don't always know the truth. [...] It is good that we are having an open discussion about these problems [...]. For a long time now, we have neglected to hold such public debates.'[49] Deployed in this way, the discussion is elevated to a symbol of openness and figures as the central cultural technique of a modern socialist society.

48 Gerlich, 'Den richtigen Partner'.

49 'Die Wahrheit ist es, die allein entscheidet. Leider kennen sie die Eltern manchmal selbst nicht. [...] Daß wir offen über die Probleme sprechen, [...] das ist gut. [...] Solche Auseinandersetzungen in der Öffentlichkeit haben wir für lange Zeit versäumt.'; Gerlich, 'Die Mär vom Klapperstorch'.

Narrative Contrast and Estrangement Effects

The actions of the 'parents' structure the films' narratives. Just as well, however, the reactions of their children and the voice-over clearly classify parents' approaches as either 'right' or 'wrong': Either they are open to discussing the 'touchy topics' of sexuality with their children, or they aren't. As in many other health education films from the first half of the 20th century, Oelschlägel's films place the two attitudes in juxtaposition. For example, in the case of Anita's and Peter's parents referred to above, the voice-over makes a clear judgement about which approach to the adolescent's problems is the right one, namely, that of Peter's parents.[50] While Peter's parents represent the good role model that, as the film shows, will be copied by the next generation (symbolized here by Peter), the future of Anita's development with her mistrusting parents is not further explored but left to the viewer's imagination. Contrasted with the positive example given by Peter and his parents, the negative path that her development will take is depicted as self-evident and without alternative.

In *Weil ich kein Kind mehr bin*, the alternatives posed by this narrative strategy are compressed into the decision that one parent has to make. A mother finds a love letter addressed to her daughter. One choice is to read it and tear it up, which would not only damage her child's trust in her, but would also force her child to lie, as everybody knows that 'the forbidden fruit is the sweetest'. The alternative is set off by a freeze-frame: The mother brings the letter to her daughter's teacher and has a discussion with him about it. The teacher's assurances that the relationship between Lilo and Bernd is 'exemplary' and 'clean' have a calming effect on the mother. He advises her to exert 'control through trust'.[51]

This is the only instance of such an open-ended narrative in the series. But, taken together with the extradiegetic voice-over, whose presence is consistent throughout the entire series, it is clear that the films' mimetic illusion is constantly being broken. The voice-over not only comments, corrects, or supports the screened actions, but also brings the audience into the narrative, using 'we' when making comments and offering viewers advice on how to translate the knowledge imparted by the film into their own lives. The estrangement effects deployed by Oelschlägel in his film series can be traced to Bertolt Brecht's Epic Theatre. The aim of the technique is

50 Bonah and Laukötter, 'Moving Pictures and Medicine'.

51 'Die verbotenen Früchte sind bekanntlich die süßesten', 'vorbildhaft', 'sauber', 'Kontrolle durch Vertrauen'.

to break through the mimetic illusion of the stage, thus provoking audience members to take a critical position on the actions depicted.[52] Applied to this pedagogical context, one might argue that, even though Oelschlägel invites his audience to copy the performed actions of the presented educators, he still ascribed the audience an agency to thoughtfully engage with the material presented. As he outlined in his discussions on his aesthetic approach (which will be discussed later), he thought that the viewer should feel involved as 'a fellow researcher' of the knowledge transmitted by the film.[53] Moreover, by using this technique, Oelschlägel set his work in dialogue with experimental films in the 1960s, which also made use of this technique in their films, to underline his artistic self-understanding and approach.

The Voice of Social Sciences

The status given to the voice-over intensifies its estranging effect. The voice comments on the characters' actions and choices from a distance and often provides additional scientific information, like the following voice-over from a scene in *Sagst du's deinem Kinde?*: 'Studies conducted at various schools have shown that only 4 per cent of pupils aged twelve to thirteen have spoken with their parents about relations between man and woman and the difficulties that go along with them. Out of 1,000 pupils 40, out of 100 only 4, in this class only one.'[54]

The voice-over also explains the actions of the psychologist holding class in *Keine Scheu vor heiklen Fragen*. The psychologist's lesson deploys images from medical science, and he even tells pupils about a sex education film being screened at the local cinema. The voice-over then undergirds the psychologist's position not only by emphasizing the latter's scientific expertise, but also by positioning itself as a sort of objective observer. In other words, the extradiegetic voice is depicted as the voice of science itself. The scientific framework not only plays a significant role in the films themselves, but was also instrumental in their production and distribution. Gerhard Witzlack from the Psychology Division of the German Institute for Pedagogy served as a technical adviser on the set of all the films in the series. Additionally, the pedagogue Sigrid Hauptvogel served as a technical

52 Walsh, *Brechtian Aspect*. Cf. also Wulff, 'Verfremdungseffekt'.

53 'Mitforscher'; Oelschlägel, 'Warum', p. 248.

54 'Untersuchungen an verschiedenen Schulen ergaben: nur 4 Prozent der Schüler des 12. und 13. Lebensjahres sind von ihren Eltern über die Beziehungen zwischen Mann und Frau den damit zusammenhängenden Problemen aufgeklärt worden. Von 1.000 Schülern 40, von 100 4, in dieser Klasse einer.'

adviser for the first three films, Heinz Grassel replacing her for the fourth. Grassel had published in the field and argued that sex education should be taught in public schools.[55] Employing academic advisers to ensure the correctness of the scientific knowledge propagated was common for such films. But, in the first half of the 20th century, this role was usually filled by medical doctors. The expansive use of psychologists and pedagogues was a new phenomenon, which can be explained by the fact that, in the post-war years, psychology and pedagogy were increasingly concerned with the practical application of their research.

Witzlack also wrote the 'Pamphlets for Educational Films' ('*Beiheft zum Lehrerbildungsfilm*') that were to be read by the professionals screening Oelschlägel's films and running the post-screening discussions. In these pamphlets, Witzlack explained the films' contents and intentions and discussed the various ways the screenings could be organized. Witzlack explicitly comments on the ways these pamphlets were supposed to be used: 'For training teachers in the fields of psychology and pedagogy and for pedagogical propaganda.'[56]

As the films themselves make the scientific nature of their treatment of the topic explicit, it seems that the scientific knowledge referred to would be made explicit as well. However, the opposite is the case. Although the films make a plea for parents and educators to be open to discussing 'touchy topics', they neither pose concrete questions about the act of sex, contraception, etc., nor do they offer any concrete answers. In the films and in the reportage on their screenings, terms like sexuality, sex, procreation, and sexual organs are not mentioned at all. The only exception is in *Keine Scheu vor heiklen Fragen*, in which a psychologist refers to a woman's vagina when discussing the female body. In another scene, during the positive father-son talk, words like 'bodily unification' and 'phallus' are used. Otherwise, the films speak of 'the problem' when addressing sex or sexual contact.[57] The reportage on the films is similar. One report discusses a 'biology teacher' who seeks to improve adolescents' knowledge about the 'problems of how people are made'.[58] In one of the discussions cited, Linda Ansorg, the law expert from Humboldt University, speaks of 'society's responsibility'. And Bernd Bittighöfer from the SED Central Committee's Institute for Social

55 Grassel and Heilbock, *Erziehung zur künftigen Liebe*.

56 'Für die Lehrerausbildung und Lehrerweiterbildung in den Fächern Psychologie und Pädagogik sowie für die pädagogische Propaganda'; Witzlack, *Beiheft zum Lehrerbildungsfilm*.

57 'körperliche Vereinigung', 'männliches Glied', 'Problem'.

58 'Probleme der Menschwerdung'; Gerlich, 'Die Mär vom Klapperstorch'.

Sciences speaks of the 'failure of social forces' when discussing the parents' false approaches depicted in the films. Details on questions of sexuality and procreation are wholly absent.[59] The same is true for the visualization of any forms of sexuality and questions of reproduction. While in the first half of the 20th century health education films were called 'hybrids' because they combined fictional stories with scientifically informed visual 'facts', Oelschlägel left out any form of precise visualization of these issues: We only see short kisses. In other words, the proclaimed openness to talk and visualize sexuality and reproduction had its limits and price. Thus, the films stress more the educative than the sexual-information aspects. The teaching on sexuality blurs into a teaching on teaching.

The Depiction of Emotions in the Series

The way knowledge about sexuality is presented in the films has an asymmetrical relation to the way emotions are thematized. While the presentation of sexual knowledge is filled with gaps, emotions are discussed intensively. The films argue for trust, understanding, empathy, for taking the feelings of adolescents seriously, and for 'true' love. Interestingly, the camera often takes up the perspective of the adolescents in a style reminiscent of *cinéma vérité*.[60] This technique was also used, for example, in French (amateur and television) films on sex education;[61] however, there is no way to verify whether there were close connections and exchanges between Oelschlägel and these French directors.[62] Yet, he might have been exposed to these documentary trends on the basis of his (and his film's) participation in film festivals with international involvement.

Additionally, the films feature recordings of real-life adolescents' conversations to fill out the feelings and thoughts of the fictional adolescent characters. Gender-specific differences are also marked: The boys are depicted as sexually active, whereas the girls are depicted as more reserved. Ria's attempts to overcome her coyness in *Weil ich kein Kind mehr bin* are the only exception, but her behaviour is portrayed as stemming from her vanity and thus as something to be avoided. In that sense, the films mirror

59 'Verantwortung der Gesellschaft', 'Die gesellschaftlichen Kräfte haben in diesem Fall versagt.'; Gerlich, 'Den richtigen Partner'.

60 Winkler, 'Biology, Morality and Gender'.

61 See the contribution by Christian Bonah in this volume.

62 *Cinéma vérité* techniques also gained attention in US televised medical dramas in the late 1960s to prove film's authenticity. See: Ostherr, *Medical Visions*, pp. 152–189.

not only contemporary gender roles, but they also express how they are emotionally evaluated.

Actions like writing 'Anita loves Peter' on the blackboard in *Sagst du's deinem Kinde?* are not condemned, but are treated as 'play' or as adolescents 'putting their feet in the water'. The films depict the adolescents as being in a sort of in-between situation, no longer children, but not yet adults. For this reason, they have to receive guidance from educators, the school, parents, pedagogues, and psychologists when trying to deal with their own emotions. The films suggest that managing emotions is the only way to ensure that adolescents make it through puberty without getting into family and school conflicts. Puberty is thus constructed as a process of transformation that needs guidance from socialist methods of education, including openness, trust, and 'independence and responsibility for oneself'.[63] The closing sequence of *Sagst du's deinem Kinde?* makes the social dimension of this education of adolescents explicit. The voice-over states: 'We know we have done a good job raising our children when their desire to be useful for others has become an essential part of their character.'[64] In other words, adolescents not only go through a biological process, transitioning from life as a child to life as an adult, but also undergo a political transformation, becoming members of a new socialist society.

Negatively assessed emotions are also depicted in the films, and are always attributed to the parents. For example, in *Weil ich kein Kind mehr bin*, the voice-over says Ria's mother 'raised her to be vain'. The voice-over also accuses another child's parents of having 'blind trust' in their child as a consequence of their self-centredness.[65] *Sagst du's deinem Kinde?* and *Keine Scheu vor heiklen Fragen* both treat a lack of trust and understanding, coupled with strictness and punishment, as counterproductive in the process of education. Moreover, the inclusion of interviews with adolescents living in youth homes in *Keine Scheu vor heiklen Fragen* underscores the consequences of parents' failure to provide their children with a good upbringing. The adolescents from youth homes talk about their traumatic childhood experiences, explaining how they were beaten, attacked with a kitchen knife, or abandoned by their parents. And they inform viewers about the after-effects of their experiences, like one adolescent who explicitly states that, because of her experiences, she doesn't think she would ever have children of her own.

63 'Selbständigkeit und Eigenverantwortung'; Witzlack, *Beiheft zum Lehrerbildungsfilm*, p. 19.

64 'Wir haben unsere Kinder dann gut erzogen, wenn ihnen das Gefühl, für andere nützlich sein zu wollen, zum Charakterbedürfnis geworden ist.'

65 'herangezüchtete falsche Eitelkeit', 'blinde Vertrauensseligkeit'.

While earlier sex education films emphasized the transmission of knowledge and treated the discussion of emotions as just another mode of communicating it, Oelschlägel's films differ because they place primacy on education about emotions themselves. As we have seen, the 'emotional education' articulated in Oelschlägel's films not only forwards the notion that adolescents must be guided by educators when dealing with their emotions. Just as well, the emotions of adults (that is, the intended audience of the films) also have to be educated.

Emotions within Oelschlägel's Aesthetics

In his films, Götz Oelschlägel emphasized the important sociopolitical role of emotions in the process of education, and in sex education in particular. Beyond that, he also thought emotions were an important political factor, an idea that informed how he directed his films and addressed his audience. His theoretical writings on film in the GDR, including 'popular science films', demonstrate this.

In an article published in 1961, Oelschlägel posed the question: 'Why are our films so boring?' ('*Warum sind unsere Filme langweilig?*')[66] The question was occasioned by the fact that the films most praised in the GDR enjoyed no resonance at international film festivals. Oelschlägel was not convinced by the argument that the films' contents were 'scientifically founded and socially useful' and that it was simply the form of the films that were 'uninteresting, uninspired, deficient', because, for him, following the 'theses of Marxist-Leninist aesthetics', form and content could not be separated, but were necessarily fused in a 'dialectical unity'. A film's underlying idea, concept, and mode of presentation were thus not issues of form, but issues of content. For him, content was 'a form of selection, ideologically-artistically conceived material, not simply material that speaks for itself'.[67] This 'aesthetic, concept-based character of content' had to be carried by an 'artistic idea': 'Without an artistic idea, a film cannot become a work of art. Without an artistic idea, a popular-science film will not be convincing.'[68] Oelschlägel

66 Oelschlägel, 'Warum'; Winkler, 'Biology, Morality and Gender'.

67 'wissenschaftlich einwandfrei und gesellschaftlich nutzbringend', 'mangelhaft, einfallslos, uninteressant', 'These der marxistisch-leninistischen Ästhetik', 'dialektische Einheit', 'gestaltete Auswahl, ist ideologisch-künstlerisch konzipierter Stoff, nicht Stoff mit Aussage schlechthin'; Oelschlägel, 'Warum', p. 247.

68 'ästhetisch-konzeptionelle Charakter des Inhalts', 'künstlerische Idee', 'Ohne künstlerische Idee wird ein Spielfilm kein Kunstwerk. Ohne künstlerische Idee wird ein populärwissenschaftlicher Film keine Überzeugungskraft haben.'; Oelschlägel, 'Warum', p. 247.

did not consider popular-science films works of art, since they were not concerned with the 'knowledge of man', but rather with 'transmitting objective laws'. Nevertheless, he thought that films of this genre also needed to have an artistic idea in order to be effective, and that previous films of the genre had worked according to a different principle.[69] In them, the topic addressed was the content, the didactic element informed the dramaturgy, and the 'message was the principle of their form'. For this reason, the films were overburdened with didactic considerations, and, as a result, they were ineffective. Accordingly, Oelschlägel continues: 'In popular science films, the artistic idea is the key to viewing the dramaturgic staging of the material as the content itself. It is the *conditio sine qua non* for the effectivity of the intended message. The essence of the artistic idea is always emotional.'[70]

In other words, for Oelschlägel, transmitting the ideals of socialist education through film was contingent upon the films' form being guided by an emotionally based artistic idea. He was thus not interested in amusing his audience or making them laugh, but in evoking feelings of 'creative pleasure, even happiness and pride' in the viewer watching objective scenes of scientific research.[71] As mentioned above, Oelschlägel's specific understanding of socialist ideals implied that the viewer should feel involved as 'a fellow researcher' of the knowledge being transmitted by the film. Thus, he asked of each and every film: 'Which artistic idea leads our creative, interested, knowledge-hungry viewer to understand the truth of the topic addressed? Which means are suited to create suspense, wake interest, and evoke joy in the production of novel, relevant, and legitimate connections?'[72]

Additionally, Oelschlägel stated that the 'author's ethical and scientific drive to communicate' manifests itself through the artistic idea as 'action', claiming that it takes an artistic idea to activate 'ideological wisdom'. He

69 'Erkenntnis des Menschen', 'Kenntnisvermittlung objektiver Gesetzmäßigkeiten'; Oelschlägel, 'Warum', p. 248.

70 'daß die Aussage zum Prinzip der Gestaltung erklärt wird', 'Die künstlerische Idee beim populärwissenschaftlichen Film ist der Schlüssel zur dramatischen Konzipierung des Stoffes als Inhalt, ist die unabdingbare Voraussetzung für die Wirksamkeit der beabsichtigten Aussage. Das Wesen der künstlerischen Idee ist immer emotional.'; Oelschlägel, 'Warum', p. 248.

71 On pleasure in socialist states, see Crowley and Reid, 'Introduction'.

72 'schöpferisches Vergnügen, ja Glück und Stolz', 'Mitforscher', 'Welche künstlerische Idee führt den Zuschauer, den interessierten, von plötzlichem Wissensdurst gepackten, von schöpferischem Vergnügen erfaßten Zuschauer zur Erkenntnis der Wahrheit unseres Themas? Welche Mittel sind geeignet, Spannung zu erzeugen, Interesse zu wecken, Spaß empfinden zu lassen beim Auffinden neuartiger, großer gesetzmäßiger Zusammenhänge?'; Oelschlägel, 'Warum', p. 248.

concluded that the sooner directors recognize this drive to communicate as a 'social responsibility', the sooner their films would have an active effect on the 'development of socialist consciousness'.[73]

Conclusion

The artistic ideas Götz Oelschlägel had in mind when producing his series *Beziehungen zwischen Jungen und Mädchen* cannot be easily reconstructed. However, this article has sought to elucidate the wide spectrum of techniques he deployed—such as discussion, narrative contrasts, estrangement effects, voice-overs as the voice of science, and the depiction of emotions—and their various functions within his films. These techniques served to 'create suspense', 'wake interest', and 'evoke joy' in adults responsible for guiding their adolescents through puberty.

The analysis also demonstrated that Oelschlägel considered puberty and the questions of sexuality and procreation bound up with it to be a special cinematic object. Although the films take their impetus from a biological process, the cinematic depiction of the difficulties of adolescence were taken as an occasion for making political statements about the education of the 'socialist subject'. At the same time, the topic made it possible for Oelschlägel to address his visions about socialist education to two different audiences: adolescents as well as their parents and educators. From this perspective, Oelschlägel's films can also be read as a form of instruction for the development of 'socialist consciousness'. It is certainly remarkable that Oelschlägel's definition of social responsibility was less guided by the concern to simply transmit knowledge and more guided by a concern to help shape viewers' emotions. This shows the extent to which emotions were seen as a key to health education at that time. Thus, the suggestive potential of films to change people's emotions by depicting emotions to be imitated has a political and performative dimension that needs to be taken into account, and not only by those working in film history.

As stated at the beginning, the series' last film, *Keine Scheu vor heiklen Fragen*, marked the end of a liberal era in the history of the GDR. In the decades that followed, Oelschlägel's call for a more open approach to politics, experimentation in film, and a filmic engagement to foster feelings such

73 'das ethische und wissenschaftliche Mitteilungsbedürfnis der Autoren', 'ideologische Weisheit', 'gesellschaftliche Verantwortlichkeit', 'Entwicklungsprozeß sozialistischen Bewußtseins'; Oelschlägel, 'Warum', p. 249.

as trust, empathy, and love for one's child was not answered. In contrast, older didactic ideas underwent a renaissance. Götz Oelschlägel, who died on 29 May 1969, likely would have resented this, as: 'One feels so much in these times!'[74]

Works Cited

Films, Television Programmes, and Recordings

Keine Scheu vor heiklen Fragen, directed by Götz Oelschlägel, DEFA, 1965.
Partner, directed by Götz Oelschlägel, DEFA, 1965.
Sagst du's deinem Kinde?, directed by Götz Oelschlägel, DEFA, 1963.
Weil ich kein Kind mehr bin, directed by Götz Oelschlägel, DEFA, 1964.

Books and Articles

Agde, Günter, ed., *Kahlschlag: Das 11. Plenum des ZK der SED 1965: Studien und Dokumente* (Berlin: Aufbau-Taschenbuch-Verlag, 1991).
Antosch, Georg, 'Farbenreiche Filmpalette: Erste Eindrücke vom VIII. Dokumentar- und Kurzfilmfestival in Leipzig', *Neue Zeit*, 20, 270 (18 November 1965), p. 3.
Bauer, Heinz, 'Eine ältere Frau heiraten?', *Junge Welt*, 10, 158 (7/8 July 1956), p. 5.
Bonah, Christian, David Cantor, and Anja Laukötter, eds., *Health Education Films in the Twentieth Century* (Rochester: University of Rochester Press, 2018).
Bonah, Christian, and Anja Laukötter, 'Moving Pictures and Medicine in the First Half of the 20th Century: Some Notes on International Historical Developments and the Potential of Medical Film Research', *Gesnerus: Swiss Journal of the History of Medicine and Sciences* 66, 1 (2009), pp. 121–145.
Bretschneider, Wolfgang, *Sexuell aufklären, rechtzeitig und richtig: Ein Ratgeber für sexuelle Erziehung* (Leipzig: Urania-Verlag, 1956).
Crowley, David, and Susan E. Reid, 'Introduction: Pleasures in Socialism?', in *Pleasures in Socialism: Leisure and Luxury in the Eastern Bloc*, ed. by David Crowley and Susan E. Reid (Evanston, IL: Northwestern University Press, 2010), pp. 3–51.
Droit, Emmanuelle, *Vorwärts zum neuen Menschen? Die sozialistische Erziehung (1949–1989)*, trans. by Michael Esch (Cologne: Böhlau, 2014)
EB, 'Beratung für Eltern', *Berliner Zeitung*, 22, 12 (12 January 1966), p. 12.

74 'Man fühlt so viel in dieser Zeit!' This statement is a quote from Oelschlägel's series *Relations between Boys and Girls*.

Eder, Franz X., 'Das Sexuelle beschreiben, zeigen und aufführen: Mediale Strategien im deutschsprachigen Sexualdiskurs von 1945 bis Anfang der siebziger Jahre', in *Fragen Sie Dr. Sex! Ratgeberkommunikation und die mediale Konstruktion des Sexuellen*, ed. by Peter-Paul Bänziger, Stefanie Duttweiler, Philipp Sarasin, and Annika Wellmann (Berlin: Suhrkamp, 2010), pp. 94–122.

'Ein Buch über Liebe: Prof. Dr. Neubert antwortet auf Fragen junger Menschen', *Junge Welt*, 10, 158 (7/8 July 1956), p. 5.

Ena, 'Seminar für Eheberatung', *Neue Zeit*, 20, 88 (16 April 1966), p. 5.

Erdmann, Horst, 'Lektion und Filmabend', *Neues Deutschland*, 20, 42 (11 February 1965), p. 5.

'Erste Gäste eingetroffen', *Neues Deutschland*, 20, 311 (11 November 1965), p. 4.

Fenemore, Mark, 'The Growing Pains of Sex Education in the German Democratic Republic (GDR), 1945–69', in *Shaping Sexual Knowledge: A Cultural History of Sex Education in Twentieth Century Europe*, ed. by Lutz D. H. Sauerteig and Roger Davidson (London: Routledge, 2009), pp. 71–90.

Fenemore, Mark, *Sex, Thugs and Rock 'n' Roll: Teenage Rebels in Cold-War East Germany* (New York: Berghahn, 2007).

'Festivale', *Neues Deutschland*, 21, 236 (28 August 1966), p. 8.

'Filme aus aller Welt: Zur VIII. Internationalen Dokumentar- und Kurzfilmwoche', *Berliner Zeitung*, 21, 314 (14 November 1965), p. 6.

'Filme für Millionen: Woche des Kurz- und Dokumentarfilms vom 2. bis 15. Oktober', *Neues Deutschland*, 19, 272 (2 October 1964), p. 4.

Gerlich, Inge, 'Den richtigen Partner gewählt?', *Berliner Zeitung*, 21, 188 (11 July 1965), p. Beilage 8 [16].

Gerlich, Inge, 'Die Mär vom Klapperstorch oder …', *Berliner Zeitung*, 20, 128 (10 May 1964), p. Beilage 3 [11].

Grassel, Heinz, and Klaus Heilbock, *Erziehung zur künftigen Liebe* (Berlin: Volk und Wissen, 1958).

Gumbert, Heather L., *Envisioning Socialism: Television and the Cold War in the German Democratic Republic* (Ann Arbor: University of Michigan Press, 2014).

Hall, G. Stanley, *Adolescence: Its Psychology and its Relations to Physiology, Anthropology, Sociology, Sex, Crime, Religion and Education*, vols. 1 and 2 (New York: Appleton, 1919).

Herzog, Dagmar, '"Das späte Menschenrecht": Auf der Suche nach einer nachfaschistischen Sexualmoral', in *Demokratie im Schatten der Gewalt: Geschichten des Privaten im deutschen Nachkrieg*, ed. by Daniel Fulda, Dagmar Herzog, Stefan L. Hoffmann, and Till van Rahden (Göttingen: Wallstein, 2010), pp. 201–230.

Herzog, Dagmar, *Sex after Fascism: Memory and Morality in Twentieth-Century Germany* (Princeton: Princeton University Press, 2005)

I.G., 'Erste "Pädagogische Woche"', *Berliner Zeitung*, 21, 34 (3 February 1965), p. 12.

'Ist Liebe ein romantischer Begriff? Partner—Ein Film für junge Leute, der Diskussionen provoziert', *Du und deine Zeit—Wochenendbeilage der Jungen Welt*, 3 (16/17 January 1965), not paginated.

Jahn, Marianne, 'Keine Scheu vor heiklen Fragen', *Elternhaus und Schule*, 13, 2 (1966), p. 28.

Jahn, Marianne, 'Partner', *Elternhaus und Schule*, 14, 5 (1965), p. 19.

Jahn, Marianne, 'Sagst Du's deinem Kinde? DEFA-Filme zur sexuellen Erziehung: Wichtig für Lehrer und Eltern', *Deutsche Lehrerzeitung*, 11, 8 (21 February 1964), p. 6.

'Keine Scheu vor heiklen Fragen', *Berliner Zeitung*, 24, 202 (24 July 1968), p. 10.

Knietzsch, Horst, 'Festival mit Niveau: Zu einigen Filmen der VIII. Internationalen Leipziger Dokumentar- und Kurzfilmwoche', *Neues Deutschland*, 20, 326 (27 November 1965), p. 4.

'Kunstpreisträger 1965', *Berliner Zeitung*, 21, 73 (14 March 1965), p. 6.

Laukötter, Anja, 'How Films Entered the Classroom: The Sciences and the Emotional Education of Youth through Health Education Films in the United States and Germany, 1910–30', *Osiris*, 31, 1 (2016), pp. 181–200, doi:10.1086/688161.

Laukötter, Anja, 'Listen and Watch: The Practice of Lecturing a Film and the Epistemological Status of Sex Education Films in Germany', *Gesnerus: Swiss Journal of the History of Medicine and Sciences*, 1 (2015), pp. 56–76.

Laukötter, Anja, 'Politik im Kino: Eine Emotions- und Wissenschaftsgeschichte des Sexualaufklärungsfilms im 20. Jahrhundert' (Habilitation thesis, Humboldt Universität zu Berlin, 2018).

Miersch, Annette, *Schulmädchen-Report: Der deutsche Sexfilm der 70er Jahre* (Berlin: Bertz, 2003).

Mönch, Regina, 'Kontrollverlust: Filme und das wirkliche Leben', in *Kamera! Licht! Aktion! Filme über Körper und Gesundheit 1915–1990*, ed. by Susanne Rößiger and Uta Schwarz (Dresden: Sandstein, 2011), pp. 78–84

Neubert, Rudolf, *Die Geschlechterfrage: Ein Buch für junge Menschen* (Rudolstadt: Greifenverlag, 1956).

Neubert, Rudolf, *Was sage ich meinem Kinde? Einige Ratschläge für Eltern* (Rudolstadt: Greifenverlag, 1961).

Niemeyer, Christin, and Ulrich Pfeil, eds., *Der deutsche Film im Kalten Krieg / Cinéma allemand et guerre froid* (Brussels: Lang, 2014).

Oelschlägel, Götz, 'Warum sind unsere Filme langweilig?', *Deutsche Filmkunst: Zeitschrift für Theorie und Praxis des Filmschaffens*, 9, 7 (1961), pp. 247–249.

Ostherr, Kirsten, *Medical Visions: Producing the Patient through Film, Television and Imaging Technologies* (Oxford: Oxford University Press, 2013).

Pelzer, Helmuth, 'Vor einer ernsten Frage: Wer spricht mit wem über die Liebe? Zu einem Erziehungsproblem', *Junge Welt*, 10 (4/5 February 1956), not paginated.

Peschke, Norbert, 'Drei Filme suchen ihr Publikum: Zu der Filmtrilogie "Begegnung mit dem anderen Geschlecht"', *Elternhaus und Schule*, 13, 3 (1964), p. 16.

Schwarz, Uta, 'Vom Jahrmarktspektakel zum Aufklärungsinstrument: Gesundheitsfilme in Deutschland und der historische Filmbestand des Deutschen Hygiene-Museums Dresden', in *Kamera! Licht! Aktion! Filme über Körper und Gesundheit 1915–1990*, ed. by Susanne Rößiger and Uta Schwarz (Dresden: Sandstein, 2011), pp. 12–49.

Steinmetz, Rüdiger, 'Television History in Germany: Media-Political and Media-Ethical Aspects', in *German Television: Historical and Theoretical Approaches*, ed. by Larson Powell and Robert Shandley (New York: Berghahn, 2016), pp. 133–154.

Ulbricht, Walter, 'Antwort auf aktuelle Fragen der Jugend: Aus der Rede von Walter Ulbricht auf dem V. Parlament der Freien Deutschen Jugend am 26. Mai 1955', *Junge Welt*, 9, 143 (18/19 June 1955), p. 3.

Walsh, Martin, *The Brechtian Aspect of Radical Cinema*, ed. by Keith M. Griffiths (London: British Film Institute, 1981).

Winkler, Anita, 'Biology, Morality and Gender: East and West German Sex Education in Films, 1945–70' (PhD thesis, Durham University, 2014).

Witzlack, Gerhard, *Beiheft zum Lehrerbildungsfilm: Begegnung mit dem anderen Geschlecht III: Weil ich kein Kind mehr bin, T-IF63*, ed. by Deutsches Zentralinstitut für Lehrmittel, Berlin (Berlin: Volk und Wissen, 1964).

Wulff, Hans Jürgen, 'Verfremdungseffekt', in *Lexikon der Filmbegriffe*, 12 October 2012, http://filmlexikon.uni-kiel.de/index.php?action=lexikon&tag=det&id=1574, accessed 20 July 2015.

Z., 'Beiträge in Edinburgh', *Neue Zeit*, 20, 205 (2 September 1966), p. 4.

About the Author

PD Dr. **Anja Laukötter** is a historian of nineteenth- and twentieth-century European history working in the field of social and cultural history and history of science. She is a researcher at the Center for the History of Emotions at the Max Planck Institute for Human Development and co-principal investigator of the ERC Advanced grant BodyCapital. In addition to other subjects, the main field of her research is the transnational/global history of media, the history of emotions, and the history of psychology and pedagogy. Contact details: laukoetter@mpib-berlin.mpg.de

8. Revealing Norms and Sowing Confusion: VALIE EXPORT's Body

Sophie Delpeux
Translated from the French by Simon Pleasance

Abstract
Created in 1968, VALIE EXPORT is a pseudonym that allows an Austrian Artist to explicitly criticize the way the art world and market exclude women then. In an advertising pastiche, she puts her own body in display to reveal the stereotypes coming with such a representation, but also how to escape from it with numerous performances, images and manifests. In this article, her body will be considered as a critical capital, enemy of Capital.

Keywords: performance art; feminism; Austria; VALIE EXPORT; stereotypes; pastiche; art market; gender; self-portrait.

A tightly composed black-and-white photograph framing the face and shoulders of a young blonde woman with her eyes closed, and a cigarette between her lips. Her left eyelid is slightly enhanced by make-up. Her right eye is invisible—in front of it, a packet of cigarettes is held aloft by the young woman, whose fingers seem blurred, cut off by the lower edge of the frame. This figure and the gesture fill the image and even give the impression of going beyond its edges. The packet of cigarettes is thus imposed on the onlooker and presents a second female face, associated with a brand, VALIE EXPORT *made in Austria*, as well as a motto: *Semper et Ubique/Immer und Überall* ('Always and everywhere'). This photograph is titled *SMART EXPORT* (Figure 8.1). It is dated 1970 and it is not so much an advertisement, as the way in which an Austrian artist introduces the new identity she has just created. In the late 1960s, Waltraud Höllinger, née Lehner, decided to abandon the names of her father and husband, and replaced them with

Bonah, C. and A. Laukötter (eds.), *Body, Capital, and Screens: Visual Media and the Healthy Self in the 20th Century*. Taylor & Francis Group, 2020
DOI 10.5117/9789462988293_CH08

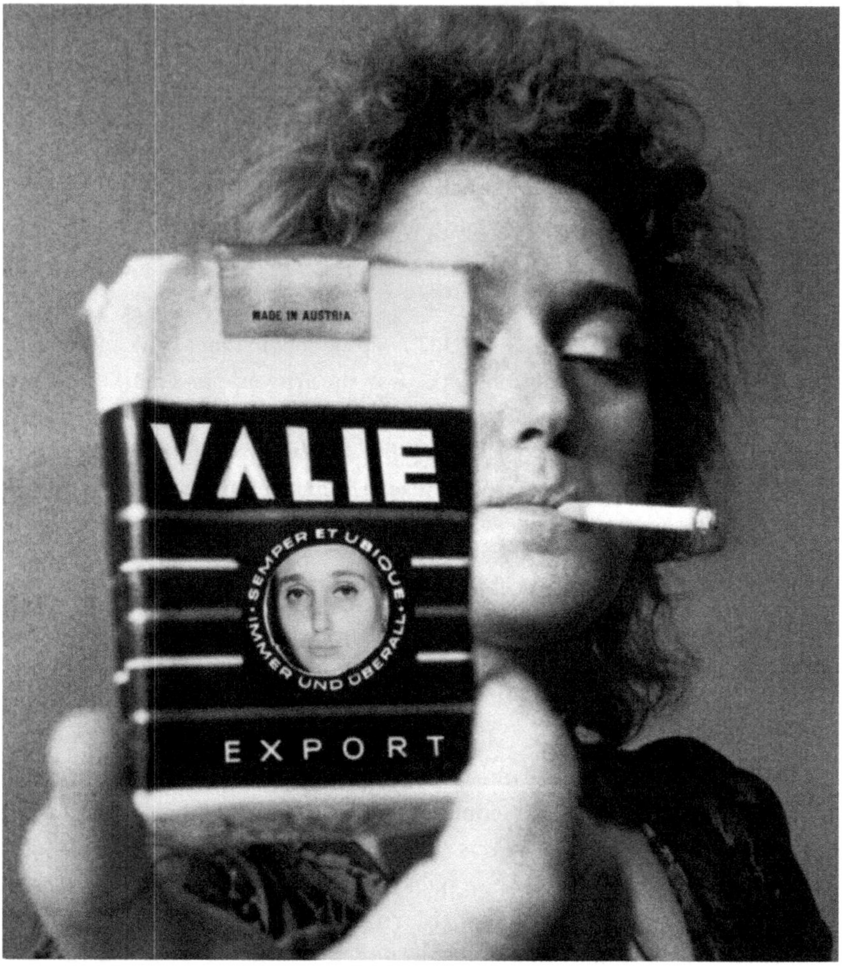

8.1. SMART EXPORT, circa 1970.

VALIE EXPORT. This pseudonym may sound like a patronymic, but let us make no mistake: What is involved is an *artistic creation*, no less. The artist says she invented it 'as if she had made a drawing'.[1] By making her own body and identity the object of her artistic research, she was part and parcel of those actionist activities that came to the fore in Vienna in 1963. It was no longer the production of a permanent work that focussed those artists' attention, but rather how art could interact with the real world through fleeting events, sometimes recorded by photography. The first New York happenings, in the late 1950s, opened up the possibility of getting into

1 'comme si elle avait fait un dessin'; Hofleitner, *VALIE EXPORT*, p. 93.

painting and having an experience within it, an experience that Austrian artists would politicize. So, VALIE EXPORT was created within a context in which the artist's body was already perceived as a critical and subversive agency—her predecessors' actions had been censored and suppressed. So for the art historian I am, analysis of these 'performance arts' that grapple with the historical and political realities of the period is tantamount to examining *strategies* which aim to upset models of bodily representation, in the broad sense, on a societal scale, and not just in the domain of art.

Emancipation through Imagery

The VALIE EXPORT avatar would enable the artist to undertake an investigation into the links between the body—in particular the female body—and its representation. She becomes involved in this, based on this image. It does not escape the attention of the keen onlooker that it is the same woman who holds the packet of cigarettes and who appears on the label on the packet. The woman who is consumed is also the woman who consumes. Here, there is a self-sufficiency which is asserted and which can be associated with the ideas put forward by the artist in her text *Women's Art: A Manifesto* two years later.[2] In that essay, the artist asserts: 'If reality is a social construction and men its engineers', this infers that women are 'dealing with a male reality.'[3] Because women 'had no access to the media', they had never managed to produce 'a self-defined image' of themselves 'and thus a different view of the social function of woman'.[4] She ends that essay with these words:

> the arts can be understood as a medium of our self-definition adding new values to the arts. these values, transmitted via the cultural sign-process, will alter reality towards an accommodation of female needs.[5]

The image titled *SMART EXPORT* seems to fit into this perspective: In it, the artist self-defines both her name and her image, a process made visible and emphasized by its division. The construction and dissemination of this image are thus a political act aimed to transform reality, so that the latter

2 VALIE EXPORT, 'Women's Art'.
3 VALIE EXPORT, 'Women's Art', p. 869.
4 VALIE EXPORT, 'Women's Art', p. 869.
5 VALIE EXPORT, 'Women's Art', p. 870.

is not just built by men, but jointly created. It remains for us to grasp why the artist makes a pastiche of an advertising image with *SMART EXPORT*.

It was actually based on the name of a Virginia cigarette, very well-known in Austria at the time—Austrian Export—that the artist created her new identity. In so doing, VALIE EXPORT moved away from the pseudonym and more towards the brand: for example, the artist demanded that it should always be written in capital letters. In this sense, the self-representation of *SMART EXPORT* also had to do with self-promotion—two notions which may seem to be removed from one another, if not contradictory at first glance. How are we to interpret this conjunction between the political issue, that is, the possibility for a woman to have her own image, and the commercial issue, not to say the marketing question? To understand this, we must go back to the economic and social situation of women in the 1970s. That was a period of awareness and of demands. Feminist movements ushered in an initial finding in the creative world: the very scant representation of artworks produced by women. This gave rise to criticism, but also to academic research; a first generation of female art historians engaged in those movements deciphered the phenomena of impediments, snags, and erasure, phenomena which barred the way to the careers of many (female) artists, both past and present. Those artists were thus long confined to amateurism and/or oblivion. One of the texts which reveals these phenomena of exclusion was written by Linda Nochlin and published in 1971 in the magazine *ARTnews*. It was titled 'Why Have There Been No Great Women Artists?'[6] In it, the author highlights the fact that this debate had always been reduced to the question of talent, hiding the other fact that it was the social and economic context which had invariably been the major obstacle to women's artistic output:

> But in actuality, as we all know, things as they are and as they have been, in the arts as in a hundred other areas, are stultifying, oppressive and discouraging to all those, women among them, who did not have the good fortune to be born white, preferably middle class and, above all, male.[7]

The idea that the art world, as it is constructed and formed, sediment-like, has always, on principle, excluded women thus became something quite obvious, shared by militant female artists all over the world, including VALIE EXPORT.

6 Nochlin, 'Why'.

7 Nochlin, 'Why', p. 150.

The Taboo about the Productive Female Worker

What we mean by the art world, in sociology, is a set of people who make it possible for a work to be identified as art, and thereby assume value, which is as symbolic as it is monetary. With *SMART EXPORT*, the artist short-circuited those intermediaries who had never been favourable to the artistic work of women, and imposed herself as an artist who was not only professional, but also offensive in the strategic way her image was broadcast—she spilled out of the frame and wanted to impose herself *Always and Everywhere*. In the context just set forth, there was, needless to say, a healthy dose of irony in this presentation: If what was at issue here was an international artistic career with the use of *export*, it barely existed for the women of that period, and the artist was fully aware of that.[8] But it did not stop there. With this image, the artist also infringed a tacit and age-old rule, consisting, since the arrival of the Academies in Europe, in the fact that the artist does not play a direct part in the sale and promotion of her work. It is precisely by the creation of intermediaries and go-betweens—dealers, for example, that craftsmanship has become art, and the craftsman/artisan an artist, once the artists was occupied with just creative work and no longer base material considerations. Raymonde Moulin, an eminent French sociologist of art, demonstrated in an article dated 1971—no coincidence—both the arbitrariness and the duplicity of this construct. The essay was titled 'Champ artistique et société industrielle capitaliste (1971)' ('Artistic Domain and Capitalist Industrial Society [1971]').[9] In it, the author wondered about the 'historical detours' that have permitted the artistic domain to become autonomous, and art objects to be radically differentiated from craftsmanship, and then from industrial products. It is worth noting that such a study was contemporary with *SMART EXPORT* and that, in these undoubtedly different fields, it was the same stereotype that was spoken out against, that idea that artistic activity was *above* economics. As much with this self-representation as with Moulin's brilliant text, economics and artists were, on the contrary, drawn together, until they were but one, because VALIE EXPORT was a brand and the sociologist was quite formal about this in her article:

> The artist is subjected to a system of organization with regard to the artistic life whose basic principle is the economic order. Slipped into

8 See Quemin, 'L'influence'. The first listings of artists date from the 1970s, and, in lists averaging a hundred or so figures, only four or five women artists appear in the bottom half of the chart.

9 Moulin, 'Champ artistique'.

> capitalist society and grappling with an ever-growing commercialization of art, artists, dealers, and art-lovers will try to disguise themselves and hide from others the economic logic which underpins their attitudes and their behaviour [...]. If the official imagery posits art as something absolute, glorifies artists, and represents the relation between the art-lover and the work as pure, unmotivated love, this is in order to mask the economic combinations to which artists are subjected.[10]

In boasting about herself and by selling herself in a direct way with *SMART EXPORT*, the artist revealed the flipside of this 'official imagery', just like Moulin, by placing economics, again just like the sociologist, at the centre of her action and her artistic appearance. This was all the more understandable because her argument was part and parcel of a feminist view (which was not the case with Moulin), which associated the financial dependence of women with the impossibility of creating art, a situation they have found themselves in up until now. In a very witty way, Virginia Woolf summed this up in 1929 in her famous essay, *A Room of One's Own*:

> If only Mrs. Seton and her mother and her mother before her had learnt the great art of making money and had left their money, like their fathers and their grandfathers before them, to found fellowships and lectureships and prizes and scholarships appropriated to the use of their own sex, we might have dined very tolerably up here alone off a bird and a bottle of wine; we might have looked forward without undue confidence to a pleasant and honourable lifetime spent in the shelter of one of the liberally endowed professions.[11]

If these ideas are about literary creation, they can be readily generalized to cover the entire field of creation. When Woolf laments the fact that women had remained poor from generation to generation, and had not had the *art* of earning money, and that, as a result, those who had enjoyed the

10 'L'artiste se trouve soumis à un système d'organisation de la vie artistique dont le principe fondamental est l'ordre économique. Insérés dans la société capitaliste et aux prises avec une commercialisation grandissante de l'art, artistes, marchands, amateurs d'art vont tenter de se dissimuler et de dissimuler à autrui la logique économique qui sous-tend leurs attitudes et leurs comportements [...]. Si l'imagerie officielle pose l'art en absolu, glorifie les artistes, représente la relation de l'amateur à l'œuvre comme amour pur et désintéressé, c'est pour masquer les combinaisons économiques auxquelles sont assujettis les artistes.'; Moulin, 'Champ artistique', p. 43.

11 Woolf, *Room*, p. 33.

independence necessary to undertake creative activity had been few and far between, the creation of the VALIE EXPORT brand resonates with this history of women. In the manner of exaggeration and a certain outrageousness, this image has a powerful symbolic content: This *art* of business which the artist plunged into was the art that was missing for her female forebears and her sisters, whose invisibility she lamented in her 1972 manifesto.

To finally assume the full measure of this self-representation, it will help to emphasize a final factor: It was her body and her face which the artist involved in this publicity pastiche. In it, she associated not only her artistic praxis, but her actual person with an economic activity. In so doing, she was once again close to what Moulin spelled out in her article. According to Moulin, the artist, in capitalist society, had become a 'productive worker', no sooner than exclusive contracts had been signed with art dealers: 'It is not only the product that finds its way into an economic circuit of supply and demand, but the producer, too, whose material means of producing depend on his capacity for inclusion in the market.'[12] This producer—read: the artist—had become more important than the object produced, which Moulin summed up thus: 'The fetishism of the author has taken over from the fetishism of the work: it is the signature that has become merchandise',[13] with the consequence that: 'From the moment when the artist has made a name for himself, his behaviour is, at every moment, and no matter what he does, the very definition of what a real artist is.'[14] The interest of the art world had thus shifted to what the artist *is*, rather than to what he or she *does*. The corollary of this was that the person, moral and physical alike, of the artist had thus become *the* guarantee of a value on the market. This, give or take, is what the *SMART EXPORT* self-representation highlights, with the artist and her attitude having become products and assuming as much: To have a career, it would seem that there is nothing else to do than to introduce yourself. VALIE EXPORT, however, is not the first to have made this phenomenon visible. To take just the most famous example, Andy Warhol realized very early on that his attitude, far more than what he produced, could be the object of a media-based and financial investment. For this

12 'ce n'est pas seulement le produit qui entre dans un circuit économique d'offre et de demande, mais le producteur, dont les moyens matériels de produire dépendent de sa capacité d'insertion dans le marché'; Moulin, 'Champ artistique', p. 42.

13 'le fétichisme de l'auteur a pris le relais du fétichisme de l'œuvre : c'est la signature qui est devenue marchandise'; Moulin, 'Champ artistique', p. 47.

14 'à partir du moment où l'artiste s'est fait un nom, son comportement est à chaque instant et, quoi qu'il fasse, la définition même de ce qu'est un véritable artiste'; Moulin, 'Champ artistique', p. 47.

reason, he took great care to construct nothing less than a mise-en-scène-like production, staged around his own persona and his studio, known as The Factory, with ever more self-portraits and shocking statements, and more and more relations with the world of show business. As never before in the history of artistic activities, Warhol became a star attracting adulation and loathing, drumming up commissions, and, at the same time, giving rise to nothing less than fascination. He also agreed—and there was nothing haphazard about this—to become associated with brands of alcohol and microcomputers, and he even went so far as to publish a list of items, with which he would accept to link his identity, in a small advertisement in *The Village Voice* in February 1966. On the list—coincidence! coincidence!—we find cigarettes.

> I'll endorse with my name any of the following: clothing, AC-DC, cigarettes, small tapes, sound equipment, Rock 'n' Roll records, anything, film and film equipment, Food, Helium, WHIPS, Money; love and kisses ANDY WARHOL. EL 5-9941.[15]

As a former advertising man well-versed in the art of selling things, Warhol highlighted, with both delight and cynicism, the secret link existing between art praxis and industrial praxis, by creating nothing less than a brand image. But, precisely where he always laconically averred that he had nothing more to say about such phenomena and, on the contrary, was pleased about that (fame and money being the two rare values that he laid claim to), VALIE EXPORT does her utmost to use this link to turn her artistic person and her artist's body into a critical body. It is not a matter, for her, of speaking out against the power (and the value) that have trapped the artist's attitude, but of making use of them to political ends—herein lies all the determination displayed by the split woman of *SMART EXPORT.*

VALIE EXPORT's Body: A Capital Enemy of Capital

It is most interesting to observe that, in the very same period, Jean Baudrillard was also interested in this issue of the body invested by capital, not within the art world, but on the scale of Western society, where, to use his own words, the body had become 'the most beautiful consumer item'.[16] He

15 The advertisement published in *The Village Voice* (10 February 1966), p. 2.
16 'le plus bel objet de consommation'; Baudrillard, *La société de consommation.*

noted that, after centuries spent 'persuading people that they did not have a body [...], people today systematically persist in *persuading them about their body*',[17] and giving them a status in such a pivotal way that, for the author, they have 'literally replaced the soul'.[18] A reflection which, needless to say, resonates with the shift from interest in the object to the artist, as mentioned above. The originality of Baudrillard's idea was that it showed that the ubiquity of the body in the 1970s and its promotion were not signs of a liberation after centuries of taboos and moral and religious prohibitions, but, on the contrary, of a new alienation, this time by profit:

> The body thus 're-appropriated' is done so right away in relation to 'capitalist' goals: in other words, if it is invested, it is to make it bear fruit. This re-appropriated body is not so treated in accordance with the autonomous end purposes of the subject, but based on a normative principle of pleasure and profitability.[19]

The interest of this analysis also resides in the fact that it puts forward a differentiated approach to women's bodies within this phenomenon. For Baudrillard, 'woman and body have shared the same bondage', and the 'emancipation of woman and the emancipation of body are logically and historically connected';[20] the consequence of this is that control is exercised more on this body, because, together with that of young people, it has 'the most revolutionary virtuality', and thus runs 'the most fundamental risk for any kind of established order'.[21] In the way in which he described emancipation as relative—what he called a 'myth of emancipation'—Baudrillard associated it with the advertising man, whose purpose is to sell things, rather than free things up: 'We give women Woman to consume, to the young Young People, and, in this formal and narcissistic

17 'à convaincre les gens qu'ils n'en avaient pas [...], on s'obstine aujourd'hui systématiquement à les convaincre de leur corps'; Baudrillard, *La société de consummation*, p. 200, emphasis in original.

18 'littéralement substitué à l'âme'; Baudrillard, *La société de consummation*, p. 200.

19 'Le corps ainsi "réapproprié" l'est d'emblée en fonction d'objectifs "capitalistes": autrement dit, s'il est investi, c'est pour le faire fructifier. Ce corps réapproprié ne l'est pas selon les finalités autonomes du sujet, mais selon un principe normatif de jouissance et de rentabilité'; Baudrillard, *La société de consummation*, p. 204.

20 'la femme et le corps ont partagé la même servitude', 'l'émancipation de la femme et l'émancipation du corps sont logiquement et historiquement liés'; Baudrillard, *La société de consummation*, p. 215.

21 'la virtualité la plus révolutionnaire', 'le risque le plus fondamental pour quelque ordre établi que ce soit'; Baudrillard, *La société de consummation*, p. 216.

emancipation, we manage to ward off their real liberation.'[22] If we follow Baudrillard, it seems clear that this false emancipation represents, on top of the age-old history of women being represented and depicted by men, a resistance to the project of self-definition and self-representation, which it is VALIE EXPORT's intention to undertake by way of the media. In this regard, the historical moment in which *SMART EXPORT* might be described as a standard is a complex one because, in it, attempts at emancipation are stifled by their being transformed into consumer products. Because this standard becomes just one of the aspects of this 'myth of emancipation' as described by Baudrillard, this liberated and slightly arrogant woman, who smokes and seems self-sufficient, can thus be reduced to the simple role of creating more consumption. Whether she is an artist or not...

It would seem that the artist was fully aware of this threat of retrieval and profitability. At the same time that she embarked upon this task of self-representation in 1968, of which *SMART EXPORT* is an example, she involved her artist's body in various acts and events, in the public place and in places given over to art. This offered her the possibility of incarnating many different aspects of femininity in real life, by way of experiences undergone, and experimental situations. She could thus identify with certain stereotypes in order to speak out against them, when she had a garter and the top of a silk stocking tattooed on her thigh in 1970 (*Body Sign Action*, 1970, Figure 8.2) or, in another vein, displayed herself in outfits and attitudes that were offbeat in relation to those norms. Three famous performances were part and parcel of this logic. The first was titled *Tapp und Tastkino* ('Tap and Touch Cinema', 1968, Figure 8.3), during which, with her torso hidden by a small portable theatre, she allowed passers-by to touch her breasts in Munich, and then in Vienna. The second, in 1969, was titled *Aus der Mappe der Hundigkeit* ('From the Portfolio of Doggedness'); in this work, she walked her friend Peter Weibel on all fours and on a leash in the streets of Vienna. For the third, which was held in that same year, she entered a cinema, armed with a mock machine-gun, and wearing a pair of jeans with a triangle cut out of the crotch to show her pubis. The performance was called *Genitalpanik* ('Genital Panic', Figure 8.4). A famous poster of the artist in that combat gear was published. In it, she appears with her hair combed back and her face unsmiling, presenting a figure of a fearsome and unusual fighter. Three

22 'On donne à consommer de la Femme aux femmes, des Jeunes aux jeunes, et, dans cette émancipation formelle et narcissique, on réussit à conjurer leur libération réelle'; Baudrillard, *La société de consummation*, p. 216.

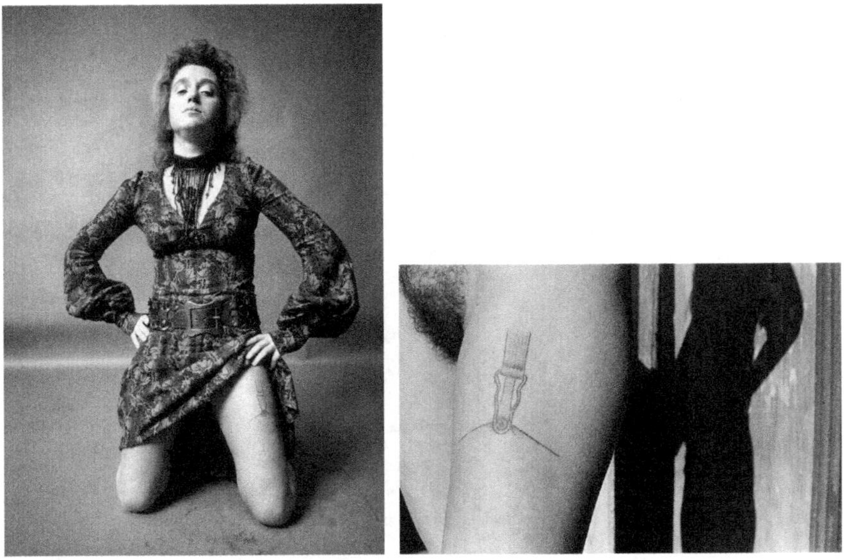

8.2. Body Sign Action—Tätonierung, 1970.

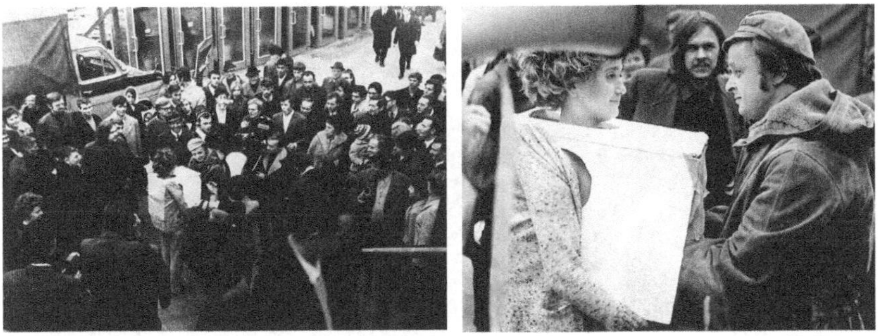

8.3. *Tapp und Tastkino* ('Tap and touch cinema'), Vienna 1968.

years later, with a performance such as *Hyperbulie*, she presented herself naked inside a structure of electrified wires confining her (Figure 8.5). The assignation to a small space, along with the issue of the danger incurred by wanting to move about freely, were emphasized. These are just a few small examples, in a far larger output, which show that the creation called VALIE EXPORT could be seductive, aggressive, commonplace, androgynous, dominating, imprisoned, and a victim, which is not an exhaustive list. If there is a question of creating a 'different social view of woman'—I am borrowing the artist's words—it would seem to be through the splitting of the VALIE EXPORT subject into various subpersonalities. Subpersonalities which permit an endless number of tests, an endless amount of role play,

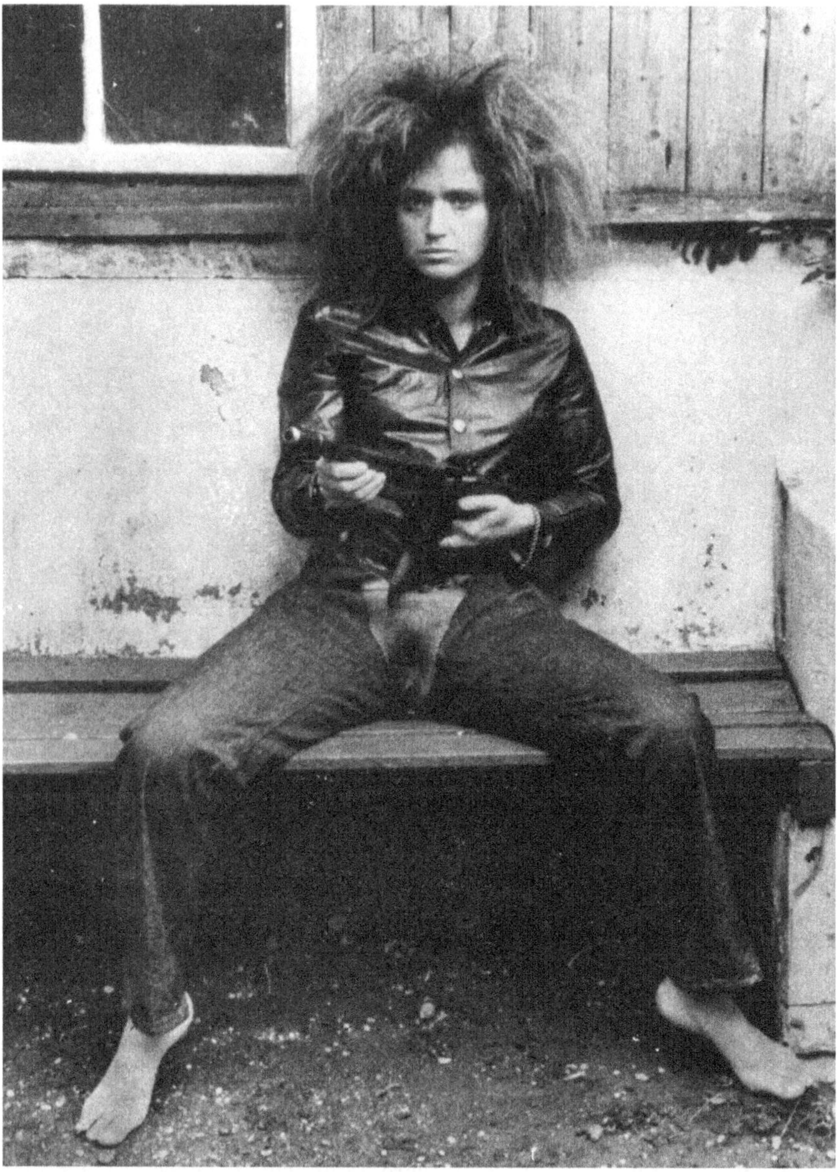

8.4. *Genitalpanik* ('Genital panic'), 1969, Poster n/b, 67 × 49.8 cm.

and an endless series of duplications. The female figure she incarnates can never be frozen in a single definition, or image.

By this yardstick, the duplication of *SMART EXPORT* is just one example of an overall increase within this artist's praxis, lending her full weight to the motto *Semper et Ubique*. In a recent interview, the artist confirms as

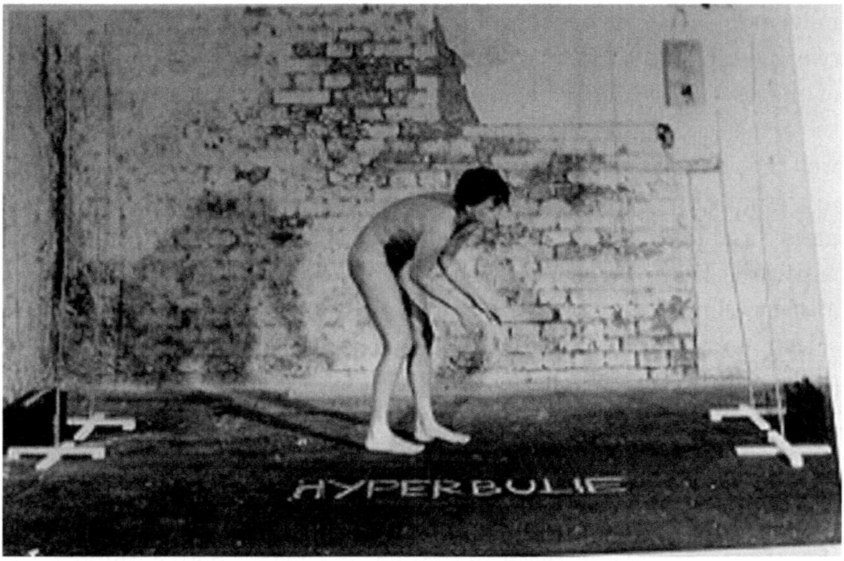

8.5. *Hyperbulie*, 1973, photographies d'action n/b, images by Herman Hendrich.

much: 'Showing the different identities of my self has always been one a concern of mine as an artist.'[23] This smithereening may be disquieting—it is probably the artist's aim to put the stereotypical representation of woman in a state of crisis. Needless to say, this ushers in a questioning about what we call the reality of a gendered identity and the way in which we can grasp it, or not. But to never be the same is also tantamount to withstanding the logic of the profitability of the artist's body: Coherence and a unique and constant face make identification easier, and thereby commerce. Here, we should think again about the way Warhol, on the contrary, cultivated a homogeneous image throughout his lengthy career to make business simpler.

I will take a last example within the VALIE EXPORT project, which further indicates that determination to create a productive body in terms of emancipation and not of capital, which seems to me to typify the artist's approach. What is involved is the film installation titled *Adjungierte Dislokationen* ('Adjunct Dislocations', 1973). Three simultaneous projections form this work: In the largest of them (a 16 mm film), the artist strolls about with two Super 8 cameras attached to her torso and back. In the other two, which are smaller, cityscapes and natural landscapes file past. Obeying a reflex, the viewer concludes that he is simultaneously looking at the

23 'Montrer les différentes identités que peut revêtir ma personnalité a toujours été une de mes préoccupations d'artiste'; Delpeux, 'VALIE EXPORT', p. 71.

movements that the artist is making with her brace of cameras and the two resulting films. Her body thus appears in the image as *also* a producer of images.[24] A division which makes us see three ways and further enables the artist to question the standards for representing the female body, as well the possibilities of her experience. To film with two cameras attached to her body, the artist is obliged to restrict her movements, in both their nature and their scope. She takes slow chassé steps, she arches her body rearwards, lies down on the asphalt, and makes all these unusual gestures at a very slowed-down pace, which is also unusual. Her entire behaviour sidesteps ordinariness, and dodges what seems usual as movements and gestures in the urban space (Figure 8.6).

The behavioural reasons are thus revealed to us, just like the low tolerance threshold which governs them. Without being as outrageous and weird as the 'silly walk' adopted by John Cleese in the famous Monty Python sketch, this different way of moving has nothing less than a disruptive potential.[25] When she refers to *Adjungierte Dislokationen*, VALIE EXPORT defines this piece as an 'investigation about the environment' undertaken 'through the body'.[26] So the artist offers us a chance to see her experiment and have contact with this experimental process. By feeling her environment in a different way, she permits herself and us to have another body, in the way in which it positions itself in space, and tries to grasp and occupy it. But there is more. If she offers us the possibility of an identification and an unlearning which liberates us from the standardized (and gendered) gesture and movement of *Adjungierte Dislokationen*, VALIE EXPORT also introduces confusion into these processes. In no time, the 8 mm images which file past do not, in any way, correspond with what the artist seems to be filming in the 16 mm film. This phase shift gives rise to another awareness: Not only has the viewer internalized standards of behaviour, but they also anticipate what seems to comply with the experience undergone by the artist in the projection on the left. This highlights our desire to predict what the experience should produce. By fooling this prediction, the artist shows us our active role in the construction of reality, the way in which we enclose ourselves in stereotypical kinds of conduct, which are repetitive and predictable. To describe this stage of the experience, she talks about an 'environmental body', a body

24 This is the subject of my essay *Le corps-caméra*, in which I propose seeing a project-based identity somewhere between performance and photographic performance image: one intervening in the field of the visible in order to subvert it; Delpeux, *Le corps-caméra*.

25 'The Ministry of Silly Walks', *Monty Python's Flying Circus*, season 2, episode 1, first aired on 15 September 1970.

26 The artist quoted in Mueller, *VALIE EXPORT*, p. 19.

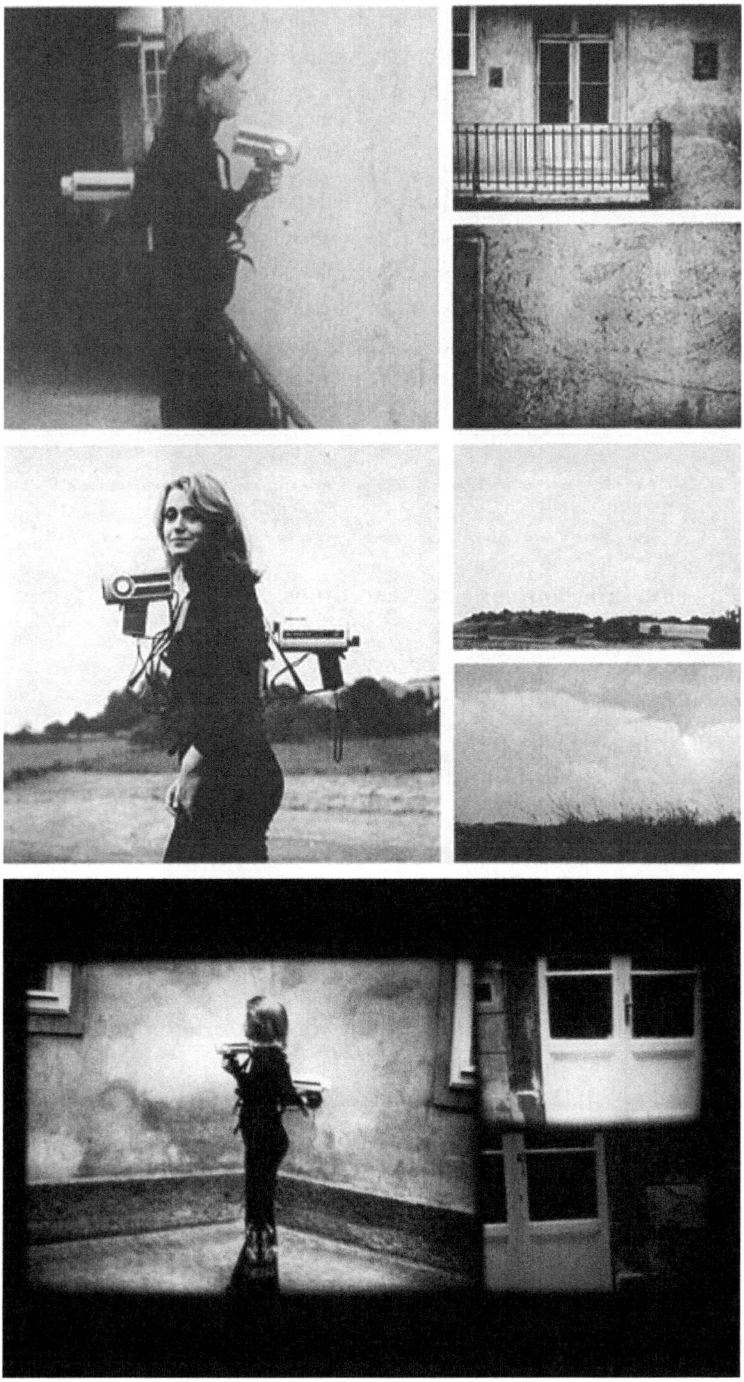

8.6. *Adjungierte Dislokationen*, 1973.

which no longer undergoes, but rather produces its environment.[27] She thus lends form to a thoroughly contemporary period, and to Jean Baudrillard's hunch: Despite the ubiquitous danger of its normalization and profitability, the body can also show itself as 'a living and contradictory agency', and, in so doing, fulfil 'its revolutionary virtuality'.[28]

This artist's body called VALIE EXPORT explores this virtuality, or so it seems to me, by means of investigations which multiply her faces and thereby render it—her body—elusive. Because they cannot be frozen in a single image, neither her gestures nor her patterns of behaviour ever have the required advertising coherence. If there is a capital which the artist wishes to assert to win her autonomy, it is as critical capital, the enemy of capital.

Works Cited

Films, Television Programmes, and Recordings

Adjungierte Dislokationen, by VALIE EXPORT, 1973.
Genitalpanik, by VALIE EXPORT, 1969.
Hyperbulie, by VALIE EXPORT, 1973.
Tapp und Tastkino, by VALIE EXPORT, 1968.

Books and Articles

Baudrillard, Jean, *La société de consummation: Ses mythes, ses structures* (Paris: Gallimard, 1970).

Delpeux, Sophie, *Le corps-caméra: Le performer et son image* (Paris: Textuel, 2010).

Delpeux, Sophie, 'VALIE EXPORT, Carolee Schneemann, erró: Le regard et l'image', *Artpress2*, sommaires, 24 (10 February 2012), pp. 63–72.

Hofleitner, Johanna, 'VALIE EXPORT: Split-reality entretien avec Johanna Hofleitner', *Blocnotes*, 12 (April/May 1996), pp. 93–97.

Moulin, Raymonde, 'Champ artistique et société industrielle capitaliste (1971)', in *De la valeur de l'art: Recueil d'articles* (Paris: Flammarion, 1995), pp. 34–54.

Mueller, Roswitha, *VALIE EXPORT: Fragments of the Imagination* (Bloomington: Indiana University Press, 1994).

27 Mueller, *VALIE EXPORT*, p. 19.

28 'une instance vivante et contradictoire'; Baudrillard, *La société de consummation*, p. 212.

Nochlin, Linda, 'Why Have There Been no Great Women Artists ?', in *Women, Art and Power and Other Essays*, ed. by Linda Nochlin (New York: Harper and Row, 1988), pp. 145–178 (originally published in *ARTnews*, January 1971).
Quemin, Alain, 'L'influence du genre dans l'accès à la notoriété: La place des femmes dans les palmarès réputationnels', in *Les stars de l'art contemporain* (Paris: CNRS, 2013), pp. 337–383.
VALIE EXPORT, 'Women's Art: A Manifesto (1972)', in *Theories and Documents of Contemporary Art: A Sourcebook of Artists' Writings*, ed. by Kristine Stiles and Peter Selz, 2nd ed. (Berkeley: University of California Press, 2012), pp. 869–870.
Woolf, Virginia, *A Room of One's Own* (London: Hogarth, 1929).

About the Author

Sophie Delpeux is a lecturer in Art History at the University Paris 1 Panthéon-Sorbonne. Former *Pensionnaire* of the French Academy in Rome (Villa Medici), she focuses her researches on Performance Art. Her Ph.D was a study about the photographic documentation of these past events (*Le corps-caméra. Le performer et son image*, Paris, Textuel, 2010) and how it opens reality to fiction through artists's bodies. The political, social but also therapeutical aspects of these art forms are at the center of her present academic works. She also writes about contemporary art.
Contact details: sdelpeux@univ-paris1.fr

9. 'Before Education, Good Food, and Health': World Citizenship and Biopolitics in UNESCO's Post-War Literacy Films

Zoë Druick

Abstract

Following its establishment in 1945, UNESCO worked to promote the aims of the UN through a range of educational mechanisms. This chapter considers the textual operations of the agency's film work in support of fundamental education, literacy and health in the late 1940s and early 1950s, arguing that some of the agency's structural and ideological contradictions are available for reading therein. Considering *The Task Ahead, Mondsee Seminar, World Without End, Books for All*, and the Healthy Village Project in relation to the UN Declaration of Human Rights (1948) and UNESCO's Statements on Race (1950, 1951), the essay explores the ways in which UNESCO filmmakers illustrated the *technobiological* and often racialized operationalization of the UN's universal humanist aims.

Keywords: United Nations; UNESCO; biopolitics; educational film; fundamental education; literacy; health; human rights; race

The Task Ahead, a short information film produced by the United Nations Educational, Scientific and Cultural Organization (UNESCO) in 1951, well expresses the enormous scope of the agency's mandate. Over the course of just seventeen and a half minutes, the film establishes that 'hunger, sickness, and misery' stalk the world's masses and posits that education, especially the transfer of technical and scientific skills, is the answer to the scourge of ignorance and war. Amidst all the progress shown in the film, including care for European children maimed in war, and Palestinian

Bonah, C. and A. Laukötter (eds.), *Body, Capital, and Screens: Visual Media and the Healthy Self in the 20th Century*. Taylor & Francis Group, 2020
DOI 10.5117/9789462988293_CH09

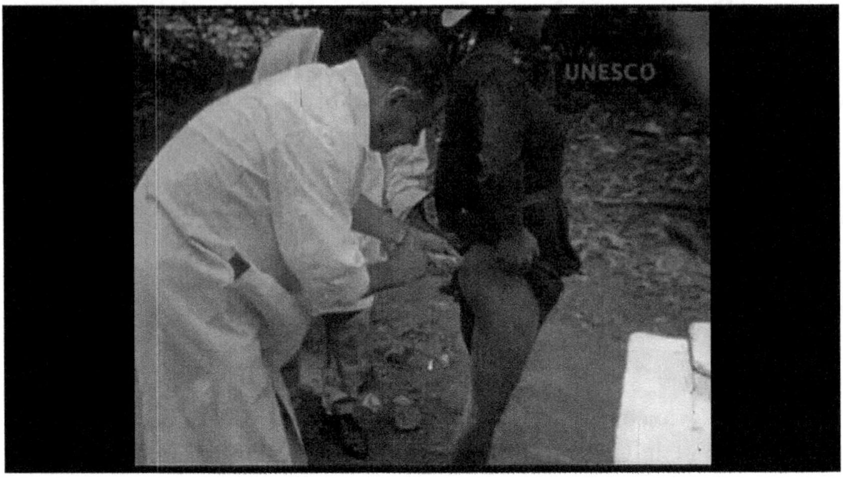

9.1. The transfer of bio-technology in *The Task Ahead* (1951).

children living in refugee camps in Gaza, the final sequence set in Haiti is perhaps the most compelling. The Marbial Valley is presented as a part of the world 'where men and women are shut off', and UNESCO workers are shown offering technical assistance and fundamental education to these, the world's neglected. In a sequence of images devoted to subsistence farming and social reproduction (a schoolhouse, women washing clothes in a river, children being fed) a barefoot young woman in a black dress and wide-brimmed white hat approaches a white doctor working at a makeshift outdoor clinic. Without any warning, the camera cuts to a close-up of her leg, which is covered with raw, open sores. The European male narrator makes no comment about her condition, speaking instead about the technical work needed in Haiti, from soil remediation and reforestation to water management. In a scene redolent of early 20th-century anthropology, her dress is perfunctorily lifted by the doctor and she is shown, in full profile, receiving a shot in the buttocks, her body objectified and rendered entirely visible (Figure 9.1). This is followed by an equally disturbing close-up shot of the diseased foot of a young boy while the narrator speaks of the need to give children the opportunities for a better life (Figure 9.2).

Two years later, a similar, but much more artfully crafted sequence of people being treated for similar nasty sores on their lower limbs (identified as yaws)—this time in Northern Thailand—appeared in the film *World Without End* (1953), a major production of the UNESCO Division of Mass Communication directed by two British documentary veterans, Basil Wright and Paul Rotha. In this version, the villagers are shown reluctantly

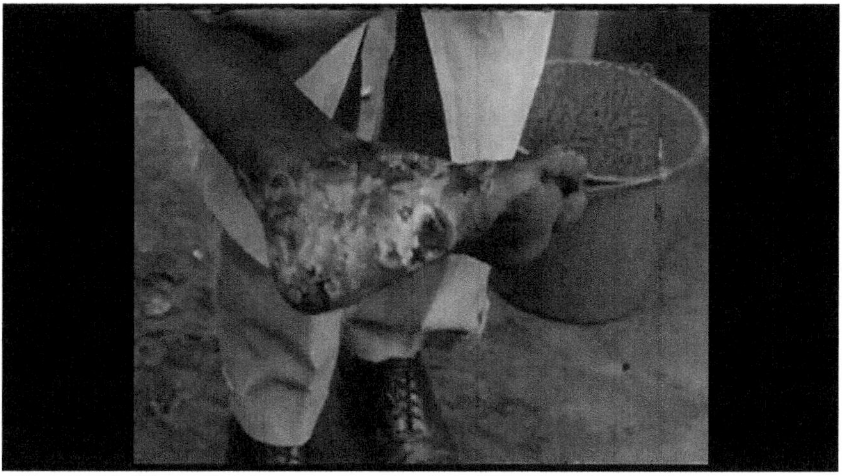

9.2. Yaws as a metaphor for the urgent need for technology transfer in *The Task Ahead* (1951).

attending a meeting with medical officers. Once one child has been given an inoculation, the villagers all approach at once, ready to be cured of their terrible affliction.

In both cases, the vivid close-ups of the diseased feet and limbs produce in the viewer a feeling of abjection associated with the bodies being shown. In neither case do we hear anything from the people, nor do we see them cured by the treatments they are shown to receive. The Haitian and Thai people are depicted as helpless to treat their own dismal afflictions. Western medical treatment is presented as a benevolent form of technology transfer, an urgent way to help. However, in both cases, the films isolate technical aid from any discussion of political or historical context. The contagious diseases on these bodies act as a visual metaphor for the deformity of the human spirit brought about by deficits in the basic provision for decent life. Without modern medicine and other technologies, these nameless individuals are presented as being abandoned to their compromised fates. However, both films emphasize that fundamental education, or the teaching of literacy, combined with hygiene and agricultural techniques, is a crucial step in the improvement of these desperate lives. Education and health are thus linked through the malleable body of the postcolonial subject. As the narrator of *Hungry Minds* (1947; a film made by the National Film Board of Canada in conjunction with the Canadian Council for Reconstruction through UNESCO) succinctly puts it, 'before education, good health and food'.

In what follows, I consider UNESCO films and other aspects of the organization's visual culture of the late 1940s and early 1950s in order to think through the ways in which, for all its lofty educational goals for peace, freedom, and cosmopolitan world citizenship, the agency often operated at the level of populations rather than publics, focussing on basic healthcare, agriculture, and literacy as precursors to higher aims. The film-making activities of the United Nations (UN), like all industrial film-making, documented and promoted the organization's activities and values, which were, for the most part, 'technobiological'.[1]

Although UNESCO didn't make many films of its own, preferring for reasons both pecuniary and philosophical to encourage the committees of member nations to sponsor their own work on the subject of the UN and its agencies, the films it did sponsor in this period, including *The Task Ahead, Mondsee Seminar* (1950), *World Without End, Books for All* (1954), and the film miniatures of the UNESCO Healthy Village Project (1949), connect in compelling ways to its major initiatives, the *Universal Declaration of Human Rights*, the *Statements on Race*, and the launch of a major programme of fundamental education. Not only the film-makers but also the producers and administrators of the Division of Mass Communication were often connected to the British Documentary film group. For instance, John Grierson, father of the British documentary movement, was followed in the position at the helm of the Division of Mass Communication by Ross McLean, formerly his deputy at the National Film Board of Canada.[2] The combination of reportage, documentary, and moral injunction in these films that so clearly follow from the British documentary tradition combine to tell a compelling story about the UN's biopolitical operations in this period. Nevertheless, as I hope to show, despite their non-self-reflexive emphasis on the supremacy of Western culture and technology, the aporias and contradictions they register are also able to provide an important key to unlock the logic of the UN, highlighting the special contributions that film analysis can make to the historiography of the organization.

UNESCO's Communicative Mandate

UNESCO, the UN's agency for education, science, and culture, was launched with much fanfare at the end of the Second World War to support the mandate of the United Nations and to promote the worthy causes of international lawfulness, the prevention of war, the support for universal human rights, and the promotion of 'social progress'. Its founding constitution charged

1 Birn, 'Backstage', p. 136; Hediger and Vonderau, 'Record'; Langlois, 'And Action!'.

2 Druick, 'UNESCO'.

the organization to build the 'defences of peace' in the minds of humankind and made the claim that ignorance in particular was a leading cause of war. Despite this somewhat idealistic premise, the organization always maintained its focus on culture in general and education for peace in particular, as alone capable of bringing about the 'intellectual and moral solidarity of mankind' that would successfully create peace where political and economic arrangements had failed.[3]

UNESCO's constitution, signed in San Francisco on 16 November 1945, endorsed three principles: equal opportunities for education, the scientific pursuit of objective truth, and the free exchange of ideas and knowledge. The document presented the assurance that, given the right conditions and the correct content, communication between peoples could lead to fuller comprehension of differences and therefore mutual understanding.[4] In Article I of the constitution, international cooperation is called upon to give the 'people of all countries access to the printed and published materials produced by any of them', and mass communication is singled out as a means to promote the free flow of ideas by 'word and image'. There is a clear suggestion that international agreements should be modified to facilitate this transmission, something that UNESCO would indeed go on to pursue during the decade.[5] All of these initiatives are part of what Donna Haraway has identified as the therapeutic understanding of communication that prevailed in the post-war agency.[6] By this logic, good communication is the route to productive social relations, while bad communication is destined to produce the reverse. Thus, communication becomes the operative level at which to accomplish social and political goals.[7]

The founding of UNESCO is thus a compelling landmark in international politics for the expression of the discursive power of culture, knowledge,

3 Numerous commentators have noted what a curious claim this is in relation to the recent war in Europe, whose causes could hardly be said to have been based on ignorance. In 1945, even UNESCO head Julian Huxley observed that Nazi Germany had been a highly literate society. Michelle Brattain notes that, in the 1950s, many social scientists, such as Theodor Adorno, questioned the precept that education could be used as an inoculant against racism (Huxley, *UNESCO*, p. 33; Brattain, 'Race').

4 United Nations Educational, Scientific, and Cultural Organization, *Constitution*.

5 For instance, in 1950, UN member states ratified the Agreement on the Importation of Educational, Scientific and Cultural Materials, which was intended to exempt such materials from duties. In 1952, UNESCO developed the Universal Copyright Convention for states that disagreed with aspects of the Berne Convention. And, in 1954, a convention was adopted related to the free movement of persons engaged in educational, scientific, and cultural activities.

6 Haraway, 'Remodelling'. See also Selcer, 'View from Everywhere'.

7 Wagman, 'Locating UNESCO'.

and information. Explicitly, it represents a moment when the liberal view of the formative power of information to create publics and constitute cosmopolitan citizens was making a play for global hegemony. In this regard, the founding of UNESCO represents the apex of liberal internationalist aspiration, a utopia of ideas.[8] Yet, UNESCO's actual on-the-ground operation at the level of practices of what often amounted to neocolonial health, labour, and education policies provides a far different perspective.

The seeds of this contradiction can be seen in the philosophy of Julian Huxley, UNESCO's first director. Huxley, a biologist, believed in the capacity of 'scientific world humanism', to dispassionately improve the lot of humans with technological advances.[9] He was also an unabashed supporter of what he termed positive eugenics, advocating for the scientific improvement of defective populations through breeding.[10] This view led him to a problematic analysis of 'race' and human accomplishment. According to his views, underdeveloped intelligence stemmed from cultural and environmental rather than biological deficiencies. Yet, even transposed to deficiencies in environment or education, Huxley's conflation of the 'dark areas' of the globe—the areas in need of enlightenment—with the places where the 'dark' people live was racist at its core.[11] In effect, regardless of the cause of compromised populations, his views insidiously reinforced a cultural hierarchy that placed Europe at its apex.[12] Proceeding from this 'scientific' position, UNESCO's projects to catalogue and promote the best of human accomplishments remained invariably Western in orientation.[13] Most generously, UNESCO's evolutionary or eugenic humanism can be said to have had a racist unconscious that positioned the agency's work in terms of a global governmentality meant to uphold the power structure of the neo-imperial order. This was the backdrop against which the agency's film-makers and designers sought to explore ways to represent the global totality.

Looking at the organization's activities rather than its rhetoric exposes the instrumentalization of the idea of knowledge that is liable to occur when its promotion is reduced to a set of techniques developed to operate on particular bodies for specific reasons. In UNESCO's films, these contradictions between word and deed are most clearly expressed, making

8 Sluga, 'UNESCO'.
9 Huxley, *UNESCO*, p. 6.
10 Huxley, 'Eugenics'.
11 Huxley, *UNESCO*, p. 18. See also Sluga, 'UNESCO'.
12 Hazard, *Postwar Anti-Racism*.
13 Duedahl, 'Selling Mankind'.

them useful sites of historical analysis. In what follows, I consider some of the literacy films made by UNESCO in its early years as a means to think about the contradictions at play in both the organization and the liberal internationalist philosophy that underwrote it.

Universal Declaration of Human Rights and the Statements on Race

The challenge for UNESCO's staff was to 'transform [...] broad mandates into workable doctrines, procedures, and ways of acting in the world', and the same might be said for the film-makers trying to find workable ways to communicate and visualize the organization's abstract principles.[14] In the late 1940s, there were two main initiatives that shaped UNESCO's focus: *The Universal Declaration of Human Rights* (1948, UDHR) and the *Statements on Race* (1950 and 1951). Both discursive exercises engaged numerous intellectuals and led to expansive discussion and debate.[15] They also figured directly in the production of the agency's visual culture. In 1949, a year after the UDHR, for instance, UNESCO sponsored a major exhibition at Le Musée Galliéra in Paris entitled *Human Rights* (*Les droits de l'homme*). Arranged as an immersive, interactive exhibit, the layout encouraged engagement with a range of photographs and text displayed on ten-foot pillars, as well as film and object installations. By focussing on a cross section of human achievement, the show attempted to demonstrate that there was a general universal tendency towards progress and human rights, even though the founding of the UN spoke rather to an 'increasingly apparent moral fragmentation'.[16] In addition, as the curators of a recent reconstruction of the show point out, 'despite [an] attempt to write the history of human rights in a global and inclusive moral language [...] the universalism that informed UNESCO's institutional discourse in the exhibition remained distinctly European', with declarations from the French and American revolutions figuring prominently.[17]

The *Human Rights* exhibition and subsequent folio publication universalize the Western notion of human rights and tell a story of world civilization as a struggle for human rights over the ages, beginning with cave-dwellers and ending with the 'free citizen of a modern democracy' living in a nuclear

14 Barnett and Finnemore, *Rules for the World*, p. 5.
15 Haraway, *Primate Visions*; Selcer, 'Beyond the Cephalic Index'.
16 Bregengaard and Prag, 'Visualizing Universalism', not paginated.
17 Bregengaard and Prag, 'Visualizing Universalism', not paginated.

family unit.[18] High points in various civilizations are presented as common heritage of a global humanity—a notion that would become an intrinsic part of the UNESCO narrative.[19] Nevertheless, Western, urban modernity is taken to be the apex of human achievement. Presumably due to its absence from the UN membership rolls at the time, the Soviet Union is visually missing from the project. This omission of a non-liberal democratic branch of industrial human organization perfectly encapsulates the provincialism of UNESCO's professed universalism.[20]

The distribution of the exhibition followed the agency's own logic, launching in Paris, where UNESCO was headquartered, and then touring around the UN's 50 member nations. The next year, 10,000 abbreviated albums of the exhibit were printed by the Department of Mass Communication. A scene of the album being distributed by UNESCO staff appears in *The Task Ahead*. The first page in the album depicts an illustration of planet Earth from space, with the continent of Africa clearly foregrounded, although Albrecht Dürer's engraving of Adam and Eve floating off to the right is somewhat obscured. Dignitaries at the exhibit are also shown looking at one of the elements that was often described as most notable: a three-dimensional map of the world superimposed on a massive diagram of population growth, and a large board with twelve portals registering the average number of 'white, brown, black and yellow children' born per second.[21] Thus, despite the show's stated objective of promoting the equal contributions to global civilization, its denouement ultimately resides in a depiction of humanity as a set of distinct, racialized populations, with white people set to be inundated through global birth rates by those with brown, black, and yellow skin.

The purpose of the travelling album of the exhibit is illustrated in *Mondsee Seminar*, in which adult educators attending the UNESCO seminar are shown to be looking at the exhibit mounted on boards on the lawn of the Kreuzstein Hotel in Austria. In the context of the film, which is concerned with the *techniques* of adult education, the content of the images is less important than the fact of its remote installation, and the whole scene is shot with a dynamic right to left travelling shot that recaptures some of the excitement, if not the scale, of the Parisian installation.[22]

18 Allbeson, 'Photographic Diplomacy'.

19 Brouillette, 'UNESCO'; Duedahl, 'Selling Mankind'.

20 Aitken, 'Provincializing Embedded Liberalism'.

21 Bregengaard and Prag, 'Visualizing Universalism', not paginated.

22 The idea of encouraging member states to undertake their own projects related to the aims of the UN was the impetus behind one of the most famous photographic exhibits of the era,

UNESCO, 'Race', and Global Governmentality

Staffed mainly by French and English nationals—who, together, held over 90 per cent of UNESCO posts in 1947—the organization's continuities with colonial administration and logistics were readily apparent.[23] Most relevant to my argument is the way in which UNESCO's initiatives in the field of visual culture operated at the level of 'race' in its pursuit of 'global governmentality'.[24] In pursuit of the lofty goals set out in its mandate, UNESCO's day-to-day activities showed that these ideals were necessarily translated into pragmatic strategies. From 'fundamental education' campaigns to the improvement of basic living conditions through the transfer of technologies, biopolitical projects figured most prominently in the organization's work.

As formerly colonized peoples of the world grappled with the imperial inheritances of the UN in general and UNESCO in particular, the organization paid lip service to a tantalizing new world of universal human rights and absolute equality.[25] In many ways, UNESCO's dizzying contradictions—imperial *and* postcolonial; global *and* Euro-American; humanist *and* technobiological; emancipatory *and* technocratic—grew out of its connection to interwar progressive education, on one hand, and the late stages of Anglo-European imperialism, on the other. The post-war focus on primary healthcare in the former colonies, for instance, was a direct link to late colonial welfare policies of the 1930s and 1940s, which had attempted to prop up dying colonial regimes through the ethical promise of improvement

Edward Steichen's *Family of Man* show, first exhibited at the Museum of Modern Art in New York in 1955, and then touring the world before selling millions of copies as a book. The UN figures prominently in the *Family of Man*, as does a liberal humanist vision that resonates with the apolitical narrative of peace through common understanding promoted by UNESCO (and seen in the earlier *Les droits de l'homme* exhibit). The links between the global family and the United Nations are made exactingly clear through the visual juxtaposition of the comparative global families depicted by the exhibit with the UN parliamentary assembly. The show promotes the idea of family as the universal form, 'a globalized, utopian family album [...] the family serv[ing] as a metaphor [...] for a system of international discipline and harmony'. Popular photography exhibits and publications of this sort were also the perfect self-reflexive promotion for UNESCO's communicative goals, with the black-and-white realist photograph presented as the quintessential form of 'universal communication'. The exhibit came to be permanently displayed at the Clervaux Museum in Luxembourg in 1994 and, in 2003, was accepted for inclusion in UNESCO's Memory of the World Register (Sekula, 'Traffic in Photographs', p. 19; Turner, *Democratic Surround*).

23 Sluga, 'UNESCO'; see also Hodge, 'British Colonial Expertise'.

24 Jaeger, 'UN Reform'.

25 Hodge, 'British Colonial Expertise'; Sherwood, 'United Nations'.

of the lot of colonial wards.[26] The League of Nations, the UN's predecessor, had pioneered in the realm of international politics by focussing on food and health rather than other, more contentious political topics.[27] Through film and other educational means, the League had also attempted to create 'self-disciplined, normal, compliant, moral, or entrepreneurial individuals'.[28] In so doing, the League had operated along the lines of the 'biologization of the social', the 'central defining characteristic of modernity', according to historian Edward R. Dickinson.[29] Picking up where the League left off, the UN's agencies, too, put their focus on the biopolitical.[30]

In the Global North, UNESCO's work was equally focussed on racialized bodies, although, there, it paradoxically took the form of debunking the concept of 'race'. Beginning with UNESCO's two statements on race in 1950 and 1951, the organization commissioned a number of studies to explore the fallacious and destructive discourse of racial hierarchies. These appeared in three series of mass-produced and widely distributed scholarly pamphlets and books by well-known social scientists (*The Race Question in Modern Science*, *The Race Question in Modern Thought*, and *Race and Society*), most famously, Claude Lévi-Strauss, whose pamphlet 'Race and History' is still considered the most popular publication ever produced by UNESCO.[31] The project led to a number of expressions in the UNESCO *Courier* as well as a picture book for children, *What is Race? Evidence from Scientists*.[32] All of this work aimed to debunk the scientific basis for racial categories and promote the modern ideal of universal rights for 'Man'. Although members of the Soviet bloc presciently pointed out that, without equality of economic status, universal rights were as good as meaningless,

26 Webster, 'Development Advisors'.
27 Pemberton, 'Changing Shape'; Staples, *Birth of Development*.
28 Jaeger, 'World Opinion', p. 594.
29 Dickinson, 'Biopolitics', p. 3.
30 Michel Foucault has identified the biological—life itself—as the sphere through which government of the modern subject occurs. According to his analysis, in liberal regimes, governmental power operates though the combination of the disciplinary constitution of the individual and the eugenic and biopolitical attention to the health of the population as a whole, with the family operating as an essential governmental hinge between individual and state. Campaigns to teach hygiene and medicalize favoured populations are thus as intrinsic to modern European government as are genocidal policies against racialized enemies. The Holocaust, which horrified the West and was so central to UNESCO's raison d'être, was, on a global scale, not a unique phenomenon. It was, rather, the application of orderly, genocidal techniques in Europe that had already been perfected in colonial settings (Arendt, *Origins of Totalitarianism*; Foucault, *Society Must be Defended*; Foucault, *Psychiatric Power*; Foucault, *Security*; Mbembe, 'Necropolitics').
31 Duedahl, 'From Racial Strangers'; Visweswaran, *Un/common Cultures*.
32 See also Bangham, 'What is Race'.

these considerations were sidelined by the Western nations, as well as some 'Third World' nations, which wanted to use the declaration of universal rights as leverage to improve their own condition as newly postcolonial states on the international stage.[33]

The concept of population presented in the UNESCO statements on race effectively made race into a malleable social and political category rather than a natural one. Thus, although universality was meant to create a new basis for politics beyond race, it ended up paradoxically replicating the neocolonial power relationships with new window dressing, as racialized populations remained marked in relation to a white, male norm and were categorically unable to obtain the status of the Western universals against which they were nevertheless perpetually measured.[34]

Visualizing UNESCO's Literacy Campaigns

The very limited original film work that UNESCO produced was largely related to the promotion of the organization's activities, especially its work on literacy, such as *The Task Ahead*, *Mondsee Seminar*, *Books for All*, and *World Without End*.[35] In two different lengths and several language versions, *World Without End* was shown extensively at film festivals and in film societies and was broadcast in several national contexts.[36] This film, which uses the UN's work in Siam (Thailand) and Mexico as a metonym of its global vision, is an excellent primer on the concept of fundamental education, the prototype of UN-based technical assistance and developmentalism, adopted as central part of UNESCO's programme in 1947.[37] It also expresses some of the contradictions at work in the output of British documentary film

33 Cmiel, 'Human Rights'; Marshall, 'Freud and Marx'. Members of the Soviet bloc also vociferously rejected the UN's universal claims for individual rights, arguing that the basis for life was much more material, centring around food, clothing, fuel, and housing. The 'universal individualism' on which the UN was built is far from universal, as has been elaborated in socialist and postcolonial critiques of the organization.

34 Despite Julian Huxley and other key players' emphasis on the neutrality and universality of science in anti-racism work, seen from another perspective, it was actually science itself that had help to establish the differential family of man discourse in the mid nineteenth century (Stepan, 'Race').

35 See Longo, 'Palimpsests of Power'.

36 Aitken, 'World Without End'; Druick, 'Visualising the World'; MacDonald, 'Evasive Enlightenment'.

37 Dorn and Ghodsee, 'Cold War Politicization'; Sluga, 'UNESCO'; Webster, 'Development Advisors'.

movement stalwarts who made claims of political progressiveness, but also readily worked within imperial and Orientalist frameworks.[38]

The fact that the film is concerned with fundamental education well illustrates its organizational character—it was made expressly to promote UNESCO's initiatives. But fundamental education itself was also the quintessential biopolitical policy of the agency. It was determined early on that the loftier (and more liberal) principle of the free flow of information was ultimately reliant on something as banal as basic literacy. Where people could not read and write (and thereby constitute a modern public), the existence of a local press was irrelevant. To educate for literacy would, by this logic, establish one of the basic conditions for democracy—with the side benefit of producing enhanced human capital.[39] The advocacy of literacy neatly avoided the discussion of content—there is no mention of enlightenment or consciousness-raising as was done by socialist literacy initiatives, for instance. This is an 'instrumentalized literacy', to use Charles Dorn and Kristen Ghodsee's phrase, with reading conceptualized as a neutral technique.[40]

However, more than this, fundamental education (FE) was part of a development theory that defined UNESCO throughout the post-war decade for teaching literacy as a means to practical social improvements, especially for peasants and small-scale farmers. According to Phillip Jones, the term, proposed by the Chinese delegate, was chosen over the alternatives 'mass education' and 'popular culture', proposed by the English and French delegates respectively, because it amalgamated and *operationalized* human rights, international collaboration, mass education, and social progress.[41] The first three FE pilot projects—in East Africa, Haiti, and China—were modelled on British colonial 'mass education'.[42] The first experiment, undertaken in the Marbial valley in Haiti in 1948, failed in a telling way. Haiti was one of only a handful of independent states with predominantly black populations eligible to be founding members of the UN/UNESCO. The project, co-sponsored by the World Health Organization (WHO) and the Rockefeller Foundation, was a multipronged affair that included teacher training as well as the establishment of rural primary schools, an agricultural school, rural clinics, a health education clinic, a library, and programmes of adult education.

38 Aitken, 'Provincializing Embedded Liberalism'.
39 Dorn and Ghodsee, 'Cold War Politicization'.
40 Dorn and Ghodsee, 'Cold War Politicization', p. 373.
41 Jones, 'Unesco', p. 48.
42 Sluga, 'UNESCO', p. 410

Yet, the project was plagued by racist treatment from UNESCO's administration and, after only a few years, was handed off to the Haitian government. Without an adequate funding plan in place, it was left to languish.[43] The Haitian pilot programme showed both the potential of global aid and the disastrous consequences that could result if funding did not follow through. Its failure was so spectacular, in fact, that it led to the cancellation of the Chinese and East African pilots as well.[44]

The Marbial sequence in *The Task Ahead*, described at the outset of this chapter, was likely edited together from footage meant to document the project. Unlike many of the other sequences, it constitutes an uncharacteristically sustained section. Positioned at almost the very end of the film, it is also the section that communicates the most concern over concrete challenges to improving the living standards of the world's poor. Unlike displaced populations from the Second World War, the Haitians are structurally poor and disadvantaged. Yet, the film contains no indication of any of the conditions that make Haiti unique. The fact of its revolution beginning with a slave revolt just two years after the French revolution and subsequent debilitating sanctions and boycotts from Europe and the United States, for instance.[45] Absent, too, is the vocal support of Caribbean nations and the National Association for the Advancement of Colored People (NAACP) in the United States for the application of the principles of universal human rights in the lead up to the UDHR.[46] This sequence acts as something of an abstraction of a very particular situation, rendering Haiti into an anyplace of the Global South in need of Western aid. The effect is made even starker by the discrepancy between the visuals and the soundtrack. The white male narrator's decision to discuss the needs of the nation rather than address what is wrong with the woman's leg indicates a kind of 'sonic colour line', as identified by Jennifer Lynn Stoever. Black people are at once highly visible and silenced, or 'soundproofed'.[47] This aesthetic strategy cannot be attributed solely to dominant conventions of narration or financial restraint, as multi-voiced narrations and other sonic experiments had already been used widely in documentary since the 1930s. Rather, it must be seen as the expression of a contradiction built into UNESCO's neo-imperialist Euro-humanist vision. Despite lip service to universal humanism, black and other non-white bodies

43 Verna, 'Haiti'.

44 Dorn and Ghodsee, 'Cold War Politicization'.

45 James, *Black Jacobins*.

46 Hazard, *Postwar Anti-Racism*.

47 Stoever, *Sonic Color Line*, p. 260.

were seen as biopolitical problems to be turned into human capital. Their histories and cultures, though considered lesser branches of the family of man, were seen to be no impediment to making them into productive economic actors. UNESCO's programme of fundamental education was a similar compromise between equality and freedom, on one hand, and pragmatism, on the other.

In an address to a London conference on 'Film in Colonial Development' given on 16 January 1948, John Grierson, Director of Mass Communications at UNESCO, parsed the difference between fundamental education and full literacy in his address on 'The Film and Primitive Peoples':

> The wider aim of Fundamental Education [...] is to help men and women to live fuller lives in adjustment with their changing environment, to develop the best elements of their own culture, and to achieve the economic and social progress which will enable them to take their place in the world. Fundamental Education should thus be designed to provide a first step to further education. While universal literacy may be a desirable ideal, the teaching of reading and writing is not the only, or even always the most immediate, purpose of Fundamental Education.[48]

According to this logic, the application of technological fixes for fundamental education became the birthplace of media literacy.[49] If you couldn't create literacy, you could still educate people with the 'illiterate media'.[50] Faced with an enormous population to be educated across the globe and very limited funds, UNESCO employees made the logical decision to mobilize technology and focus on the use of visual media in general, and educational films in particular, as the best way to jump the 'literacy hurdle'.

A good example of the emphasis on media for fundamental education can be found in The Healthy Village project, another one of UNESCO's educational initiatives, undertaken in 1949 in Pehpei, China. Film animator Norman McLaren was seconded from the National Film Board of Canada to run workshops for local artists and primary healthcare providers on how to communicate health messages through visual means. While the Red Army marched through town, his team innovated inexpensive direct application filmstrip-making techniques, scroll boxes, and two-way posters to convey

48 Grierson, 'Film and Primitive Peoples', p. 10.
49 Druick, 'Myth of Media Literacy'.
50 Carey, *Communication as Culture*, p. 9.

the simple messages about hygiene (e.g. wash your hands before handling food or touching your eyes, keep flies off your food).[51]

The five films produced by the workshop focus on making visible invisible forces such as bacteria, viruses, and nutrients. In the animated short film *Cholera*, for instance, a woman is shown washing her clothes in a river. Another woman approaches the river downstream and draws water. A close-up on a drop of water in her bucket shows that it is full of bugs—bacteria, presumably from the first woman's dirty clothes. A man drinks from the bucket and the bacteria are shown entering his system. He begins throwing up and then dies violently leaving his inadvertent killer—his wife—sobbing by his side. However, in an alternate ending, the man receives a shot that neutralizes the bacteria and is shown alive and smiling at the camera. In the short *Eat Beans, Vegetables and Fruits for Vitality*, a stick figure awakens and goes for a walk in the woods. After eating a few leafy vegetables foraged there, the figure expresses its newfound revitalization through animation drawn directly onto the 35mm film, dancing in a wildly exuberant expression of pure joie de vivre. In both cases, invisible actors—vaccines and nutrients—are demonstrated with simple animated morality tales.

The China audiovisual experiment was itself made into a filmstrip for educators as well as a publication, both of which are showcased in *Mondsee Seminar.* In one compelling scene, a group of four educators, three white and one Asian, is shown light-heartedly threading the projector and then turning off the lights in order to watch the first few frames of the filmstrip. The scene then cuts to a reverse shot of another group of four—this time three Asian women and a child—also gathered around a projector in a dark room, their attention apparently on the screen, which remains outside the frame. The film cuts back to the projected filmstrip and finally back to the original group as the lights are switched back on (Figures 9.3–9.5). In this sequence, the educators at the seminar are connected by means of the space of the projected filmstrip into a relationship with others watching the same thing, but presumably in a different context (possibly in Asia, although their location isn't made explicit. They may be attendees at the same seminar, although there are no other all-Asian groups shown at any point or any children).[52]

51 McLaren, 'I Saw'; UNESCO, *Healthy Village*.

52 The Fundamental Education programme in East Africa was tied to UNESCO's ill-fated 1946 groundnut scheme. Run in conjunction with the British government and the Overseas Food Corporation, it aimed to transform colonial subjects into modern workers by means of the production of vegetable oil. After it turned out that the region's terrain and rainfall were ill-suited to peanut cultivation, the company—and the educators—finally pulled out in 1951, leaving huge swaths of devastated land and plans to develop human capital in ruins (Sluga, 'UNESCO').

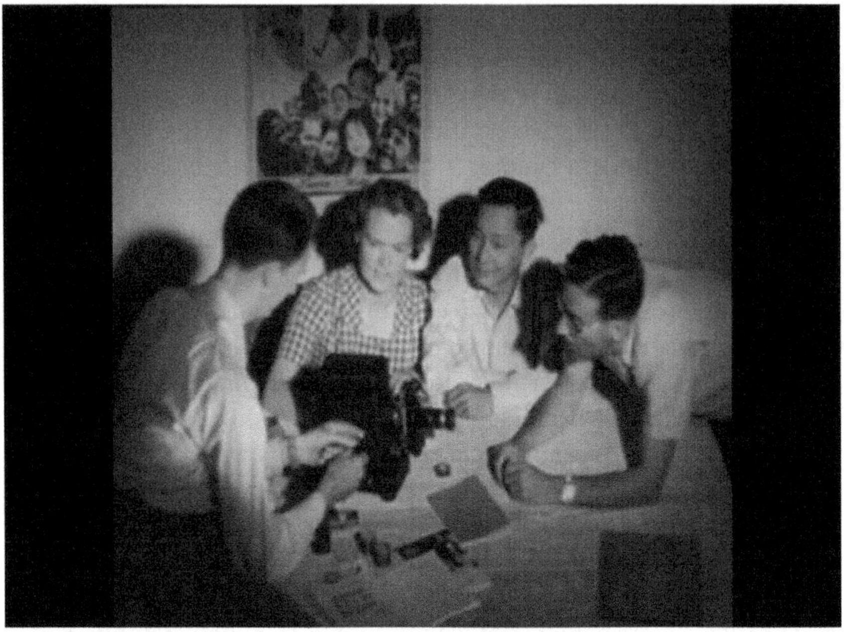

9.3. Adult educators thread up a *Healthy Village* filmstrip in *Mondsee Seminar.*

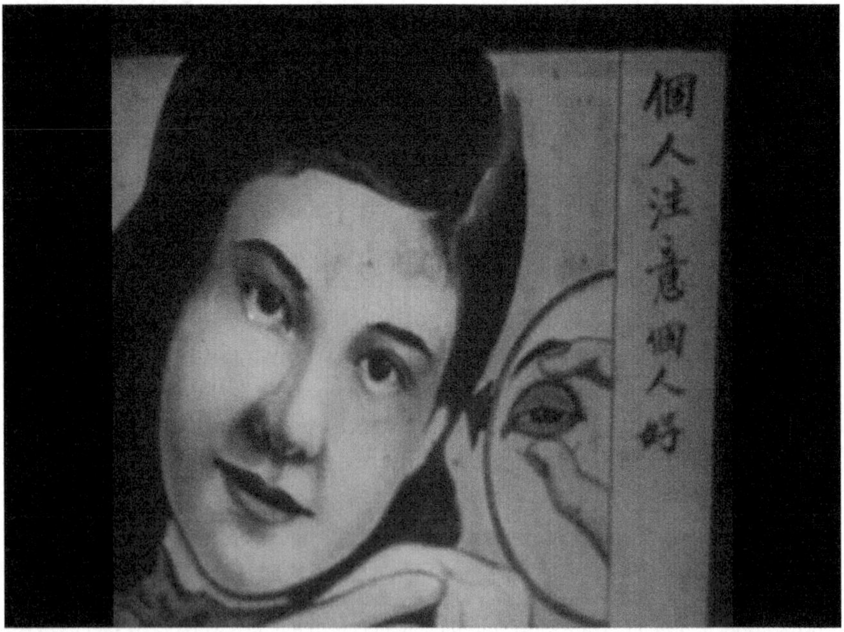

9.4. Promoting eye health from a *Healthy Village* filmstrip shown within *Mondsee Seminar.*

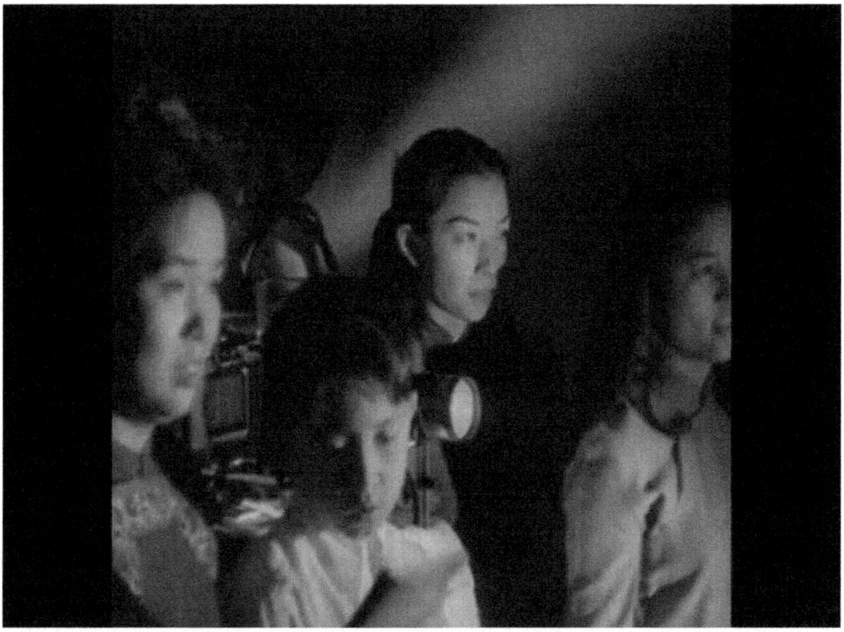

9.5. An unidentified audience watches the *Healthy Village* filmstrip in *Mondsee Seminar.*

World Without End tellingly avoids recounting any stories from Haiti, China, or East Africa and illustrates fundamental education through the use of visual aids in Mexico and a travelling library in Thailand—the places paradoxically chosen, in part, since neither country had been involved in a UNESCO fundamental education scheme—and links these communicative strategies with improvement at the level of both population subsistence and development.[53] Fundamental education is thus seamlessly woven into the project of development and modernization without dwelling on any problematic specifics. The film demonstrates the conception of the global population linked by shared space and time—a concept conveyed by an eye-line match edit connecting a Mexican peasant sitting in the dust to the UN headquarters building on 42nd street in New York City—and connects health, agriculture, and literacy projects being undertaken in each space to the benevolence and oversight of the UN (Figure 9.6).

World Without End perfectly expresses the contradictions of UNESCO's discourse of global citizenship and human rights. It is told from a Western perspective (by dint of both the sonic and the visual address to the viewer), while, at the same time, attempting to decentralize the UN project by

53 Smyth, 'Roots of Community Development', p. 419.

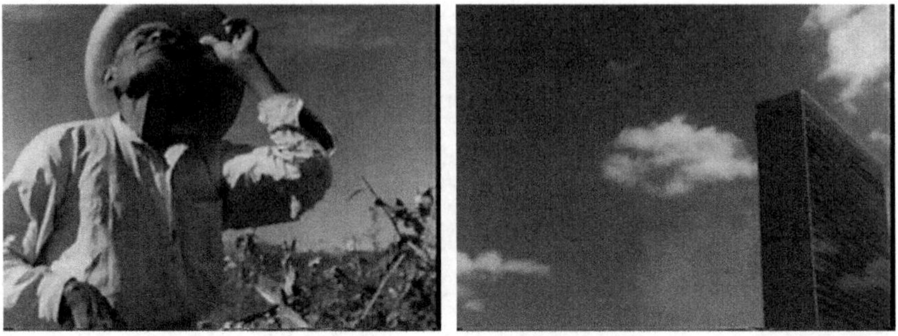

9.6. The representation of a unified global time and space in *World without End* (1953): A peasant in Mexico looks up to see the UN headquarters in New York City.

presenting all the experts shown in the film as visibly racialized people from the regions and states depicted. With the exception of the narrator, no one else is heard speaking on the soundtrack, which, instead, uses 'ethnic'-sounding folk music to signify its movement between Asia and Latin America. Thus, *World Without End* also enacts a sonic colour line keeping non-Western speakers from being heard while, nevertheless, keeping their bodies squarely within the frame.

After undertaking media health education work in UNESCO missions in China and India, Norman McLaren cryptically wrote: 'I have come to feel certain that this Fundamental Education is no more than giving aspirin for an abscessed tooth. In the long run perhaps a bad thing.'[54] It seems likely that McLaren is referring to the discrepancy between the inflated promises of literacy and health campaigns, on the one hand, and the lack of financial resources and political will to carry them through in a way that would fully benefit the people being targeted, on the other. He thus came to the realization of many literacy workers who, much as they may have wanted to 'reinforce indigenous values', likely realized that, through their 'help' to achieve Western modernization, they ended up contributing to the structural undermining of traditional cultures—often with disastrous results.[55]

54 Cited in Dobson, 'Norman McLaren', p. 34.

55 Watras 'UNESCO's Programme', p. 237. There were numerous problems with the concept of fundamental education, many of which stemmed from its provenance in colonial educational policy. For instance, UNESCO experts tended to demand competency in a student's national language. But, in many of the countries being modernized, such as the Philippines, there were numerous indigenous languages. The fundamental education regime thus became implicated in the imposition of national languages, sometimes against the will of speakers of other languages. In other cases, literacy programmes were directly tied to Christian evangelism, with all that entailed. It was clear to many that UNESCO's conception of literacy was a stark contrast to the

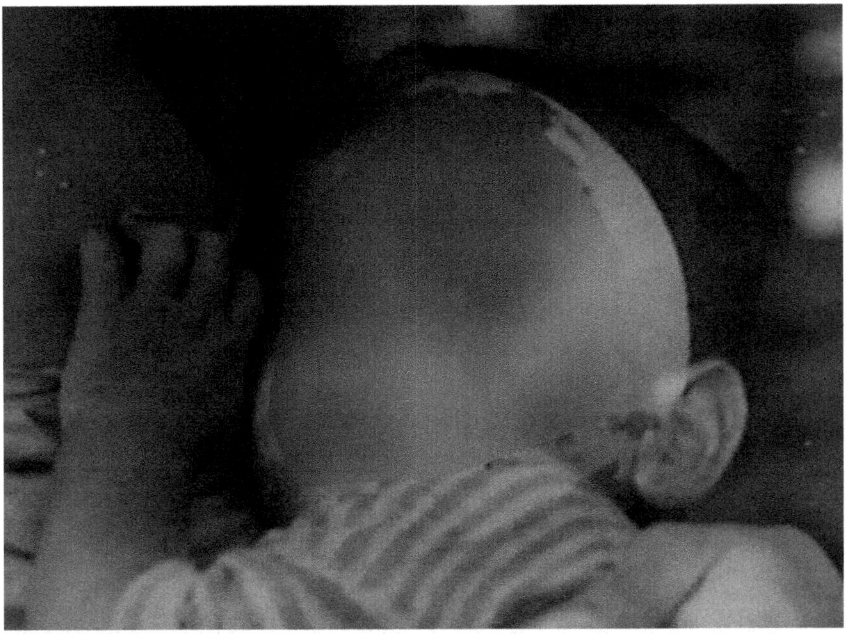

9.7. The globe, one of the favourite images for representing the 'family of man', superimposed on the face of a distressed baby in *World Without End*.

Despite the film's support for fundamental education, UNESCO's ambivalence about globalization is clearly depicted in the final section of *World Without End*, in which the narrator anxiously declares that the world's people are suddenly very close together and that the needs of the Global South can no longer be ignored. The film's final image is of an upset Asian child at his mother's breast who turns to confront the camera with an unblinking and unsmiling gaze while an image of the globe is superimposed onto his face (Figure 9.7). Coming as the culmination of a short sequence of images of nine children from different cultures, the image conveys the idea that the world is at a crucial moment, and the film encourages the Western viewer to consider supporting the UN and its agencies as a bulwark against global chaos that will inevitably ensue if the world's peoples are not provided for. Through the relay of gazes between the child, his mother, and the camera/

socialist literacy programmes that linked peasant literacy to 'pedagogies of the oppressed', focussing on consciousness-raising and empowerment rather than labour markets. See Jones, 'Unesco'; Watras, 'UNESCO's Programme'; Dorn and Ghodsee, 'Cold War Politicization'. For more on the presumed links between literacy and social progress, see Graff, 'Literacy Myth', and Druick, 'Myth of Media Literacy'.

viewer, the sequence sutures the viewer to the film's subjects in a single homogenous space and time, making it a perfect example of UNESCO's one-world organizational logic.

Orchestrating Diversity

In the UNESCO films under examination here, common strategies for visualizing the world include showing massive crowds, an image of the globe, or the flags of the member states of the UN. With the totality in mind, each film finds a way to focus on one particular group, geographical location, or national context, either through zooming in on one part of the globe or one national flag, or by using musical cues to indicate a shift in location.

World Without End's ending, with the image of the child's face superimposed on the globe, balances its opening image of a spinning globe, over which the narrator says: 'I am a man myself. And I think that everything which has to do with human beings has something to do with me, too.' This normative expression of humanism (everything human is important to all humans) is resonant with the sentiment of UNESCO's *Statement on Race* (1950), which ends with the statement: 'For every man is a piece of the continent, a part of the main, because he is involved in mankind.'[56] UNESCO's visual culture attempted to find ways to represent this sentiment of unity in diversity through the lens of humanism. Often, this involved a dialectical relationship between the universal and the particular, or a database logic that enabled the comparison of the compendium of ways of human life across different contexts.

Books for All (1954), a televised film about literacy made to celebrate the opening of the UNESCO-sponsored public library in Delhi, includes one of the most ingenious strategies for integrating a database of global examples into the film's structure. The eleven-minute film begins with a full four-minute montage of people—mainly adults—in classrooms around Asia and Africa being taught how to read and write. In lieu of the narration found in *The Task Ahead* and *World Without End*, a montage of musical styles cues the viewer's virtual travel around the globe. At the four-minute mark, the film changes tack and begins to focus exclusively on shots of Delhi and the opening of the library by President Jawaharlal Nehru. The film goes on to chronicle the many spaces, patrons, and activities of the library until, 60 seconds before the end, a film is threaded, the lights are dimmed, and an

56 UNESCO, *Statement on Race*, p. 347.

audience of children watches an abbreviated version of the global montage that opened the film, only this time without the focus on literacy. The film thus takes the viewer from being in the typical position of an educational film audience to being—via the film within the film—once removed from that position, the film's own rhetorical strategies laid bare.[57]

The correlate of the visual dialectic between the universal and the particular seen in the visual illustration of many of UNESCO's undertakings is the strategy of placing spatially disparate peoples in the same time frame. Central to UNESCO's visual culture was an attempt to orchestrate the world's diversity into a common cause. By placing everyone in the world within a unified time and space—however illusory—and making many of the projects comparative, the work often relies on the cross-section strategy that evolved in the interwar period.[58] The two groups watching the same filmstrip in *Mondsee Seminar*, the peasants in Thailand and Mexico in *World Without End*, and the literacy learners around Asia and Africa in *Books for All*, are all elements of the cross-section strategy seen most fully in the 1955 *Family of Man* photography exhibit. More than the feeling of a global village, this strategy addresses the world's diversity on a comparative humanist grid. Ironically, as Lévi-Strauss pointed out in his essay 'Race and History', the contact through colonialism, travel, commerce, and the media of globalization would inevitably reduce the diversity UNESCO purported to celebrate.

Human Rights and Biocapital

As this exploration of UNESCO's film and visual media work of the late 1940s and early 1950s indicates, in the immediate post-war world, biopolitics—the

57 *The Task Ahead*, *World Without End*, *Hungry Minds*, and *Article 55* (1951, United Nations Film Board) all use the motif of the globe. *Books for All*, *The Task Ahead*, and *World Without End* use the motif of large crowds in motion seem from above. *World Without End* and *The Price of Peace*, a United Nations newsreel from 1951 that features short speeches from representatives to the United Nations, use the motif of the crescent of flags of member nations to represent a global comity.

58 Cowan, *Walter Ruttmann*. As I have argued elsewhere, this visualization of statistics creates a kind of fiction at the heart of documentary, breathing life into what are, after all, only arbitrary categories to begin with (Druick, *Projecting Canada*). At the national level, this is a form of 'government realism', not unlike what James C. Scott has called 'seeing like a state' (Scott, *Seeing*). At the international level, this operates as a new form of governmentality, potentially placing everyone in the world into the same comparative grid. Children were often used to depict the promises of the new world order. See Rabin, 'Social History'.

governance of populations—brushed up against the promotion of culture and learning in intriguing ways, lending a disciplinary dimension to the liberal humanism being expounded. Modernization, democratization, and health were all explicitly tied to techniques of communication that were meant to forge the modern citizen in a global public sphere. The world was presented as newly globalized—seemingly through the neutral mechanism of technology—and this, in turn, was seen to have facilitated the movement of people and ideas. The opposing systems of the post-war world's superpowers were equally obscured by the studied apoliticism of UNESCO's functionalist rhetoric. The health of the population was explicitly linked to the use of science to debunk the divisive and meaningless concept of 'race' and to unite humanity. And the emphasis on public-formation often belied the fact that the figures through which the discourses of human rights were acted out appear to be the docile bodies of biopolitical regimes, often little more than anonymous archetypes in the family of man.

Even though the family of man discourse emphasizes the universality of the human condition, UNESCO's tendency in practice was to bifurcate its representational strategies between north and south. Despite the fact that civilization is repeatedly framed in UNESCO materials as common and universal, in its films, people in the Global South—such as the woman receiving the treatment in Haiti—are mainly shown to be complying with the modernization plans of the Global North, which are presented as a disinterested means of human progress. Meanwhile, in the Global North, the recent conflicts are reframed as misunderstandings based on the lack of knowledge about the value of cultural diversity. Yet, even as the category of 'race' is being debunked and disavowed by UNESCO's public statements, it is renewed nonetheless—if unconsciously—through the relationship of north to south being reinscribed into both the media texts and the media flows. This is something that, with the expansion of the ranks of postcolonial nations, would become the subject of the decolonizing work of the late 1950s and after.[59]

As I've explored here, in the first post-war decade, UNESCO's visual education projects quickly evolved their global biopolitical tenor. While presenting itself as an organization neutrally supporting the use of

59 The Non-Aligned Movement of African and Asian UN member nations met for the first time in Bandung, Indonesia in 1955, and later pushed for a project of international understanding that led to the establishment of the Major Project on the Mutual Appreciation of Eastern and Western Cultural Values—in many ways, the beginning of the postcolonial movement at the UN (Wong, 'Relocating East and West').

media to promote human rights in a newly crafted global public sphere, UNESCO's mandate took shape in the application of technological fixes and the development of human capital in a global biopolitical regime. As I've tried to indicate, UNESCO's actual programmes tended to take place at the most practical of levels. The films thus show people packing books into crates or threading a projector, ploughing a field or receiving an inoculation. For all the talk of humanism, then, UNESCO's representational practices tended along much more prosaic lines. Thus, although UNESCO was putatively engaged with ideas—with education, science, and culture—it can actually be seen alongside the UN's other 'technobiological' agencies operating at the disciplinary level of bodies. This explains why inoculation and farming techniques were the subjects of its films as often as was the genius of scientists and artists. Paradoxically, in order to bring about macro-level improvements, the operation of cultures and civilizations needed to be statistically mapped and improved at micro levels that were often fundamentally dehumanizing. To consider an individual as a vector of disease, for instance, is not usually, at the same time, to present them as the subject of history and the bearer of human rights. The universal values of humanism were often held apart from the actual processes of modernization and technology transfer thought to be the first steps in the establishment of human rights.

UNESCO's public relations and educational film work is telling, then, in terms of both what it displays and what it obscures. Discourses of individualism, freedom of expression, communication, and human rights were mobilized to justify the use of technical expertise in development. Yet, the emphasis on universalism only barely obscures the Eurocentrism that informed the organization; its express debunking of 'race' is complicated by the visual treatment of non-Europeans as bodies in need of disciplining in relation to the global system.

Global images of the sort produced under the auspices of UNESCO mapped a complex vision encompassing the lofty goals of world civilization, on one hand, and formation of human or biological capital, on the other. After the war, UNESCO lent moral authority to a transition from colonialism to globalization. Its philosophy also sparked a racist backlash in the United States and fostered disillusionment in the activists and progressive educators from around the world who had tried to believe in its promise.[60] That the prefigurative politics of the agency were not totally obscured by its imperial legacies and aggressive capitalist futures, is testament to their deep and

60 Hazard, *Postwar Anti-Racism*.

abiding utopian promise. UNESCO partakes in a complex international history, to be sure. But the contradictions involved in attempts to operationalize ideas of universalism, anti-racism, and peace through technical assistance and to transform colonial regimes into liberal democratic ones in the post-war years lives on in the visual records of the biopolitical initiatives sponsored by the agency.

Works Cited

Films, Television Programmes, and Recordings

Article 55, United Nations Film Board, 1951.
Books for All, UNESCO, 1954.
Cholera, by Norman McLaren, 1949.
Eat Beans, Vegetables and Fruits for Vitality, by Norman McLaren, 1949.
Hungry Minds, directed by Tom Daly, NFB/UNESCO, 1947.
Mondsee Seminar, UNESCO, 1950.
The Price of Peace, UN, 1951.
The Task Ahead, UNESCO, 1951.
World Without End, directed by Basil Wright and Paul Rotha, UNESCO Division of Mass Communication, 1953.

Books and Articles

Aitken, Rob, 'Provincializing Embedded Liberalism: Film, Orientalism and the Reconstruction of World Order', *Review of International Studies*, 37, 4 (October 2011), pp. 1695–1720, https://www.jstor.org/stable/23025572.
Aitken, Rob, 'A "World Without End": Post-War Reconstruction and Everyday Internationalism in Documentary Film', *International History Review*, 35, 4 (2013), pp. 657–680, doi:10.1080/07075332.2013.813863.
Allbeson, Tom, 'Photographic Diplomacy in the Postwar World: UNESCO and the Conception of Photography as a Universal Language, 1946–1956', *Modern Intellectual History*, 12, 2 (2015), pp. 383–415, doi:10.1017/S1479244314000316.
Arendt, Hannah, *The Origins of Totalitarianism* (San Diego: Harcourt, 1976).
Bangham, Jenny, 'What is Race? UNESCO, Mass Communication and Human Genetics in the Early 1950s', *History of the Human Sciences*, 28, 5 (2015), pp. 80–107, doi:10.1177/0952695115600581.
Barnett, Michael, and Martha Finnemore, *Rules for the World: International Organizations in Global Politics* (Ithaca: Cornell University Press, 2004).

Birn, A.-E., 'Backstage: The Relationship between the Rockefeller Foundation and the World Health Organization, Part I: 1940s–1960s', *Public Health*, 128 (2014), pp. 129–140, doi:10.1016/j.puhe.2013.11.010.

Brattain, Michelle, 'Race, Racism, and Antiracism: UNESCO and the Politics of Presenting Science to the Postwar Public', *American Historical Review*, 112, 5 (December 2007), pp. 1386–1413, https://www.jstor.org/stable/40007100.

Bregengaard, Katrine, and Eva Prag, 'Visualizing Universalism: The UNESCO Human Rights Exhibition, 1949–1953', https://static1.squarespace.com/static/521fa71ae4b01a79785 66e1e/t/570fd84240261d1195924e33/1460656201979/Universalism_pamphlet.pdf, accessed 31 August 2018.

Brouillette, Sarah, 'UNESCO and the World-Literary System in Crisis', *Currents* (December 2015), pp. 1–18, http://amodern.net/article/unesco-brouillette/, accessed 16 November 2017.

Carey, James W., *Communication as Culture: Essays on Media and Society* (New York: Routledge, 1992).

Cmiel, Kenneth, 'Human Rights, Freedom of Information, and the Origins of Third-World Solidarity', in *Truth Claims: Representation and Human Rights*, ed. by Mark Philip Bradley and Patrice Petro (New Brunswick, NJ: Rutgers University Press, 2002), pp. 107–130.

Cowan, Michael, *Walter Ruttmann and the Cinema of Multiplicity: Avant-Garde—Advertising—Modernity* (Amsterdam: Amsterdam University Press, 2014).

Dickinson, Edward Ross, 'Biopolitics, Fascism, Democracy: Some Reflections on Our Discourse about "Modernity"', *Central European History*, 37, 1 (2004), pp. 1–48, https://www.jstor.org/stable/4547381.

Dobson, Terence, 'Norman McLaren: His UNESCO Work in Asia', in *Animation: Art and Industry*, ed. by Maureen Furniss (Herts: John Libbey Publishing, 2012), pp. 27–38.

Dorn, Charles, and Kristen Ghodsee, 'The Cold War Politicization of Literacy: Communism, UNESCO, and the World Bank', *Diplomatic History*, 36, 2 (April 2012), pp. 373–398, doi:10.1111/j.1467-7709.2011.01026.x.

Druick, Zoë, 'The Myth of Media Literacy', *International Journal of Communication*, 10 (2016), pp. 1125–1144.

Druick, Zoë, 'UNESCO, Film, and Education: Mediating Postwar Paradigms of Communication', in *Useful Cinema*, ed. by Charles Acland and Haidee Wasson (Durham, NC: Duke University Press, 2011), pp. 81–102.

Druick, Zoë, 'Visualising the World: The British Documentary at UNESCO', in *The Projection of Britain: A History of the GPO Film Unit*, ed. by Scott Anthony and James G. Mansell (London: Palgrave Macmillan, 2011), pp. 272–280.

Druick, Zoë, *Projecting Canada: Government Policy and Documentary Film at the National Film Board* (Montreal: McGill-Queen's University Press, 2007).

Duedahl, Poul, 'From Racial Strangers to Ethnic Minorities: On the Socio-political impact of UNESCO, 1945–60', in *Current Issues in Sociology: Work and Minorities*, ed. by Gregory A. Katsas (Athens: Athens Institute for Education and Research, 2012), pp. 155–166.

Duedahl, Poul, 'Selling Mankind: UNESCO and the Invention of Global History, 1945–1976', *Journal of World History*, 22, 1 (March 2011), pp. 101–133, http://www.jstor.org/stable/23011680.

Foucault, Michel, *Security, Territory, Population: Lectures at the Collège de France, 1977–78*, ed. by Michel Snellart, trans. by Graham Burchell (Basingstoke: Palgrave Macmillan, 2007).

Foucault, Michel, *Psychiatric Power: Lectures at the Collège de France, 1973–74*, ed. by Jacques Lagrange, trans. by Graham Burchell (Basingstoke: Palgrave Macmillan, 2006).

Foucault, Michel, *Society Must be Defended: Lectures at the Collège de France, 1975–76*, trans. by David Macey (New York: Picador, 2003).

Graff, Harvey J., 'The Literacy Myth at Thirty', *Journal of Social History*, 43, 3 (Spring 2010), pp. 635–661, https://www.jstor.org/stable/20685428.

Grierson, John, 'The Film and Primitive Peoples', in *The Film in Colonial Development: A Report of a Conference*, ed. by British Film Institute (London: British Film Institute, 1948), pp. 9–15.

Haraway, Donna [J.], *Primate Visions: Gender, Race, and Nature in the World of Modern Science* (New York: Routledge, 1989).

Haraway, Donna J., 'Remodelling the Human Way of Life: Sherwood Washburn and the New Physical Anthropology, 1950–1980', in *Bones, Bodies, Behavior: Essays on Biological Anthropology*, ed. by George W. Stocking, Jr. (Madison: University of Wisconsin Press, 1988), pp. 206–259.

Hazard, Jr., Anthony Q., *Postwar Anti-Racism: The United States, UNESCO, and 'Race', 1945–1968* (New York: Palgrave Macmillan, 2012).

Hediger, Vinzenz, and Patrick Vonderau, 'Record, Rhetoric, Rationalization: Industrial Organization and Film', in *Films That Work: Industrial Films and the Productivity of Media*, ed. by Vinzenz Hediger and Patrick Vonderau (Amsterdam: Amsterdam University Press, 2009), pp. 35–49.

Hodge, Joseph M., 'British Colonial Expertise, Post-Colonial Careering and the Early History of International Development', *Journal of Modern European History* 8, 1 (2010), pp. 24–46.

Huxley, Julian, 'Eugenics in Evolutionary Perspective', *Nature*, 195, 4838 (21 July 1962), pp. 227–228.

Huxley, Julian, *UNESCO: Its Purpose and Its Philosophy* (Washington, DC: Public Affairs Press, 1948 [1945]).

Jaeger, Hans-Martin, 'UN Reform, Biopolitics, and Global Governmentality', *International Theory*, 2, 1 (March 2010), pp. 50–86, doi:10.1017/S1752971909990182.

Jaeger, Hans-Martin, '"World Opinion" and the Founding of the UN: Governmentalizing International Politics', *European Journal of International Relations*, 14, 4 (2008), pp. 589–618, doi:10.1177/1354066108097554.

James, C. L. R., *The Black Jacobins: Toussaint L'Ouverture and the San Domingo Revolution*, 2nd rev. ed. (New York: Vintage Books, 1963).

Jones, Phillip W., 'Unesco and the Politics of Global Literacy', *Comparative Education Review*, 34, 1 (February 1990), pp. 41–60, https://www.jstor.org/stable/1188554.

Langlois, Suzanne, 'And Action! UN and UNESCO Coordinating Information Films, 1945–1951', in *A History of UNESCO: Global Actions and Impacts*, ed. by Poul Duedahl (New York: Palgrave Macmillan, 2016), pp. 73–95.

Lévi-Strauss, Claude, 'Race and History', in *The Race Question in Modern Science: Race and Science*, ed. by UNESCO (New York: Columbia University Press, 1961), pp. 219–259.

Longo, Regina, 'Palimpsests of Power: UNESCO-"Sponsored" Film Production and the Construction of a "Global Village", 1948–1953', *Velvet Light Trap* 75 (Spring 2015), pp. 88–106, doi:10.7560/VLT7507.

MacDonald, Richard, 'Evasive Enlightenment: World Without End and the Internationalism of Postwar Documentary', *Journal of British Cinema and Television*, 10, 3 (2013), pp. 452–474, doi:10.3366/jbctv.2013.0150.

Marshall, James, 'Freud and Marx at UNESCO', *American Scholar*, 16, 3 (July 1947), pp. 304–311, https://www.jstor.org/stable/41204921.

Mbembe, Achille, 'Necropolitics', trans. by Libby Meintjes, *Public Culture*, 15, 1 (Winter 2003), pp. 11–40.

McLaren, Norman, 'I Saw the Chinese Reds Take Over', *Maclean's Magazine* (15 October 1950), pp. 10–11 and 73–76.

Pemberton, Jo-Anne, 'The Changing Shape of Intellectual Cooperation: From the League of Nations to UNESCO', *Australian Journal of Politics and History*, 58, 1 (March 2012), pp. 34–50, doi:10.1111/j.1467-8497.2012.01622.x.

Rabin, Lisa M., 'A Social History of US Educational Documentary: The Travels of Three Shorts, 1945–1958', *Film History*, 29, 3 (2017), pp. 1–24.

Scott, James C., *Seeing Like a State: How Certain Schemes to Improve the Human Condition Have Failed* (New Haven: Yale University Press, 1998).

Sekula, Allan, 'The Traffic in Photographs', *Art Journal*, 41, 1 (Spring 1981), pp. 15–25, doi:10.2307/776511.

Selcer, Perrin, 'Beyond the Cephalic Index: Negotiating Politics to Produce UNESCO's Scientific Statements on Race', *Current Anthropology*, 53, Supplement 5 (April 2012), pp. S173–S184, doi:10.1086/662290.

Selcer, Perrin, 'The View from Everywhere: Disciplining Diversity in Post-World War II International Social Science', *Journal of the History of the Behavioural Sciences*, 45, 4 (Fall 2009), pp. 309–329, doi:10.1002/jhbs.20394.
Sherwood, Marika, 'The United Nations: Caribbean and African-American Attempts to Influence the Founding Conference in San Francisco in 1945', *Journal of Caribbean History*, 29, 1 (1995), pp. 25–58.
Sluga, Glenda, 'UNESCO and the (One) World of Julian Huxley', *Journal of World History*, 21, 3 (September 2010), pp. 393–418, https://www.jstor.org/stable/40985023.
Smyth, Rosaleen, 'The Roots of Community Development in Colonial Office Policy and Practice in Africa', *Social Policy & Administration*, 38, 4 (August 2004), pp. 418–436, doi:10.1111/j.1467-9515.2004.00399.x.
Staples, Amy L. S., *The Birth of Development: How the World Bank, Food and Agriculture Organization, and World Health Organization Changed the World, 1945–1965* (Kent, OH: Kent State University Press, 2006).
Stepan, Nancy Leys, 'Race, Gender, Science and Citizenship', in *Cultures of Empire: Colonizers in Britain and Empire in the Nineteenth and Twentieth Centuries: A Reader*, ed. by Catherine Hall (Manchester: Manchester University Press, 2000), pp. 61–86.
Stoever, Jennifer Lynn, *The Sonic Color Line: Race and the Cultural Politics of Listening* (New York: New York University Press, 2016).
Turner, Fred, *The Democratic Surround: Multimedia and American Liberalism From World War II to the Psychedelic Sixties* (Chicago: University of Chicago Press, 2013).
UNESCO, *Final Act of the London Conference: Constitution: Instrument Establishing a Preparatory Commission* (Ottawa: Canadian Council for Education for Citizenship, 1945).
UNESCO, *The Healthy Village: An Experiment in Visual Education in West China* (Paris: UNESCO, 1951).
UNESCO, *Statement on Race* (Paris: UNESCO, 1950).
UNESCO Department of Mass Communication, *What is Race? Evidence from Scientists* (Paris: UNESCO, 1952).
Verna, Chantalle F., 'Haiti, the Rockefeller Foundation, and UNESCO's Pilot Project in Fundamental Education, 1948–1953', *Diplomatic History*, 40, 2 (2016), pp. 269–295.
Visweswaran, Kamala, *Un/common Cultures: Racism and the Rearticulation of Cultural Difference* (Durham, NC: Duke University Press, 2010).
Wagman, Ira, 'Locating UNESCO in the Historical Study of Communication', in *The International History of Communication Study*, ed. by Peter Simonson and David W. Park (New York: Routledge, 2016), pp. 71–89.
Watras, Joseph, 'UNESCO's Programme of Fundamental Education, 1946–1959', *History of Education*, 39, 2 (March 2010), pp. 219–237, doi:10.1080/00467600903043282.

Webster, David, 'Development Advisors in a Time of Cold War and Decolonization: The United Nations Technical Assistance Administration, 1950–59', *Journal of Global History*, 6, 2 (July 2011), pp. 249–272, doi:10.1017/S1740022811000258.
Wong, Laura Elizabeth, 'Relocating East and West: UNESCO's Major Project on the Mutual Appreciation of Eastern and Western Cultural Values', *Journal of World History*, 19, 3 (September 2008), pp. 349–374, https://www.jstor.org/stable/40542619.

About the Author

Zoë Druick is Professor of Communication at Simon Fraser University. Her research considers histories, theories and trajectories of documentary and reality-based media with an emphasis on their intersection with biopolitical projects. She is author or editor of five books and is currently working on a history of UNESCO's media work.
Contact details: druick@sfu.ca

10. From Colonial to Global: Visuals and the Historiography of Body Government beyond Europe

Jean-Paul Gaudillière

Abstract

The chapter considers the dialectics of body government from the perspective of the recent historiography of health outside Europe, and its *decentring* of the Eurocentric gaze on modernity. It proposes to distinguish between a colonial, a subaltern, and a global historiography in order to discuss the ways in which these genres can engage in a more significant dialogue with the history of visuals. Commenting a small set of films, the chapter argues that such engagement is possible since colonial offices, industrial firms, the WHO, multinational pharmaceutical firms, decolonized nation-states, anthropologists or NGOs have produce diversified mediascapes, which do not only document colonial or postcolonial health interventions but also the visions and agency of subaltern subjects.

Keywords: modernity; subalterns; global history; international health; colonial medicine; visual anthropology.

Introduction

Farm to Pharmacy is a documentary shot in 2011 in India, in the state of Orissa. Four images illustrate its plea for the modernization of traditional uses of medicinal plants. The first one is shot in a greenhouse where women—who formerly engaged in collecting plants in the wild—now cultivate some of them, following the advice of an evidently non-tribal expert from Sambanth, a local health organization (Figure 10.1a). The second one shows the administration of an herbal formula against stomach pain by a

Bonah, C. and A. Laukötter (eds.), *Body, Capital, and Screens: Visual Media and the Healthy Self in the 20th Century*. Taylor & Francis Group, 2020
DOI 10.5117/9789462988293_CH10

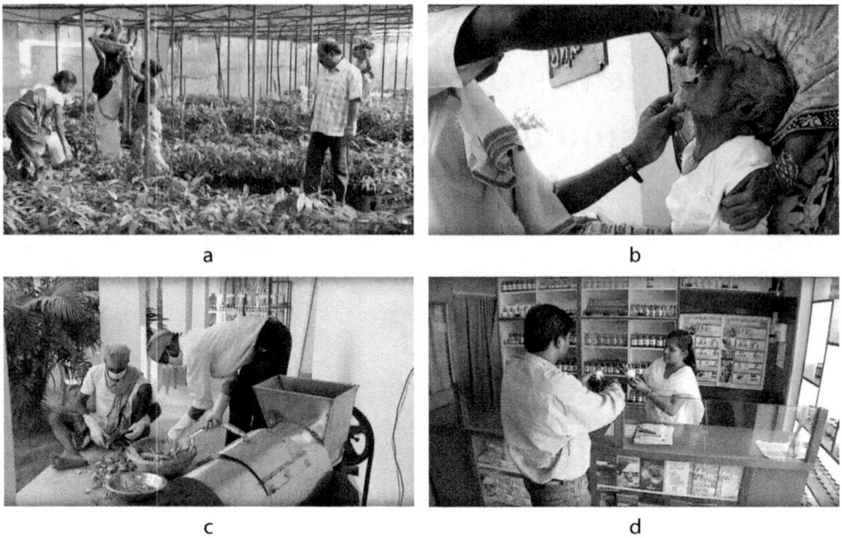

10.1. Stills taken from *Farm to Pharmacy*—a: shifting the supply of medicinal plants from collection to cultivation under the supervision of state experts, 02:57 minutes; b: turning plant mixtures into stabilized and ready-to-use combinations, 05:07 minutes; c: processing plant parts in a controlled, quick, and germ-free way, 03:50 minutes; d: selling the community-made remedies in pharmacies, 05:50 minutes.

vaidya, a practitioner of Ayurveda, who belongs to the teams of healers the non-governmental organization (NGO) has organized to improve access to care (Figure 10.1b). The third image shows the mechanical processing of stems in order to prepare a whole plant extract in good manufacturing conditions, evidenced by the masks and caps the workers wear (Figure 10.1c). The fourth shot illustrates the economic success of the project with a store where the community sells the products of its cooperative production unit and brings in new income that is 'equitably distributed' (Figure 10.1d).

The film promotes the activities of a local NGO called Sambanth, whose employees work with tribal communities in order to advance a 'holistic, participatory, sustainable' model for the revitalization of local health traditions based on modernized uses of medicinal plants. The film thus portrays remote and impoverished people whose ancient knowledge and plant resources are vanishing, now benefitting from the expertise of the NGO to build a non-biomedical system of care and pharmaceutical production.

Farm to Pharmacy is therefore a misnomer, as the title refers only to the final status of medicinal plants. A better name could have been *From Healing Traditions to Industrial Holistic Remedies*, since the film links two patterns of transformation of the local knowledge: its integration in a formal arrangement articulating healing and pharmacy, on the one hand, and the modernization of its practices to sell remedies while conserving the botanical resources, on the other. *Farm to Pharmacy* thus conveys a strong visual argument about bodies (tribal, sick, expert), care (holistic, traditional, ethno-pharmaceutical), and capital (manufacturing, commercial, human).

Body, capital, and screens: The association of these three words, the editors of this book explain, points to the role that modern visual mass media played in the transition from a national biopolitical public-health paradigm at the beginning of the nineteenth century—characterized by collective bodies, a workforce, and labour society—to societal forms of the late 20th century, where normality for better and healthier individual life is increasingly shaped by market forces and fundamentalism.[1]

This is not an isolated claim. Over the past 20 years, many authors in the history and/or the social studies of science and medicine have argued for similar grand transformations of the relationship between biology, human bodies, and the social fabric of society—even though they have not addressed the question of media production. To take one well-known example, Nikolas Rose's book *The Politics of Life Itself*, insists on the idea that a new regime of discourses and practices characterizes contemporary body politics with the new centrality given to the government of (biological) risk.[2] Rose argues that this regime has roots in three major trends: the molecularization of biomedicine; the subjectification of biopolitics (the new identities of patients, users, or consumers becoming responsible for their health, i.e. managers of their personal risks); and the convergence of health and economics through the development of bio-capital, risk prevention markets, and globalization.

Rose's approach owes much to Michel Foucault's famous lectures on 'Naissance de la biopolitique' at the College de France, which—since their publication—have puzzled historians of health.[3] In spite of the lectures' title, Foucault did not delve into the government of populations but focussed rather on the advent on neoliberalism, German ordo-liberal economics, and what he perceived to be major shifts in the relationship between the state and the market. Biopolitics was, however, not far away. The new politico-economic order Foucault was struggling to describe was linked, in many ways, to another transition he had previously explored, namely, the diversification of biopolitics into a regime of *discipline* and sovereignty, on the one hand, and a regime of *regulation*, insurance, and probabilistic control of conducts on the other.

1 Introduction to this volume, p. 1.

2 Rose, *Politics of Life Itself.*

3 Foucault, *Naissance de la biopolitique*.

By pointing to the new roles of genetics, its molecularization, and its links to the government of risks, and labelling his new regime a 'politics of life itself', Rose echoed Foucault's approach of regulation and pointed to the intimate relationship neoliberalism was creating between markets, bodies, and their self-regulation. However, while Foucault insisted on the synchronic relationship between disciplinary and regulatory technologies, Rose critically introduced a diachronic dimension in line with the core hypothesis of this book.

To a perspective already centred on body practices, *Body, Capital, and Screens: Visual Media and the Healthy Self in the 20th Century* adds a strong interest in the social life of markets *and* the media, that is, a strong interest in the relationship between the actions of economic actors, consumers, companies, marketers, or regulatory institutions alike, as well as the production of visual discourses. The following chapter considers the dialectics of body government from the perspective of the recent historiography of health outside Europe, and its *decentring* of the Eurocentric gaze on modernity. We argue that this historiography, with its diverse approaches to the changing relationship between knowledge, economies, and government, raises the question of how we—as historians—can approach the neoliberal management of health with its cortège of market logic, performance, individual responsibility, and choices, and thus open venues for enhanced dialogue with the history of visuals.

Three Historiographies of Health beyond Europe: Empires, Subalterns, World

If anything can count as a massive, unambiguous, and all too often highly destructive form of disciplinary government of health and bodies, it is the nineteenth- and 20th-century form of globalization associated with the making of the French, British, German, Dutch, and Belgian empires in Africa and Asia. Healthy bodies, markets, and empires then came together around several patterns of action that recent historiography has sought to disentangle. The first mode of existence of colonial medicine was around the problems Europeans were facing when they moved to the 'tropics': their lack of adaptation to the places and their inhabitants, including their inability to resist fevers, to adjust to the local food, and to endure the heat and humidity.[4]

4 Harrison, *Public Health in British India*; Harrison, *Medicine in an Age*; Pati and Harrison, *Health, Medicine and Empire*.

The existence of a common—humoral—episteme shared by the Hippocratic European tradition and the elite medicines of Asia initially reinforced the idea that indigenous and European bodies were not essentially different and therefore that Europeans had much to learn and to borrow from the practitioners of non-Western corpuses of medical knowledge. This radically changed during the last decades of the nineteenth century in a context of increased competition between European powers, struggle for the natural resources that a booming industry was consuming, and mounting racialization of social groups at home and abroad, in conjunction with major changes in European medical knowledge (the rise of both clinical medicine and the laboratory). The result was a profound divergence rooted in different ontologies of bodies and diseases, and the defence of a hegemonic status for Western medicine.

The second mode of existence of colonial medicine emerged out of different concerns regarding the colonial subjects and their value for the empire. Serious concerns for the fate of indigenous bodies emerged around the time of the First World War. What resulted was the invention of *mise en valeur* and development that, in practical terms, remained limited to efforts to maintain a healthy labour force and to instil (often through forcible means) a work ethic in the colonized as the backbone of rational colonial exploitation. More broadly, it did, nevertheless, also still mean the modernization of the so-called primitive or barbaric worlds and their inhabitants through the construction of new cities, the education of colonial subjects, the recovery of infertile soil, and the establishment of new institutions that sought to 'civilize' according to the ideals of republican and/or democratic virtue.[5] The policies designed to control sleeping sickness in Africa from the 1930s onwards exemplify the importance that vertical programmes then gained in the practice of colonial management.[6] Inoculation campaigns aimed at eradication through the treatment of people identified as carriers of parasites. They relied on the creation of devoted squads visiting villages, and on the standardization of quick microscopic detection that could be applied with a few instruments and at a large scale. Last but not least, they involved rudimentary assessment of treatment productivity based on the ratio between staff involved and inoculations performed.

In order to better characterize this historiography of imperial health, it is useful to take into account the issues historians have focussed on, the actors they study, the forms of capital and forms of knowledge they consider, and

5 Keller, *Colonial Madness*.

6 Lachenal, *Le médicament*.

	Imperial historiography	Subaltern historiography	World historiography
Issues	Exploitation (labour, nature), disciplinary order	Hegemony, resistance, nationalism, hybridization	Circulations, geopolitics, development, neo-liberalism
Main actors	Military, colonial administration and experts, settlers	Peasants, workers, indigenous elite	NGOs, enterprises, U.N. system, nation-states
Form of capital	Imperial, industrial, and extractive	Native, land & commerce	Multinational, financial, and industrial
Priority health problems	Epidemics, reproductive health	Epidemics, famine, and malnutrition	Emerging and neglected epidemics, reproduction
Forms of knowledge	Bacteriology, health statistics	Traditional medicine, healing & rituals	Economics, epidemiology
Sources	Colonial archives	Local and private records, oral history, ethnography	International archives

Table 10.1. Health, bodies, and government beyond Europe: Three modes of historical analysis.

the nature of the sources they have tapped into (Table 10.1). The imperial historiography of the government of bodies then appears as the history of a disciplinary order aiming to exploit both nature and subaltern people. Its main actors were the colonial agents—that is, settlers, military men, physicians, missionaries, and administrators. The capital involved came primarily from the metropolis. It was industrial in the sense that it focussed on the resources—raw materials as well as food—needed 'at home' in order to pursue the process of industrialization, and it was extractive in nature. Priority health problems were those affecting populations as such—epidemics and reproductive health with the consequence that colonial or tropical medicine as a corpus of knowledge was a combination of bacteriology and vital statistics. Finally, the sources explored were almost exclusively colonial archives, which were read 'against the grain' as Arlette Farge once put it.

In the 1980s and 1990s, a new historiography emerged outside Europe, revisiting colonial and postcolonial times from the vantage point of the native subjects. What may be called the subaltern historiography of health has indeed revealed the extent to which modernization outside Europe was grounded in non-Western views and practices that were cultural as well as material. This is powerfully illustrated by the work of the Indian Subaltern Studies Collective, which emerged as an attempt to renew the nationalist and Marxist historiography of colonial India, using Gramsci's concept of hegemony expanded along different lines during the two decades of its existence. The collective's first wave of studies focussed on the ways in which *subalterns*, that is, peasants, women, members of low caste, or workers experienced and resisted the colonial order, in congruence with or opposition to a mounting nationalist movement.[7] This was very much in line with the kind of history that emerged in the 1960s and 1970s under the label 'history from below'. During the late 1990s and early 2000s, the publication of Partha Chatterjee's *The Nation and its Fragments* and Dipesh Chakrabarty's *Provincializing Europe* signalled an important shift, as these books no longer documented and analysed the life of the subalterns but returned to elite debates on modernity and its Western origins.[8] Alternative modernity was thus important in Chakrabarty's critique of Western historiography, highlighting two responses, two modes of 'provincializing Europe': the writing of history of—and from—non-Western perspectives; and a revision of Europe's own history revealing its roots in—and connections with—non-European historical trajectories.

The history of health and body politics was far from being marginal in this *decentring*. It provided a unique nexus for analysing the status of Western knowledge, its putative incommensurability with 'Indian' counterparts, the tensions undermining colonial politics, or the defence and transformation of (reinvented or rediscovered) traditional practices. David Arnold's *Colonizing the Body* is one of the most influential books originating in the subaltern collective. His analyses of British sanitary interventions in India contrast with the imperial historiography, not in terms of objects and issues (the book is, for instance, still focussed on the management of infectious diseases, i.e. cholera, smallpox, or plague), but rather in the way he posits colonial policies in relation to the reactions and views of the people they targeted.[9]

Smallpox management is an especially interesting example since the longue durée of vaccination policies in Europe and India makes the gradual divergence between colonial and native medical systems visible. Before 1830, when orientalism nurtured a real interest in the practices of Ayurveda or Unani physicians, vaccination against smallpox was a terrain of encounter, a practice perceived as analogous to the local (Indian) custom of transferring pustules from affected to healthy bodies in order to appease the goddess Sitala and restore the balance of bodily humours. After the failed Indian uprising of 1857, in a context of racialization of British perceptions, smallpox

7 Chakrabarty, *Rethinking*.

8 Chakrabarty, *Provincializing Europe*; Chatterjee, *Nation and its Fragments*.

9 Arnold, *Colonizing the Body*.

vaccination lost its resonances with the local medical culture. It became a policy broadly enforced through inoculators recruited and trained by colonial medical officers, while elite families were courted to display their acceptance of the procedure. Smallpox vaccination was thus turned into a symbol of both the superiority of Western scientific medicine and its incommensurability with natives' medical cultures.

The legacy of the subalterns in the history of health beyond Europe has been quite significant. Recent works are, however, less concerned with hegemony and the colonization of bodies, than they are interested in the complex encounters and circulations that participated in the making of alternative medical modernity. In the case of India, two aspects of the latter have been investigated: 1) the transformation of 'traditional' practices to constitute medical systems perceived as decisive elements of an Indian national heritage; 2) the adaptation to—and borrowing of—European practices by Indian physicians who accordingly created hybrid medical cultures. Guy Attewell's exploration of the world of Ayurveda and Unani doctors in the late nineteenth and early 20th centuries is a good example of the first.[10] In *Nationalizing the Body*, Projit Mukharji, in turn, offers a convincing history of hybridization based on the practices of Bengali *daktari*, practitioners with or without qualifications who built a go-between medical world for a modern and unified India through the appropriation of biomedicine and its combination with indigenous knowledge.[11] Having collected texts and pamphlets written by Bengali doctors, most of them conserved in private hands, Mukharji traces the making of a nationalized body that emerged in parallel with Arnold's colonized body. He thus brings to the fore a different mode of subaltern agency than the latter's combination of hegemony, resistance, and compromise.

How can we summarize the shifts this subaltern historiography has performed? In terms of issues (Table 10.1), hegemony replaced exploitation, bringing in not only the idea that power is based on acceptance of the dominant discourses and practices, but also the fundamental idea that the subjects of power are not passive. The agency of subjects led not only to patterns of resistance but also to appropriation. This shift in the issues to consider is the consequence of choosing the subalterns as the main actors. The history is now written on the basis of what the 'natives' thought. This implies that the forms of capital considered are less metropolitan than local, more strongly associated with land and commerce than with industrial

10 Attewell, *Refiguring Unani Tibb.*
11 Mukharji, *Nationalizing the Body.*

production. The shift evidently required the mobilization of sources alternative to the colonial records in order to capture these voices in a more direct manner than reading institutional archives against the grain. These sources are not only less formal with written documents generally found in private collections but also ethnographies and interviews documenting the memories and legacies of the past. This has brought history into a deeper dialogue with other social sciences, and primarily with anthropology. In terms of content, the subaltern historiography of health is concerned not only with the management of epidemics (although they still figure prominently in the published works), but also with issues that, though barely discussed by the colonial administration, became major challenges for the local modernizers and the nationalists, for instance, famines and nutrition, changes in family life, or what was perceived as a 'weakening' of the colonized bodies. In parallel, the centrality of alternative modernization implies that the sources of knowledge taken into account are 'hybrid', with a critical role of reinvented and secularized medical traditions. Subaltern studies thus oscillate between 'history from below', with the emphasis initially placed on restoring the voices of the subjected, and therefore the religious dimension of healing powers, and capturing 'alternative modernity' with its unique dialectics of adaptation and opposition that grounded the rise of nationalism as the main framework to secularize and improve the practices of the local elite rather than the orally transmitted traditions of local healers.

In parallel with the rise of a subaltern historiography, another genre gained visibility in the 1990s: world history. The first issue of the *Journal of World History* thus explained:

> During the past two or three decades [...] historians have become increasingly aware of some inherent limitations in historical writing focused on national communities. [...] Many powerful historical forces simply do not respect national or even cultural boundary lines, but work their effects instead on a regional, continental, or global scale. To name but a few, these forces include population movements, economic fluctuations, climatic changes, transfers of technology, the spread of infectious and contagious diseases, imperial expansion, long-distance trade, and the spread of religious faiths, ideas, and ideals. In their efforts to analyze [...] these forces, scholars have generated a body of literature increasingly recognized as world history—historical analysis undertaken not from the viewpoint of national states, but rather from that of the global community.[12]

12 Bentley, 'New Forum', pp. iii–iv.

Since then, initiatives have been multiple, and 'global history', 'global studies', and 'history of globalization' have become reference terms for a specific mode of historiography insisting not only on the necessity of bringing together the histories of Europe and those of the rest of the world, but also on historicizing globalization, on the long-term existence of worldwide circulations and exchanges, and therefore on the multiple ways in which national or imperial histories have been connected.

Health is a highly relevant topic in this respect, not only because of the longue durée of multiple connections between Europe, the Americas, Africa, and Asia that the historical trajectory of cinchona, quinine, and malaria treatments over three centuries powerfully illustrates, but also because *global health* has—over the past 30 years—become a field in itself with its actors, institutions, programmes, and forms of knowledge that have a problematic relationship with previous patterns of interventions beyond the scale of one nation or one state.

The global is, however, a problematic category and point of entry. The historian Frederick Cooper thus writes in *Colonialism in Question* about the tyranny of the global.[13] Here, the tyranny comes in three forms. First, the global is an integral part of several hegemonic discourses (those of the financial economy, of the despaired progressive politicians, and of the postmodern 'dance of flows and fragments' that academics have taken up). Second, the global entails a dictate of 'presentism' such that history begins with contemporary issues, and is therefore barely compatible with approaches of the past for its own sake. Third, the global is always the global of a situated someone and it often goes with ungrounded generalization and the pretence of seeing from above and from nowhere, a syndrome shared with discourses of modernization.

World history has nonetheless addressed the challenge of inscribing the recent and transnational transformations of health in the past. The most visible strategy has been to write an international history focussing on the life of organizations, networks, enterprises, and individuals whose mere existence and field of action extend beyond national boundaries. Development aid, intergovernmental initiatives, and the UN system established after the Second World War are, in this respect, paramount. The current historiography tends to see their policies in deep continuity with those of colonial empires.

A good example is provided by the post-war malaria campaigns. Marcos Cueto argues that the malaria campaigns were typical outcomes of the

13 Cooper, *Colonialism in Question*.

controversial logic of a vertical programme favoured by a US-dominated international public health. They relied on a 'technological dream', focussing on a quick and single fix (Dichlorodiphenyltrichloroethane, DDT).[14] They equally built on strong confidence in short-term quasi-military interventions, led by foreign experts who mobilized operational research rather than clinical knowledge, and did not consider that specific knowledge of the local and social factors contributing to the transmission of the disease was needed. In addition, the malaria campaigns surfaced in the 1950s as Cold War attempts to use social investments to contain communism. Their termination was not only the result of mounting technical difficulties, but also of a shifting imperial agenda with the 1960s' growing commitment of US bilateral aid to population control. Finally, even if these campaigns were intergovernmental ventures grounded in the 'cooperation' between nation states, they continued the colonial policies of development based on technology transfer and medicalization designed by experts from the Global North.

Geopolitics is thus central in the narrative. In 2006, Theodore Brown, Marcos Cueto, and Elizabeth Fee published a seminal article entitled 'The World Health Organization and the Transition from International to Global Public Health'.[15] The change is seen as a political phenomenon to be placed in a large-scale context of geopolitical tensions, development strategies, and rivalry between international organizations. On that basis, global health appears as a response by prominent actors in international health—from US universities to WHO—crafted in order to adapt a rapidly changing international order as a consequence of: a) neoliberal reforms (the debt crises and structural adjustments, the creation of World Trade Organization [WTO], the globalization of intellectual property rights); and b) the fall of the Soviet bloc. This context helps to understand why the 1980s pleas against the Alma-Ata strategy, and for the return of vertical programmes, were backed by new actors like the World Bank or corporate philanthropy and became so powerful.

Not all global histories align on this pattern. Environmental history has, for instance, led to very different work when addressing industrial pollution or climate change with stronger interests in local sites and practices.[16] When it comes to health, the global has de facto favoured macroanalysis, placing geopolitics at the centre. The result (Table 10.1) is a historiography

14 Cueto, *Cold War.*
15 Brown et al., 'World Health Organization'.
16 Isenberg, *Oxford Handbook.*

based on international archives, which focusses on geopolitics and the general issues of development targets and strategies, neoliberal governance, and public-health policies. This has resulted in strong interest in the life of institutions, ranging from UN organizations to NGOs and nation states' administrative bodies, with insights into the processes of expertise, decision-making, and implementation. Within such a perspective, post-war programmes figure prominently, with important work done on the control of epidemics (malaria, smallpox), population control, and maternal/infant care. The forms of knowledge explored thus concern, in the first place, epidemiology, economics, and operational research. The forms of capital involved are almost exclusively those related to the rise of multinational enterprises: industrial capital and, for the most recent period and to a lesser extent, financial capital.

With all its richness of analysis and documentation, the global history of health thus seems to fall into the traps Frederick Cooper points out in his essay: running the risk of leaving out the practices of intervention, their contextual and localized nature, and the problematic generalization that accompanies the contemporary fabric of the global.[17] Thinking about alternatives, Cooper insists on the importance of circulation and transnational/connected histories showing that globalizations have been and are multiple. Historians should therefore target objects and issues that are more local and less global, looking at regional flows, networks, and diasporas, as well as territories, boundaries, and hindered moves. In order to open up the gaze and circumvent the asymmetry of archives and sources, historians should combine history and anthropology.[18]

Films and the Historiography of Health Government from the Colonial to the Global

Having put in place these different genres of historiography and the need for a stronger engagement between history and anthropology, it is striking that visual media appear to be missing, apart, maybe, from a significant but essentially illustrative use of photography. The question is therefore whether this situation is a matter of 'conjuncture', originating in historians' habits as they developed for a couple of decades, or a 'structural' matter,

17 Cooper, *Colonialism in Question.*

18 For a similar plea in the context of the history of health and medicine, see Harrison, 'Global Perspective'.

that is, linked to the very nature of films and their conditions of production, which result in their absence or their inappropriate status for a decentred history of health outside Europe and North America. In other words, could there be a visual colonial, subaltern, or world history of health and bodies, or is a visual rendering of the trilogy as a consequence of differing visual mediascapes in the Global South impossible?

Mere absence is clearly not the issue. The inventory of actors involved in the production of films about health and bodies in the 20th century includes colonial offices, industrial firms, the Health Organization of the League of Nations (and, later, the WHO), international health societies, multinational pharmaceutical firms, the World Bank, experts commissioned to visit developing countries, or anthropologists conducting individual as well as collective projects. Their genres are equally varied, from 'raw' documents in a research corpus to the personal souvenirs of prominent individuals, not to mention the impressive production of educational material.

Up to a recent period, however, most of this production (with the possible exception of untapped but most likely rare private sources) was not only institutional but Euro-American in origin and viewpoint. Just like imperial or global institutional archives, such films may be analysed against the grain and provide critical insights in the perspective and contradictions associated with 'external' interventions on the health and lives of others.

Films of the colonial period have often been associated with the presentation/promotion of specific campaigns or interventions. Directly echoing the events described by Guillaume Lachenal, the aforementioned *La mission Jamot au Cameroun* was produced in 1939 by the Pasteur Institute, using footage shot during the sleeping sickness control mission that Dr. Jamot led in the region of Ayos from 1926 to 1932.

The strong visual identity of the film first originates in the display of tropical medicine with its three mandatory dimensions: epidemiology, microbiology, and pathology. Epidemiological knowledge surfaces in two different ways. The first, at the beginning of the film, is the abstract display of numbers of deaths and affected persons (visible on-screen and spoken by a voice-over) and maps. The second is the sequence showing intervening teams establishing neighbourhood maps of incidence. Microbiology is, however, the iconic ingredient of the performance: Successive sequences include microscopes and technicians, slides preparation and colouring, inserts of (often drawn) images of cells and parasites, and close-ups of mosquitos.

The strong presence of pathology and clinical knowledge is the most specific aspect of *La mission Jamot*, with a long presentation of the training of African nurses (all males) received at the project's headquarters located in Ayos's hospital where, as the commentary explains, hundreds of affected patients gathered. Images of long lines waiting for examination thus precede a teaching sequence in which typical 'cases' of the different clinical syndromes associated with sleeping sickness are 'presented'. Moving images are 'doing the job' with no commentary. They reveal how the disease affects movements, how bodily control is lost with trembling patients, tics, falls, and finally paralysed patients (*grabataires*). Clinical knowledge is, to a large extent, a matter of diagnosis. In such a colonial context, it takes a rather specific form since it is always practised on collectives, that is, as screening. In *La mission Jamot*, diagnosis is based both on physical and on microscopic examinations. Sampling for blood and lymph fluid are presented as central tasks, with long shots of lymph and dorsal punctures practised on lines of waiting natives, while a commentary insists that the procedures have become routine ('two million performed in three years') and that they are demanded by the people.

This '*medicine de masse*' resonates with an aesthetics of mass campaigning. *La mission Jamot* powerfully presents the administrative and organizational nature of colonial medical ventures. It is not only that patients are almost exclusively forming lines; the interventions themselves are carried out by squads and mobiles units. These operate according to a well-defined division of labour and, in parallel, just like work on assembly lines. Microscopy is practised in groups (Figure 10.2), lymph node examination is a matter of a few standardized gestures, and record-keeping and delivery of medical cards is finally done by a specialized 'writer nurse' (*écrivain*) at the bottom end of the operating line. Unsurprisingly, performance is the outcome. It comes in the film with a final sequence bringing back the maps and numbers from the introduction but focussing on figures like the number of microscopic slides examined and the estimated number of lives saved (100,000) during the three years of the mission.

This penultimate sequence, however, fuses into the image of a laughing *Docteur Jamot*, happy to have 'awakened' Cameroon from its sleep. *La mission Jamot* is therefore also about this contrast of white characters and black bodies. Throughout the film, the difference and the hierarchy are visually made and remade: White doctors are carried along the way when squads move; with the exception of the trained African nurses, black bodies are barely clothed and are never subjects of the action. The apex of this display of disciplinary management of subaltern bodies is the practice of marking the results of diagnoses (T for trypanosomiasis) and the treatment dosage (ciphers of quantity to be inoculated) with white paint on patients' chests before they are sent to the *écrivain* (Figure 10.3).

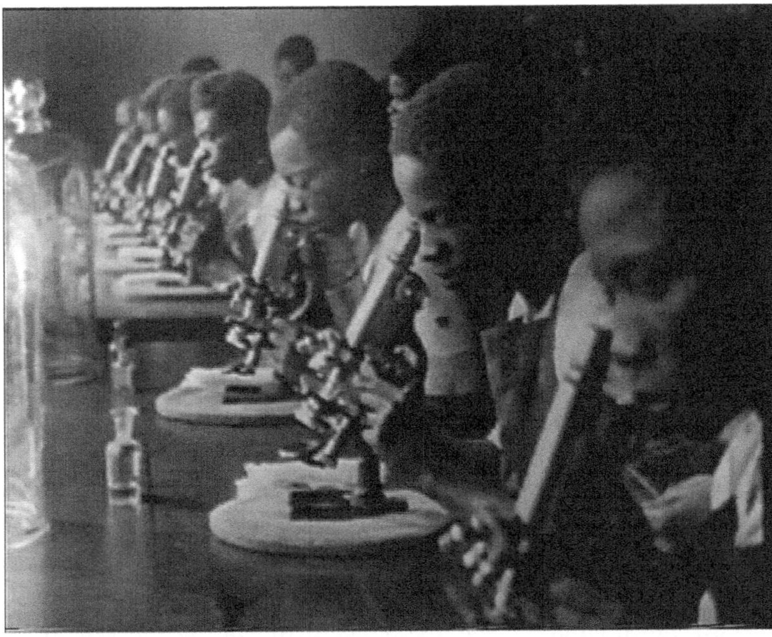

10.2. The mass diagnosis of sleeping sickness: microscopes and natives agents working in line, still taken from *La Mission Jamot*, 03:39 minutes.

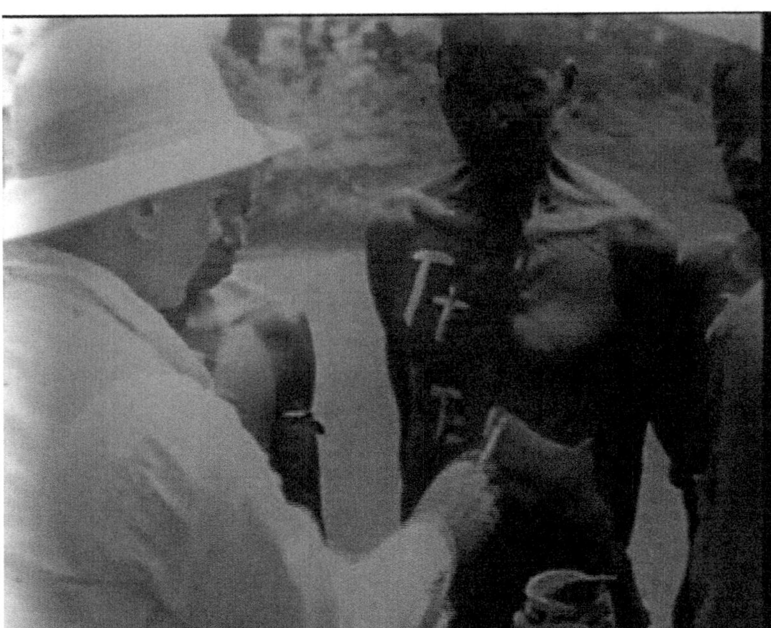

10.3. Black bodies, white doctors: painting the diagnosis' result and the treatment's dosage, still taken from *La Mission Jamot*, 14:47 minutes.

The relatively vast corpus of post-war malaria films could be used to explore the continuities of this visual culture of health campaigns before and after independence. Malaria films systematically mobilized the same elements: images of microscopes, working technicians, and microscopic shots to speak about the vectors and their cycle; long sequences of visiting teams at work, that is, sampling, examining bodies, and spraying DDT; technical artefacts ranging from DDT containers to spraying equipment and trucks; African bodies in lines or observing the intervening units.[19]

As the post-war era unfolded, significant shifts in modes of representation emerged. They challenged any scenario equating colonial projects, nation-state-based development programmes, and global health interventions in the name of outside, techno-centred, and disciplinary interventions. Research remains to be conducted in a careful and systematic way but one can—as a working hypothesis—consider two periods of significant shifts regarding both health programmes and body representations. The first one is post-war decolonization and the advent of development as a major paradigm used to think and organize *inter-national* government of health; the second one is the late 20th century and the neoliberal reshuffling of the political order.

Decolonization and the development era brought about major shifts, starting with the coming to the fore of 'Third World' nation states, which were capable of producing their own documentaries advocating for the alliance of nationalism, technology, and progress. But they also conveyed a new understanding of what the hegemony of the North might mean, with a vision of 'cooperation' under the umbrella of techno-commercial partnerships to free the world from diseases and organize a rational handling of populations and labour forces. These films thus highlight the transition from colonial *mise en valeur* to another regime of modernization and an unequal North-South relationship central to the historiography of global health: development.

A good example of the pervading presence of development aid in the postcolonial government of bodies is a 1958 documentary called *India's War against Malaria*, commissioned by the Indian Ministry of Health. It includes all the items of colonial tropical medicine campaigns, but differs from *La mission Jamot* in three ways. First, it originates with a state initiative and shows a *national* venture organized by the newly independent Indian state from the beginning to the end, even if the cooperation with the United States is acknowledged in the first sequence (but only as supplier of

19 For further discussion of this visual culture, see Bonah, 'Health Crusades'; Bonah, 'In the Service'.

massive amounts of DDT). Second, the documentary discusses not Western (European) science but the training of an *Indian* force which masters all the technologies of interventions, from microscopy to village surveys and training. Third, medical (clinical) knowledge is replaced with technologies in the most direct and physical sense of the term: the film barely shows villagers and instead focusses on operators handling laboratory instruments, trucks, DDT powder, and spraying material, and advocates one single control procedure, mosquito eradication, thus leaving out all questions of diagnosis and treatment.

Germany has a special place in this story as it faced a major challenge: redeeming itself from Nazi racism and its colonial forerunners. *Brücken der Hilfe* ('Bridges of help'), produced in 1952 by the chemical-pharmaceutical company Bayer, on the control of malaria may serve as an example as it radically departs from the standard malaria documentary in two decisive ways. First is the total absence of white people in non-European locations. Even if it follows malaria campaigning in Ghana, *Brücken der Hilfe* does not show a single white expert. All the qualified actors visible in the film are African technicians, nurses, and doctors who conduct surveys, look in microscopes, examine the bodies of their fellow countrypeople, distribute drugs, and spray insecticide. Moreover, the lines and assemblages of (black) bodies typical of *La mission Jamot* have disappeared, to be replaced by individuals, families, or informal gathering of village communities. The one exception relates to the conduct of blood sampling for diagnostic purposes, which shows a line of smiling women and children associated with an off-screen voice commenting on the fact that these women have no anxiety and were not '*kommandiert*' (commanded), but willing to participate in what is claimed to be a performance. *Brücken der Hilfe* thus constructs an image of health intervention as a local venture, organized by Africans for Africans, who willingly consent because they share the project's common goals. Spraying for mosquitoes is shown less as a procedural success and more as an interaction: While the visiting team prepares the insecticide solution, they are observed by the village assembly and the editing alternates between shots of working technicians and smiling, curious inhabitants. Similarly, in contrast to the rash entry of spraying units into houses, displayed in most malaria films, here, the indoor spraying sequence begins with a conversation between the team and the family whose house is treated (Figure 10.4).

If eradication is a matter of African mobilization for the benefit of Africans, where is development aid? This is the second level of discontinuity operating in *Brücken der Hilfe*: It reveals how a new division of labour is emerging, with Africans as performers and Europeans still the bearers of

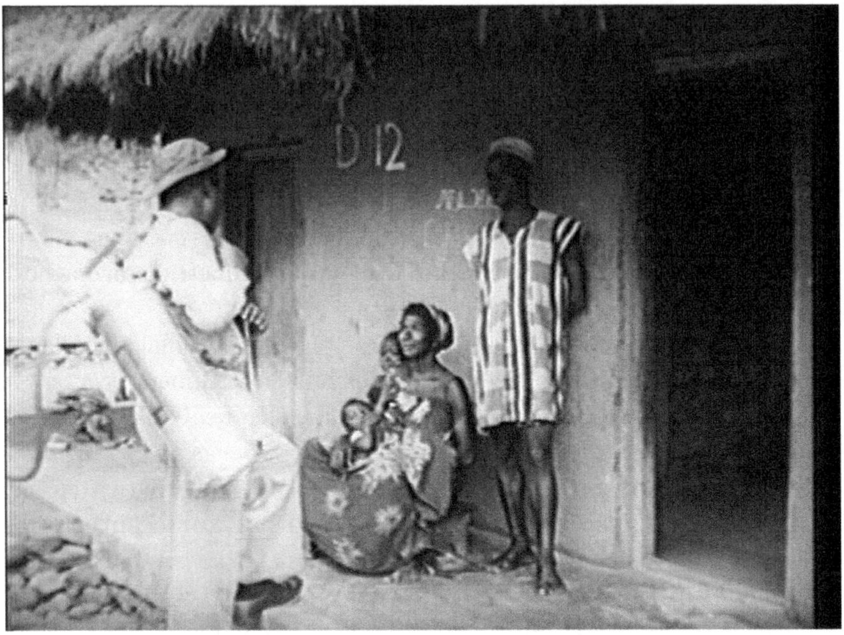

10.4. *Brücken-der-Hilfe*-Spreading units negotiating access to a village house with its inhabitants, still taken from Brücken der Hilfe, 11:26 minutes.

knowledge. As producer of the documentary, Bayer figures prominently in its narrative. Bayer and its factories (there is a long panoramic of the Leverkusen plants viewed from the sky at the end of the film) appear not as a *commanding* centre but as a *research* centre and a (tacitly market-oriented) supplier of chemical substances. In the middle of the film, a long sequence (five minutes out of a total of thirteen) narrates the history of anti-malarial drug research in Bayer's in-house laboratories. The oral listing of chemicals, trials, and effects is superimposed on images of laboratory work and production machinery that depict only chemistry and its power: technicians filling glass vessels, filtering preparations, holding measurement apparatuses, working on the background of a library of chemicals with several dozen storage vessels (Figure 10.5), testing the effects on chickens. It ends with a new miracle insecticide powder flowing out of machines.

This promotion of pharmaceutical research and development (R&D) leads up to the concluding narrative when—after the presentation of spraying teams—the films returns to Germany in order to discuss the problem of the increasing resistance of mosquitos. Far from shying away from the problem or advocating the then common response in terms of speed and enlarged mobilization to achieve eradication, the commentary—again, against the

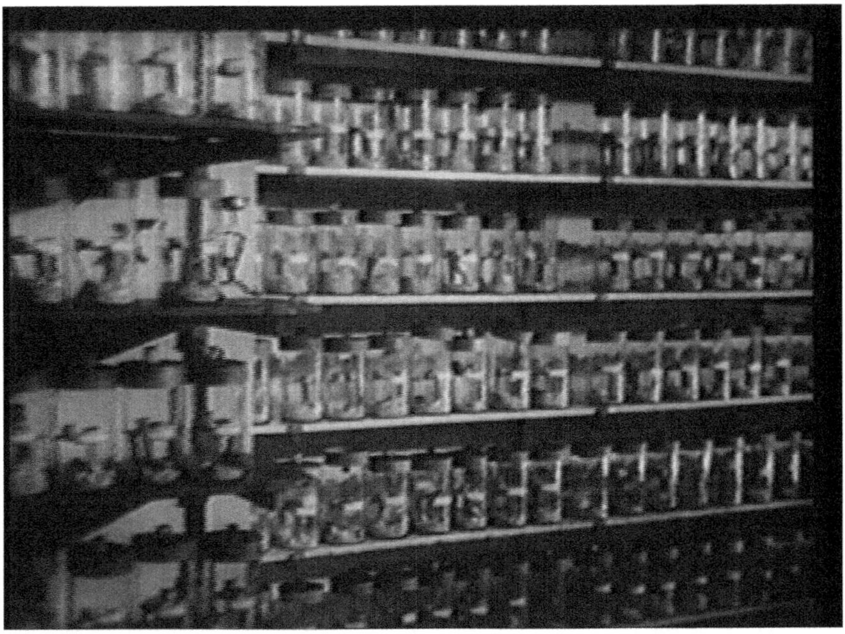

10.5. The search for molecules as main contribution of Bayer to development aid, still taken from *Brücken der Hilfe*, 06:31 minutes.

background of chemical laboratory images—highlights the ability of the German chemical industry to search for new molecules that will be tested and employed in the South in order to win the global race of 'research versus resistance'. Beyond the colonial/development transition, *Brücken der Hilfe* thus points to continuities between development and the present imagery/imaginary of global health.

Given the scale of this institutional production of films, there is little doubt that imperial and world historiographies of health, bodies, and capital beyond Europe would benefit from a more decisive and systematic reliance on media sources and their historiography. The most difficult question our typology raises is, however, that of a possible subaltern historiography, since the latter centres on voices that are much more difficult to hear in a corpus produced almost exclusively by actors from the Global North. However, one peculiar genre is equivalent to the anthropological sources subaltern historians have revisited and used, namely the small but significant production of ethnographic documentaries, which started in the interwar period and grew rapidly after the war.

Jean Rouch is, in this respect, an obligatory passage point. In *Les maîtres fous*, shot in 1955 in Accra (Ghana), Rouch explored one of the many rituals

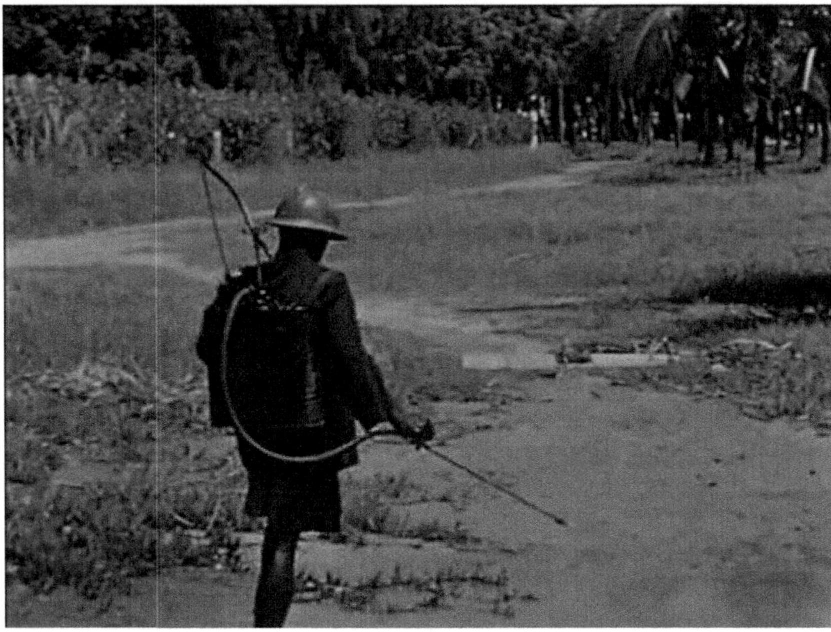

10.6. Modernization agents at work in Accra: the hygiene boy, still taken from *Les maîtres fous*, 03:00 minutes.

of possession that he would later follow with his camera. Rouch insisted on the indispensability of images, not only to better capture the complexity of actions and the centrality of bodies and movements, but also as the only way to convey something of events that Western words and categories could barely render.

The film starts with shots of Accra, one of the massive urban centres then growing in Africa ('*une Babylone noire*' says the voice-over), with images of streets, crowd assemblies, and a long sequence displaying workers: carriers, smugglers, bottle boys, timber boys, gold mine workers, and 'hygiene boys' spraying insecticides (Figure 10.6). The intent is to show the challenge the new urban order poses to all those who join it, coming from the northern rural areas. How would they survive the noise, the agitation, the painful and harsh working conditions? The possession rituals are ingredients of the response Rouch is investigating, and the camera follows members of the *haouka* sect on their way to a distant plantation.

The second and longest section of the film presents the possession ritual itself with its different phases: the presentation of new members, the public confession, the display of personalities acquired as an effect of being possessed by one of the *houakas* ('the gods of the city, of technology, of power,

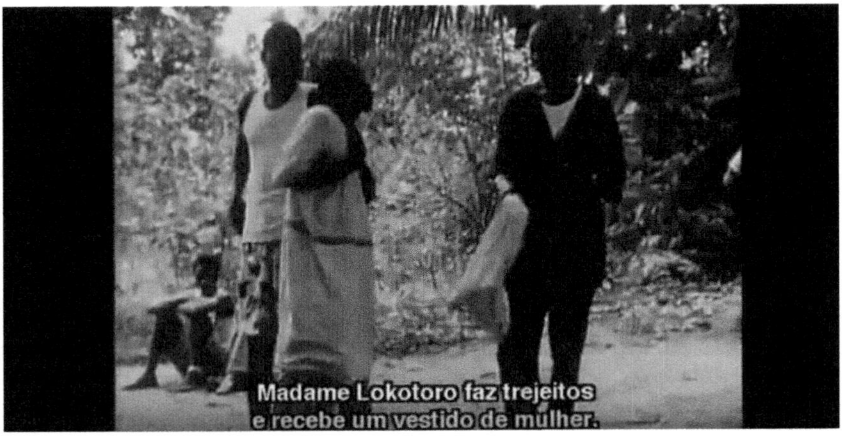

10.7. Mrs. Lokotoro, key character of the *haoukas'* possession ritual, still taken from *Les maîtres fous*, 14:45 minutes. The subtitle says 'Mrs. Lokotoro makes fits and receives a woman dress'.

of "the force"', says the voice-over), and finally the sacrifice and eating of a dog. Although the film was attacked for its display of hallucinating, 'crazy' Africans as well as the violence of some scenes, Rouch's images and commentary support a social-science reading of the situation. Entering the plantation, the camera focusses on the artefacts used: pieces of cloth displayed as flags (*Union Jacks*), a termite nest painted in black and white (*the governor's palace*), pith helmets, wooden rifles, commanding scarfs, etc. The most revealing sequence is, in that respect, the shots showing the possessed men and their respective *haouka*—most of them military characters (a lieutenant, a corporal, a general, the governor himself) or linked to the masters' technology with an engine driver and Mrs. Lokotoro, the doctor's wife (Figure 10.7)—who enact protocols of inspection, parade, surveillance, conferences, or round tables. The ceremony is mimicking the colonial order, combining mockery and appropriation of the white people's own rituals. In order to make this reading more convincing, Rouch even inserts a sequence of images of a British army corps in Ghana saluting the flag. The third section follows the participants of the ritual the next day, after they have returned to Accra and resumed their normal activities. Ironically, the leading *haoukas* are waterworks employees digging trenches in front of the local psychiatric hospital. The last comment of the voice-over thus suggests that these men are such good workers because—with possession rituals—they have found 'a remedy not to become abnormal', a remedy that European medicine neither has nor understands.

Even if Mrs. Lokotoro, the doctor's wife, could be incorporated into a narrative of colonial government of health (and of its hijacking), the most important aspect of Rouch's cinema for our discussion is not its direct documentary value but the positioning it reveals. In a vein similar to postcolonial histories like Nancy Rose Hunt's recent work on health rituals, insurgencies, medicalization, and population management in Congo, for which she decisively uses oral stories, songs, rumours, and diaries, Rouch seeks to capture otherwise unrecorded voices, and oscillates between two registers of interpretation. The first one, which prevails throughout the commentary, is that of rationalization, with the idea that the members of the *haouka* sect have invented a form of moral resistance: Mimicking the rituals of British rulers is at once a way to disempower them and to capture their symbolic power. From this perspective, possession is both foreign as a form and familiar as a process. It may be accounted for in the same way that the social sciences have secularized and read Christian rituals, and this preserves the view from outside that the voice-over perfectly instantiates.

The second register of interpretation echoes the Subaltern Studies Collective's warning that such rationalization can remain a master discourse since it dismisses the actors' own motives and explanations for their actions and turns the ritual into a symbolic event, denying the existence of *haoukas* and possession as such. When David Arnold discussed the indigenous ritual of smallpox transfer in colonial India, he argued that what was inacceptable in the British transformation of the practice into vaccination was its secularization, the erasing of all links with the goddess Sitala. Rouch tries to avoid this very same trap in the last scenes of the film when the commentary introduces a different reading of possession, speaking of a 'remedy' through which the colonized subjects confront the madness of living in Accra, can perform their duties as workers without losing their minds, and thereby gain agency. The *haoukas* are therefore not only real *for them* but they are real *for us* since they make possible something—a form of cure or a mode of socialization—that European societies have either lost or never found in the first place.

Les maîtres fous thus offers the same response to the problem of hegemony and its critical reading as the subaltern historiography does, namely, balancing recording and retelling, to promote decentred voices. Such strategy might well have become commonplace in ethnographic filming after the Second World War when the divorce with imperial anthropology was consumed. Rouch was, however, never fully satisfied with the commenting voice, and he was also ready to let things go in a more profound way, rewriting scenarios with the performers he was studying, or handing the camera to them. This transfer of agency acquired institutional dimensions with the establishment of a film section within the new social-science institute created in Niamey after independence, that Rouch directed and where a whole generation of Nigerian ethnographers and film-makers emerged.

Although a subaltern historiography of body capital in the period from the 1930s to the 1970s may tap into the corpus of ethnographic documentaries, it is important to point out the diversification of possible sources when production in the Global South diversified from the early 1960s onwards. *Farm to Pharmacy* mentioned above, along with its promotion of a 'neo-traditional' vision of health, bodies, and capital, is not an isolated example. A history of global health and its relations to the neoliberal mode of body government could thus rely on a palette of visual sources in addition to the documentaries that Northern players made to promote their new agenda of health for growth, risk management, sustainable development, and community participation.

Conclusion

Michel Foucault's famous lessons on the birth of biopolitics did not delve much into the government of populations but focussed on the advent on neoliberalism and what he perceived to be major shifts in the relationship between the state and the market. The new politico-economic order that Foucault sought to identify may be seen as the most recent step in the transition from a regime revolving around disciplines and sovereignty, to a regime of governmentality revolving around norms of conduct, regulation, and individuals' choices.

Echoing this distinction, this chapter has discussed the recently decentred historiography of the body and health practices, focussing on the ways in which writing a history of health government beyond Europe has shifted our understanding of the local and the global (and thus the relationship between history and anthropology), the status of Western and non-Western health practices, and the dialectics between discipline and regulation. It thus distinguishes three modes of writing about bodies, health, and capital (Table 10.1): colonial history with its focus on empires, processes of diffusion from the centre to the periphery, and mass-campaigning; postcolonial and subaltern history, which seeks to 'provincialize' Europe through local stories of hegemony, resistance, and alternative modernity; and global history with its interest in geopolitics, international arenas, flows, and development.

Such a classificatory exercise is always schematic, as it operates on the basis of a limited set of categories and does not do justice to the forms of historical writing that fail to match, or that blur, the neat arrangement of types. Typology is nonetheless helpful in: a) emphasizing the relative coherence of each mode of historiography, as the grid helps to reveal its strengths and blind spots, as well as its relationship to peculiar periods in the 20th-century trajectory of health government; b) highlighting the benefits of new ways of articulating these three modes, and thus furthering our understanding of the critical role of neoliberalism—including its limitations—in the contemporary dialectics of capital, bodies, and government.

Having put in place these different genres of historiography, it is striking that visual media barely play a role in their operations. The first claim of this chapter is therefore that a more decisive engagement with the history of visuals will greatly benefit our understanding of the changing relationship between capital, bodies, and government beyond Europe. This perspective, however, raises the difficult issue of sources. Decentring implies access to sources beyond those produced by the 'big actors' of imperial, international, or global health. Up to a recent period, most of the production of films and visuals was not only institutional but Euro-American in origin and viewpoint. Such films provide critical insights into the perspective and contradictions associated with 'external' interventions on the health and lives of others. A subaltern historiography of body capital should, however, tap into alternative corpuses, which may include not only ethnographic films but also the multiple visuals produced in the Global South from the early 1960s onward. Since the latter production has rarely figured in studies of (non-fiction) films, its existence grounds the second claim of this chapter, namely, that the historiography of visuals may benefit from a double decentring: provincializing Europe and North America, as well as big players.

Works Cited

Films, Television Programmes, and Recordings

Brücken der Hilfe, produced by Bayer, 1952.

Farm to Pharmacy: A Modern Approach for Traditional Medicine, Umbrella Programme on Natural Resource Management India, 2011, https://www.youtube.com/watch?v=BeF4HyIUNKU, accessed 14 August 2018.

India's War against Malaria, India Ministry of Health, 1958, https://www.youtube.com/watch?v=nD8kFvedkJo, accessed 14 August 2018.

Les maîtres fous, directed by Jean Rouch, 1955 in Jean Rouch, *Le geste cinématographique*, 4-DVD-Edition (Paris: Editions Montparnasse, 2005).

La mission Jamot au Cameroun (1926–1932), Institut Pasteur, 1939, http://medfilm.unistra. fr/wiki/La_mission_Jamot_au_Cameroun, accessed 14 August 2018.

Books and Articles

Arnold, David, *Colonizing the Body: State Medicine and Epidemic Disease in Nineteenth- Century India* (Berkeley: University of California Press, 1993).

Attewell, Guy N. A., *Refiguring Unani Tibb: Plural Healing in Late Colonial India* (New Delhi: Orient Longam, 2007).

Bentley, Jerry H., 'A New Forum for Global History', *Journal of World History*, 1, 1 (1990), pp. iii–v.

Bonah, Christian, 'In the Service of Industry and Human Health: The Bayer Corporation, Industrial Film, and Promotional Propaganda, 1934–42', in *Health Education and Film in the Twentieth Century*, ed. by Christian Bonah, David Cantor, and Anja Laukötter (Rochester: Rochester University Press, 2018), pp. 85–142.

Bonah, Christian, '"Health Crusades": Environmental Approaches as Public Health Strategies against Infections in Sanitary Propaganda Films, 1930–60', in *Environment, Health and History*, ed. by Virginia Berridge and Martin Gorsky (London: Palgrave Macmillan, 2012), pp. 154–177.

Brown, Theodore M., Marcos Cueto, and Elizabeth Fee, 'The World Health Organization and the Transition from International to Global Public Health', *American Journal of Public Health*, 96, 1 (2006), pp. 62–72, doi:10.2105/AJPH.2004.050831.

Chakrabarty, Dipesh, *Rethinking Working Class History: Bengal 1890–1940* (Princeton: Princeton University Press, 1989).

Chakrabarty, Dipesh, *Provincializing Europe: Postcolonial Thought and Historical Difference* (Princeton: Princeton University Press, 2000).

Chatterjee, Partha, *The Nation and its Fragments: Colonial and Postcolonial Histories* (Princeton: Princeton University Press, 1993).

Cooper, Frederick, *Colonialism in Question: Theory, Knowledge, History* (Berkeley: University of California Press, 2005).

Cueto, Marcos, *Cold War, Deadly Fevers: Malaria Eradication in Mexico, 1955–1975* (Baltimore: Johns Hopkins University Press, 2007).

Foucault, Michel, *Naissance de la biopolitique: Cours au Collège de France (1978–1979)* (Paris: Gallimard-Seuil, 2004).

Harrison, Mark, *Public Health in British India: Anglo-Indian Preventive Medicine 1859–1914* (Cambridge: Cambridge University Press, 1994).

Harrison, Mark, *Medicine in an Age of Commerce and Empire: Britain and its Tropical Colonies, 1660–1830* (Oxford: Oxford University Press, 2010).

Harrison, Mark, 'A Global Perspective: Reframing the History of Health, Medicine, and Disease', *Bulletin of the History of Medicine*, 89, 4 (2015), pp. 639–689, doi:10.1353/bhm.2015.0116.

Isenberg, Andrew C., ed., *The Oxford Handbook of Environmental History* (Oxford: Oxford University Press, 2017).

Keller, Richard C., *Colonial Madness: Psychiatry in French North Africa* (Chicago: University of Chicago Press, 2007).
Lachenal, Guillaume, *Le médicament qui devait sauver l'Afrique: Un scandale pharmaceutique aux colonies* (Paris: Découverte, 2014).
Mukharji, Projit Bihari, *Nationalizing the Body: The Medical Market, Print and Daktari Medicine* (London: Anthem, 2011).
Pati, Biswamoy, and Mark Harrison, eds., *Health, Medicine and Empire: Perspectives on Colonial India* (Hyderabad: Orient Longam, 2001).
Rose, Nikolas, *The Politics of Life Itself: Biomedicine, Power, and Subjectivity in the Twenty-First Century* (Princeton: Princeton University Press, 2007).

About the Author

Jean-Paul Gaudillière is historian of science and medicine and senior researcher at Inserm. His recent work focuses on the history of pharmaceutical innovation and the uses of drugs on the one hand, the dynamics of health globalization on the other hand. Since 2014 he has been leading the ERC project 'From international to global: Knowledge, disease and the post-war government of health'.
Contact details: jean-paul.gaudilliere@cnrs.fr

11. Zika Virus, Global Health Communication, and Dataveillance

Kirsten Ostherr

Abstract
Through analysis of media produced by the World Health Organization (WHO) in response to the Zika virus outbreak of 2016, this chapter demonstrates how distributed digital communication networks such as social media platforms have created significant challenges for the WHO's top-down model of information management. Unlike disease outbreaks of the past, Zika virus media circulated through mobile, social digital networks shaped by invisible algorithms and filter bubbles that helped generate counter narratives opposing the communications of official health organizations. This chapter examines Zika virus media through the analytical frames of datafication, dataveillance, and data-making to explain how diverse sources of information and social contexts of interpretation pose new challenges for global health communications.

Keywords: World Health Organization; Zika virus; health communication; datafication; dataveillance; data-making; contagion; social determinants of health; YouTube; WhatsApp; Facebook

Introduction

In the years immediately following the creation of the World Health Organization (WHO) in 1948, several films were made that presented the aspirations of this new initiative to audiences around the globe. One of those films, *The Eternal Fight* (United Nations [UN]/WHO, 1948), offered a rhetorically and stylistically sophisticated narrative of humankind's failed efforts to conquer disease through the ages. The story culminates with the creation of the WHO as a turning point in the ongoing battle

Bonah, C. and A. Laukötter (eds.), *Body, Capital, and Screens: Visual Media and the Healthy Self in the 20th Century*. Taylor & Francis Group, 2020
DOI 10.5117/9789462988293_CH11

against infectious diseases worldwide. Through a combination of live-action footage, animation, melodramatic musical score, and booming voice-over, *The Eternal Fight* dramatizes the global threat posed by highly contagious diseases such as plague and cholera. Using animated world maps, the film pointedly traces the flow of disease from less developed parts of the world to the congested urban centres that facilitate population-scale pandemics. Highlighting the role of global transportation in spreading disease and the role of global communications in halting their spread, *The Eternal Fight* presents a vision of a technologically mediated planet in need of mastery by the tools of modern surveillance and containment. The film's vision of WHO as the planet's centralized command and control headquarters conveys a tone of benevolent paternalism mixed with imperialist civilizing mission, modified by a somewhat incongruous claim of fraternalism, as the voice-over proclaims, 'All peoples of every race and belief will be helped by doctors from all races and nations. A tremendous movement of world solidarity is now born'.

As an audiovisual expression of the WHO's mission, *The Eternal Fight* captures the organization's top-down perspective on health promotion and disease eradication. Experts would assemble, analyse problems, identify solutions, and implement them in the field. In cases of sudden outbreaks, health workers would be rapidly dispatched to halt the spread of infection. Local communities would benefit from the expert knowledge made available to their territories, and, once the health problem was contained, the experts would leave. The centralized, hierarchical, and unidirectional model of knowledge dissemination in this film mirrors that of WHO and most large organizations in the post-Second World War era. Just as motion pictures were a closed form of communication that could send a sealed message in one direction to a receptive audience, the WHO was an assembly of health experts who sent professional guidance and relief to hotspots around the world with no possibility of dialogue, debate, or multidirectional exchange.

The principles and aesthetics embedded in *The Eternal Fight* illuminate the historical specificity of the approaches to health promotion and health communication of the post-war era, while also highlighting the transition from international to global health frameworks for imagining the processes of disease interventions.[1] By comparing this example to recent media productions by WHO in response to the Zika virus outbreak of 2016, we can see how changes in peer-to-peer connectivity based on distributed digital

1 Brown et al., 'World Health Organization'. See also the contribution by Jean-Paul Gaudillière in this volume.

communication networks such as social-media platforms have created significant challenges for the WHO's formal, top-down model of information management. The entry of Zika virus into global awareness has been a highly visual and digitally intermediated phenomenon, characterized by both familiar and novel contagion iconography. Unlike disease outbreaks of the past, Zika virus media circulated through mobile, social digital networks shaped by invisible algorithms and filter bubbles that helped generate counter-narratives opposing the communications of official health organizations. This chapter examines Zika virus media through the analytical frames of datafication, dataveillance, and data-making to explain how diverse sources of information and social contexts of interpretation pose new challenges for global health communications. The essay explores how datafication and narration of disease outbreaks has changed from the post-Second World War era to the present, with attention to the ways that emerging digital health platforms for health communication give rise to new concerns about the intersections of personal and global health data. These practices of health datafication create new forms of body capital that provide opportunities for alternative collectivities to emerge, while also contributing to the persistence of certain types of post-war subject formations. As an emblematic post-war use of visual material to convey the ideals of the WHO, *The Eternal Fight* captures a moment in the history of screen-based media that expands from celluloid projections to globally disseminated and increasingly personalized screens. The chapter concludes with a commentary on a short public-service cartoon, *Misión Zika* (2016), a recent co-production by the Cartoon Network, WHO, Pan American Health Organization (PAHO), and United Nations Children's Emergency Fund (UNICEF) that captures the aesthetic adaptation to digital screen culture of 21st-century health communication.

Health Datafication

Ordinary citizens around the world have begun to play an important role in collecting data about health and disease. With mobile connectivity around the world averaging 112 per cent (reflecting a total above 100 per cent due to cases of individual ownership of multiple devices), citizens' daily lives have become experiments 'in the wild', whose digital traces offer new kinds of information about human behaviour and exposures outside of the controlled settings of lab-based studies.[2] Step counters, continuous heart

2 Kemp, 'Digital in 2018', p. 91.

rate monitors, sleep trackers, calorie counters, and other types of activity trackers are popular features of wearable devices that are marketed directly to consumers. These devices contribute to a practice known as 'datafication', that is, the conversion of real-world measurements into digital constructions of reality.[3] Datafication has been further described as the process of 'rendering into data aspects of the world not previously quantified'.[4] This transformation of existing data into actionable forms generates diverse and unevenly distributed kinds of value for their producers and consumers.[5] As a result, historian Dan Bouk argues, 'individuals generate many data doubles that are commodified, capitalized, collected, celebrated, and often out of the control of those they represent'.[6] In this context, we can see health datafication as a new form of body capital that uses new techniques for measuring and counting the behaviours and exposures of daily life, generating novel forms of value when coupled with data analytics, as I will discuss below. In addition, contemporary practices of health datafication occur both within and beyond clinical settings, posing challenges to traditional understandings of agency and ownership of medical data. Consequently, these practices also challenge traditional approaches to health communication.

Current statistics about digital connectivity around the world highlight the globe scale of this phenomenon, illuminating the uneven distribution of datafication, while nonetheless showing annual trends indicating steady growth. As of January 2018, 53 per cent of the earth's human population used the internet, and 68 per cent used mobile devices.[7] Much of the world is hyper-connected through the mobile web-based devices that are constantly producing digital footprints and creating conditions of possibility for datafication of ever more aspects of daily life, including health datafication. For example, in the Asia-Pacific region, the single largest market for wearables in the world, mobile connectivity is at 102 per cent.[8] Not surprisingly, internet use globally is growing more slowly than mobile. These newer technologies leapfrog over the old wire and cable infrastructure of the internet to make new kinds of distributed networks of data that, in their untethered mobility, displace older models of state control of disease surveillance. In many low- and middle-income countries, mobile networks create new opportunities for disease surveillance through digital connectivity that previously were

3 Mayer-Schönberger and Cukier, *Big Data*.
4 Kennedy et al., 'Data and Agency', p. 1.
5 van Dijck, 'Datafication'.
6 Bouk, 'History and Political Economy', p. 85.
7 Kemp, 'Digital in 2018', p. 7.
8 Carter, 'Why Wearables Have'.

not possible in the absence of wired telecommunications infrastructures.[9] While the new paradigm relocates datafication within corporate power structures in many instances, it also remains subject to state control of information and communication. In contrast to lower overall rates and high global variance in internet connectivity, most of the planet is near or above 100 per cent mobile connectivity.[10]

In many parts of the world, at least 50 per cent of the population also uses social media, signalling that this form of communication is neither fully dominant, nor irrelevant as a source of images and narratives about current events, including disease outbreaks.[11] The most widely used social-media platforms around the world are Facebook, YouTube, WhatsApp, Facebook Messenger, WeChat, Tencent QQ, Instagram, Tumblr, Ozone, Sina Weibo, and Twitter.[12] As the world becomes increasingly digitally mediated, everything that users do on mobile, social networks becomes part of the process of datafication. Moreover, the vast data sets that are generated from the casual activities of everyday life are being combined with other data sets, and the assembled purchases, travel, communication, geography, banking, and other kinds of data are used to create digital profiles of users that shape the reality reflected back to them online.

The rise of 'user-generated content' (UGC), that is, voluntarily contributed data such as hotel ratings, purchase feedback, or homemade videos from ordinary internet users, has enabled individual citizens' digital footprints to collectively add up to very large, and potentially very valuable data sets.[13] As the health relevance of UGC became obvious to researchers and marketers in the early years of the 21st century, incidental data from mapping apps using global positioning systems (GPS), mobile shopping, restaurant reservation, and rating apps, as well as the data from social-media platforms became part of a complex digital-profiling system with significant influence on mobile health communications.[14] In addition, the growing popularity of wearable health and wellness trackers from Apple, Fitbit, Xiaomi, Garmin, and Huawei (the top five wearables companies worldwide), has created an abundance of user-generated health data. For the year 2017, total wearable device shipments worldwide reached 115.4 million units, up 10.3 per cent from

9 Wallis et al., 'Integrating mHealth'.
10 Kemp, 'Digital in 2018', pp. 29, 95.
11 Kemp, 'Digital in 2018', p. 51; World Health Organization, *Global Diffusion*, p. 127.
12 Kemp, 'Digital in 2018', p. 59.
13 Krumm et al., 'User-Generated Content'; Van Dijck, 'Users Like You'.
14 Ostherr et al., 'Trust and Privacy'; Ostherr, 'Facebook Knows a Ton'.

the 104.6 million units shipped in 2016.[15] This means that at least 115 million people were counting steps, checking their heart rates, and tracking other data, in addition to generating a multibillion-dollar industry worldwide. Yet, these devices are consumer products accessible only to those who can afford to purchase them and maintain their functionality through internet access and up-to-date smartphone interfaces. In this way, digital tracking and counting reproduces the uneven global distribution of information, capital, and health training that is present throughout the history of body capital. Importantly, like the incidental health data derived from GPS or social media, user-generated health data are produced, shared, and exploited under poorly defined privacy and ownership policies.[16] For example, the terms of use for most wearables stipulates that the company can sell the data collected by the device to third parties in the course of business deals.[17]

In terms of implications for public health, these vast data sets are widely seen as providing new sources of insight from exposures 'in the wild', creating possibilities for hypothesizing new kinds of correlations or even causations between behaviours, exposures, and health outcomes. Yet, as the healthcare industry has begun to embrace big data, a problematic adaptation of Ackoff's hierarchy has taken hold: more data equals more knowledge equals better health outcomes.[18] Ubiquitous environmental and lifestyle data from wearable technologies and mobile apps promise to uncover new indicators of health and illness from outside of traditional clinical settings. But there are many assumptions embedded in this equation. What new kinds of knowledge might these insights reveal, and for whom might they improve outcomes? The novel achievements of user-generated health data rely heavily on participants' willingness to share their data, even when doing so may not serve their own best interests.[19] The question of who benefits from big health data is therefore entangled with questions about data ownership, sharing, trust, and privacy. Under conditions of health datafication, individuals often produce data without knowing that they are doing so.

Could these new data sources help to address Social Determinants of Health (SDOH)? Public health-orientated researchers have long argued that biomedical constructs must expand to include SDOH in order to address the complex, multidimensional lived experience of disease rather than the

15 International Data Corporation, 'Global Wearables'.
16 Lupton, *Quantified Self*; Neff and Nafus, *Self-Tracking*.
17 Ostherr, 'Privacy'.
18 Ackoff, 'From Data to Wisdom'; Strasser and Edwards, 'Big Data'.
19 Leaf, 'Biggest Share'.

narrowly defined pathophysiology of disease.[20] The World Health Organization defines SDOH as 'the conditions in which people are born, grow, work, live, and age, and the wider set of forces and systems shaping the conditions of daily life'.[21] In light of its capacity to shape the conditions of daily life, I would argue that we now need to consider datafication as an element of SDOH, both for those individuals and communities who are considered 'data rich' and those who are considered 'data poor'.[22] Individuals and communities with the resources to engage in self-tracking behaviour that generates large quantities of health data can be considered 'data rich', while those with limited access to tracking devices might be understood as 'data poor'. These definitions must be nuanced, as self-tracking behaviour does not equate to the ability to gain value from that data, and, in some cases, may only result in increased dataveillance.[23] Similarly, absence of self-tracking does not prevent other forms of dataveillance on those individuals and communities, and the meaning of fainter digital signals emitting from specific groups is not self-evident, particularly for socially marginalized groups. That is, some communities may prefer to leave less 'digital exhaust' in order to evade detection by government and other authorities.[24] Health datafication as seen through the lens of SDOH is therefore a complex nexus of power relations. It offers potentially life-saving benefits for patients with chronic diseases, as well as those faced with emerging infectious diseases. At the same time, datafied SDOH can contribute to practices of surveillance and control, while creating opportunities for medico-corporate profit and exploitation. If wearable health technologies capture SDOH, can they democratize access to care? Or will they exacerbate health disparities? Or both?

Visual Iconography of Contagion: Zika Virus

By examining the visual iconography of Zika virus communications in 2016 in relation to the concept of health datafication, we can see how long-standing

20 Dahlgren and Whitehead, *Policies and Strategies*.

21 World Health Organization, *Social Determinants*, not paginated [p. 1].

22 boyd and Crawford, 'Critical Questions'.

23 'Dataveillance' is discussed at length below, but the term can be provisionally defined as 'an increasingly preferred way of monitoring citizens through social media and online communication technologies'; Van Dijck, 'Datafication', p. 204, citing Raley, 'Dataveillance and Countervailance'.

24 Zuboff, 'Big Other'; Raley, 'Dataveillance and Countervailance', p. 131, quoting Giddens, *Nation-State*.

modes of representing contagion intersect with digital network effects, thereby transforming contemporary practices of health communication. A significant feature of this mediascape is the interplay between the content of the images and their modes of transmission. This section will analyse how health datafication in the context of Zika virus has enabled the emergence of powerful counter-narratives to official health communication scripts through reinterpretation of Zika media. Such narratives based on 'alternative facts' have viral transmission capacity that can destabilize traditional knowledge hierarchies in healthcare.[25]

Historical analysis of Zika media provides a contextual framework for understanding the role of visual imagery in shaping ideas about disease. Attention to this domain of meaning-making is critically important in part because it has a long, influential history of reflecting and shaping social norms and reinforcing moralistic attitudes about social responsibility and contagion.[26] Additional importance derives from the fact that digital media information and communication networks that provide the substrata of datafication are heavily image-based. Indeed, many scholars have argued that the digital age is characterized in part by a shift from text- to image-based forms of communication, though those images of course carry highly significant textual metadata along with them.[27] Recall that YouTube and Instagram are among the most used social platforms worldwide.[28]

Since the virus came to global public awareness during the lead up to the summer Olympics in Rio de Janeiro, Brazil in 2016, Zika has been a highly visual and digitally intermediated phenomenon, drawing on both familiar and unfamiliar visual iconography that spread rapidly through Brazil's networked population, with its 113 per cent mobile connectivity rate.[29] Prominent representational tropes with historical antecedents include close-ups of mosquitoes,[30] global and local maps of contagion (including transmission pathways and localized prevalence),[31] travel advisories,[32] health workers in face masks or biohazard space suits spraying for mosquitoes,[33]

25 Shtulman, 'In Public Understanding'.
26 Ostherr, *Cinematic Prophylaxis*.
27 Baudrillard, *Simulacra and Simulation*.
28 Statista, 'Most Popular'.
29 Kemp, 'Digital in 2018', p. 97.
30 McNeil, 'Houston Braces'.
31 BBC Mundo, 'Cómo el virus zika'; World Health Organization, 'History of Zika Virus'.
32 LaMotte and Goldschmidt, 'CDC Considers'.
33 Upton, 'Scientists Tease out'; Allen, 'Miami Steps Up'.

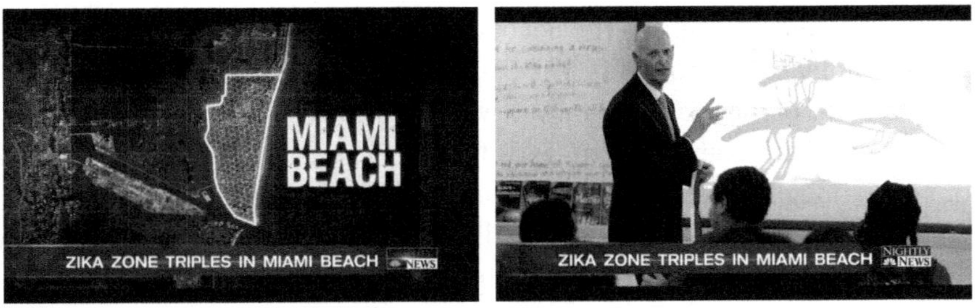

11.1. Two stills from 'Zika Zone Triples in Miami Beach', *NBC Nightly News* with Lester Holt, 17 September 2016.

aerial spraying by airplanes,[34] microscopic images of the virus (including computer-generated imagery), and doctors in white coats.[35] A televised segment on NBC News in the United States (29 September 2016) demonstrates the montage techniques historically associated with news reportage of contagion outbreaks.[36] This brief, 90-second news segment combines visual images of workers spraying insecticide, maps of transmission zones, close-ups of mosquitoes, Zika testing in laboratories, aerial spraying from airplanes, and anti-insecticide protesters at a city commissioner's meeting, all rapidly edited together, accompanied by a newscaster voice-over. This montage of iconography familiar from past outbreak narratives highlights the extent to which public perceptions of risks from emerging infectious diseases develop according to well-established rhetorical tropes.

New iconography emerging from Zika virus representations include high-tech medical imaging of infants and foetuses in utero through computed tomography (CT) scans and sonograms,[37] photographs of newborn babies with microcephaly,[38] and images of people in affected areas staring intently at smartphone screens,[39] their primary source of up-to-date information about the outbreak and risk mediation. The consistency of contagion media over time demonstrates the resilience—or inertia—of official medical media techniques for public communication about disease outbreaks. The militarized 'attack on disease' imagery of the airplanes spraying, the medicalization of the mosquito sprayers, the othering of brown faces, the pathologization of victims, and the world maps using arrows to place blame all resonate with

34 Belluck, 'Patch of Miami'; Staletovich, 'Air Attack'.
35 McNeil, 'How the Response'.
36 Holt, 'Zika Zone Triples'.
37 Dana, 'Zika Virus Takes'; McNeil, 'Zika Cases'; McNeil, 'How the Response'.
38 Worth and Osborn, 'How Brazilians Use'; World Health Organization, 'History of Zika Virus'; Firger, 'New Evidence'.
39 Worth and Osborn, 'How Brazilians Use'.

outbreak media dating to the Second World War and earlier.[40] All of this iconography can be found in *The Eternal Fight*, and in many other public-health films of the post-war era. Yet, when contrasted with the images newly associated with contagion imagery, featuring smartphones and advanced medical imaging technology, we see a conversion of the human, embodied, and social experience of disease into digital formats, rendering a clinical form of health datafication. In addition, the inclusion of footage from protesters points to a new form of contagion iconography that draws from emergent practices of dataveillance. As I will demonstrate below, the intersection of entrenched imagery with new counter-narratives has become a serious liability for health communications efforts in the age of health datafication.

From Surveillance to Dataveillance

As the practices of global public health become increasingly intermediated with techniques of health datafication, some scholars have argued that the concept of 'surveillance', a fundamental principle of epidemiology, should be reframed as 'dataveillance'. This approach is proposed to better capture how distributed networks of digital sensors and other tracking tools interface with algorithms designed to predict future behaviours and patterns. As Ruckenstein and Schüll have argued, the concept of 'surveillance' can be understood as 'too optically freighted and centrally organized a phenomenon to adequately characterize the networked, continuous tracking of digital information processing and algorithmic analysis' in contemporary practices of dataveillance.[41] That is, surveillance implies visual observation from above, as exemplified by the legions of closed-circuit television cameras conducting surveillance on the citizens of Beijing, London, and many other world cities.[42] In contrast, dataveillance emerges from diverse sources, and the resulting information is distributed to multiple interested parties, as in the 'Social Credit System' under development in China that draws from social media, financial records, gaming and entertainment, and other habits.[43] In the case of health data, sources might include narrowly defined health data as well as all the incidental social, environmental, and behavioural data routinely captured by smartphones and their apps. Dataveillance

40 Ostherr, *Cinematic Prophylaxis*.
41 Ruckenstein and Schüll, 'Datafication of Health', p. 274.
42 Lewis, 'You're Being Watched'.
43 Botsman, 'Big Data Meets'; Raley, 'Dataveillance and Countervailance'.

highlights the fact that practices of datafication are always running in the background of technologically mediated life in the 21st century, scooping up the traces of users' online, mobile interactions. Importantly, the robust global data brokering economy ensures that any number of entities can observe our digital habits and exert invisible forms of algorithmic control, regardless of which entity originally captured the data.

In addition to the decentralized and distributed forms of power expressed through dataveillance, the predictive orientation of digital 'tracking' practices signal an important shift for several scholars.[44] When used by digital health companies whose apps provide personal monitoring and control of chronic disease, these patterns can be understood as the datafication of Social Determinants of Health.[45] The case for updating the concept of 'surveillance' with 'dataveillance' is compelling, particularly in light of the growing role of digital profiling in healthcare and other sectors.[46] However, it is worth noting that the aim of epidemiological surveillance has long included pattern detection and prediction in order to halt or prevent the spread of diseases, and that practice has long used both visual and non-visual technologies of surveillance.[47] That is, the critique of surveillance as overly focussed on visual monitoring to observe events as they occur does not fully account for the more precise definition of disease surveillance as practised in public-health fieldwork, where, at present, older practices of surveillance and newer techniques of dataveillance are deeply intermediated.[48]

Therefore, while the critique of surveillance may have limited use in illuminating the applied practice of disease surveillance, the concept of dataveillance is broadly useful for analysing challenges in global health communication today. For example, the concept of dataveillance describes the work of doctors in Brazil who used the decentralized, unofficial WhatsApp network to share their findings and suspicions across diverse field sites to collectively identify the Zika virus outbreak.[49] Significantly, while those doctors were already discussing Zika in August of 2015, the Pernambuco State Secretariat of Health (an epicentre of the outbreak in Brazil) did not learn of their discoveries until two months later, in mid October.[50] By using

44 Ruckenstein and Schüll, 'Datafication of Health'; McQuillan, 'Algorithmic Paranoia'; Van Dijck, 'Datafication'.

45 Mason, 'Dear Silicon Valley'.

46 Ostherr, 'Risk Media in Medicine'.

47 Rothman et al., *Modern Epidemiology*.

48 Propeller Health, 'Outcomes'.

49 Worth and Osborn, 'How Brazilians Use'.

50 Worth and Osborn, 'How Brazilians Use'.

a service like WhatsApp, with no gatekeeper and no search function, these new, distributed forms of knowledge creation and dissemination circumvent the official, top-down, centralized command-and-control channels of health communication of the past. They are impossible to monitor, and therefore, whether intentionally or accidentally, they create alternate forms of sociality that challenge the authority of traditional forms of medical media expertise.

Moreover, because WhatsApp is used by 87 per cent of doctors in Brazil, and a similar messaging service—WeChat—is used by 50 per cent of doctors in China to communicate with their patients, the disruptive potential of this new form of health communication is significant.[51] In an effort to push back against their declining authority, the Pernambuco and Recife health departments in Brazil, two of the critical sites in the Zika outbreak, started using WhatsApp networks to send out their official messaging, consisting of traditional public-health posters with awareness and prevention information.[52] Apart from the novel use of social-media distribution networks, this strategy is otherwise consistent with centralized, top-down health media techniques dating back to the Second World War era that used posters featuring giant images of vectors like mosquitoes, with cartoon imagery instructing recipients how to behave in the face of the emerging epidemic.[53] The use of social media to distribute one-way messaging demonstrates the health departments' limited acknowledgement of the shifting paradigms of health communication in the digital age. Use of the new platform may have aided in expanding the scope of the audience, yet the monologic communication strategy of health posters suggests that the 'social' part of the novel approach was underutilized.

Some participants in the Quantified Self and e-patient movements seek to transform the processes of dataveillance and health datafication into a process of health 'data-making' that generates value for the individuals whose bodies generate the data, rather than solely for the corporations who manufacture those devices or provide formal healthcare services to those bodies.[54] It is unclear how fully citizens might resist dataveillance under current regimes of corporate and state power that monopolize data-mining practices worldwide. However, several examples emerged at the opposite end of the official health communications spectrum, when WhatsApp Zika virus support groups for mothers of babies with microcephaly emerged

51 Wieczner, 'Why WhatsApp'.
52 Worth and Osborn, 'How Brazilians Use'.
53 Ostherr, *Cinematic Prophylaxis*.
54 Pybus et al., 'Hacking the Social Life'.

across Brazil. Participants in one group created by a mother of two older children with non-Zika related microcephaly described the range of peer-to-peer healthcare practices as including emotional support and suggestions for developmentally appropriate toys and exercises for affected babies.[55] Another group formed among mothers who met in a clinic waiting room. They called themselves 'Super Mães Especiais', or 'Super Special Moms'. Researchers who spoke with group members noted the profound difference between the care that the clinic's medical team could provide, and the social, psychological, and logistical support that only the mothers could offer one another.[56] In Giddens's and Raley's terms, this activity could be considered as a form of 'countervailance' that contrasts with official forms of medical observation that measured and quantified but provided limited real value to the caregivers.

Clinicians who cared for the babies of the 'Super Mães Especiais' also found that the meta-clinical forms of care provided by the WhatsApp group played a critically important role in ensuring the mothers' sustained engagement in care for their children.[57] The value of peer-to-peer healthcare in this instance supports the observation of researchers who found a mismatch between the content of official medical communications about Zika virus and the information sought and provided by caregivers. In a study of a live tweetchat hosted by the Centers for Disease Control and Prevention (CDC), Glowacki et al. found that caregivers and health officials were both concerned with information about how to control the spread of Zika, yet they noted that the CDC 'did not appear to respond to concerns about consequences for newborns and pregnant women'.[58] Instead, the CDC followed the established practice of disseminating educational materials.

Official health organizations have recognized the value of communicating through social-media channels. Indeed, a recent survey found that nearly 80 per cent of responding WHO Member States used social media to share health messages with the public.[59] Yet, the approach taken usually follows the top-down model of older health communications media, thereby limiting the effectiveness of the WHO's deployment of social media. While some public-health researchers have recognized that social media plays a critically important role for patients and caregivers beyond providing health

55 BBC News, 'Mother Creates'.
56 Lovero and Cardoso, 'Super Special Moms'.
57 Lovero and Cardoso, 'Super Special Moms'.
58 Glowacki et al., 'Identifying the Public's Concerns', p. 1711.
59 World Health Organization, *Global Diffusion*, p. 127.

information during crises, most organizations have not adapted to the novel communicative norms that characterize common practice on these platforms.[60] In a study of Zika communications on Twitter, Fu et al. found that users clearly indicated their preference for health information generated by other users like them, which Pybus, Coté, and Blanke have called citizen data-making, 'rather than those of the government authorities'.[61] Glowacki et al. suggested that the CDC's failure to allow the public's interest to direct discussion in their Zika virus tweetchat may have been a deliberate tactic to redirect the conversation away from 'fear-ridden tweets'.[62] Yet, in the age of dataveillance, authoritarian control over communications during infectious disease outbreaks only fuels scepticism about health officials' trustworthiness.

As described above, in Brazil, WhatsApp functioned as a digital disease detection and epidemiological surveillance network, and as a social support network.[63] In what sense might we understand this phenomenon as citizen data-making? Would it be accurate to state that the WhatsApp participants benefitted from big data-driven redefinitions of health and disease? In this instance, does putting health measurement and quantification into the hands of ordinary users become a democratizing force that challenges traditional doctor-patient or state-citizen power and knowledge hierarchies? Alternatively, might health datafication potentially disrupt health infrastructures that citizens have come to depend on? Does it make users vulnerable to third-party exploitation? What factors might tip the scales in one direction or another?

Datafication and Disease Detection

One method for analysing the effects of datafication and dataveillance on health communications is a media industries approach that analyses financial transactions as critical components of communications infrastructures.[64] In this context, Facebook's purchase of WhatsApp for US $19 billion in October 2014 provides some relevant framing, particularly in light of the company's current use of the messaging app's data to target its

60 Lovero and Cardoso, 'Super Special Moms'.
61 Fu et al., 'How People React', p. 1700.
62 Glowacki et al., 'Identifying the Public's Concerns', p. 1711.
63 BBC News, 'Mother Creates'.
64 Parks and Starosielski, *Signal Traffic*.

advertisements better, and thereby boost profits.[65] One of the keys to this value stream is Facebook's acquisition of users' phone numbers through their WhatsApp accounts.[66] This form of corporate integration produces a deep digital intermediation effect, closing loopholes that had previously allowed users to avoid digital profiling based on their activities in social networks. WhatsApp's pre-Facebook terms and conditions promised that it would not share the user's phone number and personally identifiable information for commercial or marketing purposes without their consent. Although users can currently limit some of what Facebook does with their data, the mechanism for doing so is less than obvious and doesn't stop the data going to Facebook.[67] These practices of cross-platform data integration enable corporate and state powers with access to these data streams to derive value from doctors' networks, mothers of babies with microcephaly, and average citizens seeking health information online. One might argue that the citizens themselves still gain knowledge and, through that, a certain kind of power. But financial profit clearly benefits the corporate entity, not the citizens whose data gives life to the platform.

It is not surprising that Facebook wants to profit from the digital health market; so do Amazon, Google, Apple, Uber, and all of the other major technology companies.[68] The datafication practice of digitally profiling users through application of analytics to vast data sets of user behavioural data is the primary strategy for both user engagement and financial profit. Microsoft also has a digital health initiative relevant to the Zika case, in its emerging infectious disease dataveillance programme called 'Project Premonition'. The goal of this initiative is 'to detect pathogens before they cause outbreaks—by turning mosquitoes into devices that collect data from animals in the environment'.[69] The three core components of the project are: 'Find mosquito hotspots by drone', 'Collect mosquitoes with robots', and 'Detect pathogens by gene sequencing'. Project Premonition aims to automate and thereby scale up the efficiencies of human epidemiological surveillance by capitalizing on a wide range of new datafication, dataveillance, and automation techniques. But, at the opposite end of the technology-intensive solutionism spectrum,[70] a citizen science project in Spain called 'Mosquito Alert' has recently shown that 'citizen science

65 Covert, 'Facebook'; Lomas, 'WhatsApp'.
66 Lomas, 'WhatsApp'.
67 Haselton, 'Facebook's First Response'.
68 Finley, 'Embattled Tech Companies'.
69 Microsoft, 'Project Premonition'.
70 Morozov, *To Save Everything*.

costs less than traditional methods and provides early warning information and human–mosquito encounter probabilities of comparable quality with larger geographical coverage'.[71] Unlike the technology-driven approach represented by Project Premonition, these initiatives show the importance of considering socio-ecological dynamics affecting health outcomes. Citizen science, an approach enabled by the distributed networks of non-expert participants, here demonstrates that mosquito control hinges as much on an understanding of human beings as it does on an understanding of insects.

An app-based public-health initiative called 'Kidenga' was developed at University of Arizona in the United States with a similar goal of engaging children in citizen science vector surveillance. The website notes that the app 'uses an anonymous disease detection map inside of the app and is entirely community-based'.[72] While promoting the ideals of citizen science, the description of disease detection protocol resonates with dataveillance practices:

> Once a week, the Kidenga app will ask you to report whether you are healthy or sick, and mosquito activity near your home. Then visit the app to see other user reports in your area, get the latest news on Zika, dengue, and chikungunya, and learn how to protect yourself, your family, and your community from diseases spread by mosquitoes. Users in Arizona, Texas, and Florida will be able to check which counties in their states have people with Zika.[73]

While Kidenga and Mosquito Alert both use locative technologies to collect their data through mobile media platforms, they reassure participants that their data will be anonymous. However, in light of the widespread digital profiling practices enacted by Facebook and facilitated by WhatsApp data, it is reasonable to question whether the citizens engaged in these efforts are fully aware of the different types of dataveillance they may be enacting, including upon themselves.[74] Moreover, computer scientist Latanya Sweeney's research group has shown that most mobile apps share data with third parties without users' awareness.[75] Sweeney has also shown that true anonymization of data is virtually impossible.[76] Therefore, even

71 Palmer et al., 'Citizen Science', p. 3.
72 Kidenga Team, 'Download the Kidenga App'.
73 Kidenga Team, 'Download the Kidenga App'.
74 Ostherr, 'Facebook Knows a Ton'.
75 Zang et al., 'Who Knows What?'
76 Sweeney, 'Only You'.

if Kidenga disease surveillance activities only intend to provide benefits to public health, the project's use of dataveillance techniques potentially puts citizen scientists' data at risk. As this example shows, while citizen science offers a counter-narrative to technological solutionism, these practices are commonly enmeshed in the very practices of datafication they have been created to challenge. Other kinds of digitally intermediated narratives have also emerged from Zika media, particularly in reaction to public concerns about the reach of dataveillance practices. These narratives of conspiracy form the focus of the following section.

Counter-Narratives of Contagion

Practices of dataveillance generate new types of health data that expand beyond many of the infrastructures and actors traditionally involved in healthcare and health decision-making, opening up the possibility for large-scale counter-narratives to circulate in the same domain as official health communications. Data and practices of datafication have become sites of contestation between government and corporate health agencies and individual citizens. In this context, the use of mobile apps as tools for data collection and research can raise concerns over citizen scientists becoming tools of dataveillance. At the same time, practices of self-quantification may be seen as providing new opportunities for self-care or even self-governance that traditional infrastructures do not provide. The tensions between these models of dataveillance and citizen data-making are evidenced by the hundreds of people protesting in Puerto Rico in July of 2016, after the Centers for Disease Control and Prevention endorsed aerial spraying of the insecticide Naled, which is toxic to bees, birds, and fish.[77] In this instance, the official narrative that health organizations must spray insecticide to protect the human population was countered by an ecological narrative that linked harms to the environment to harms to human health.

Among publics already accustomed to social-media networks as primary sources of information, epidemiology narratives that include sources, vectors, and patterns of distribution are easily appropriated for alternative purposes. Algorithmic digital profiling creates filter bubbles and feedback loops that reinforce the plausibility of such counter-narratives.[78] A narrative of epidemiology in the context of health datafication thereby easily becomes

77 McNeil, 'Zika Cases'.

78 Pariser, *Filter Bubble.*

a narrative of conspiracy, and research has shown that the conspiracy narratives get more 'likes'.[79] A group of researchers collected data for one week in June 2016 to determine the most popular videos posted on Facebook related to Zika virus. The researchers classified all videos as either 'relevant' or 'misleading' information or news.[80] While number of likes or views is an imprecise measure of the impact of the media and the substance of the engagement, the results nonetheless highlight a significant asymmetry of exposure that is consistent with other findings on health communication through social media.[81]

The most popular relevant information post, a World Health Organization press conference by the Emergency Committee on Zika virus, had 43,000 total views.[82] The full title of the film is *WHO-BROLL—14 June 2016: Press Conference after the 3rd Meeting of Emergency Committee on Zika and Observed Increase in Neurological Disorders and Neonatal Malformations*. The main presenters, apart from members of the press who appear only briefly on the sidelines of the shot and staffers who are occasionally glimpsed, are Dr. David Heymann, Chair of the Emergency Committee on Zika and Dr. Bruce Aylward, Executive Director ad interim of the Outbreaks and Health Emergencies cluster. The film duration is listed at almost 50 minutes, and the cinematography consists of a single-camera, uncut recording of the two WHO officials presenting the findings of their committee and responding to questions. The film was not edited in post-production and used no music or other special effects, resulting in a dry, scientific, factual presentation of the known facts regarding Zika virus. In contrast to the resources demonstrably invested in *The Eternal Fight* almost 70 years earlier, the WHO press conference was not staged as a carefully created piece of persuasive media, but rather as a minimalist, emergency communication in response to a global health crisis. The earlier film engaged viewers through images and sounds created by prominent European animation studios, coupled with a narrative built on persuasion, not facts. In contrast, the WHO Zika film presented all of the available scientific evidence, but little by way of persuasion.

The most popular misleading post, a conspiracy film called *10 Shocking Reasons Why Zika Virus Fear Is another Fraudulent Medical Hoax and Vaccine Industry Funding Scam*, had 535,000 views.[83] The conspiracy film was only

79 Sharma et al., 'Zika Virus Pandemic'.

80 Sharma et al., 'Zika Virus Pandemic'.

81 Gyenes and Seymour, 'Public Health Echo'.

82 *WHO-BROLL*.

83 *10 Shocking Reasons*.

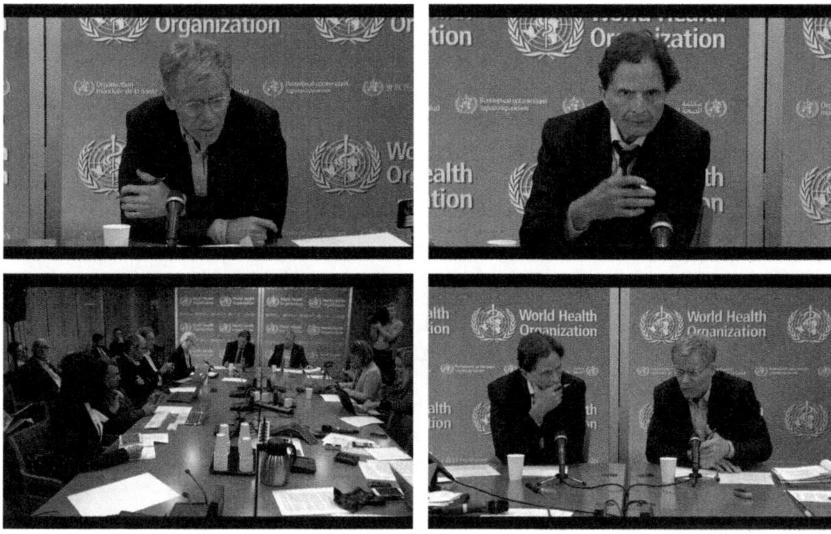

11.2. Four stills from WHO-BROLL—14 June 2016: *Press Conference after the 3rd Meeting of Emergency Committee on Zika and Observed Increase in Neurological Disorders and Neonatal Malformations*, World Health Organization, 15 June 2016.

two minutes long, and consisted of a rapidly edited montage sequence, accompanied by melodramatic music and sensationalistic intertitles presenting an argument to support the conspiracy theory in the title of the film. The tone of this film was emotional and rhetorical, not scientific and rational. Many of the iconographic images in Zika virus media (close-ups of mosquitoes, babies with microcephaly, aerial spraying from airplanes, maps) were appropriated and reinterpreted in the film to construct a counter-narrative centred on a thesis of media manipulation. The video opens with an enlarged close-up of a mosquito that fills the screen. Cutting to a montage of babies with microcephaly, the film begins its ten-point argument with the first claim, 'The microcephaly cases (shrunken heads) in Brazil were caused by larvicide chemicals, not by Zika'. The second point expands the scope of the conspiracy, stating, 'Even according to the CDC, which is aggressively pushing false Zika fear, nearly all Zika infections are harmless [...]'. Moving deeper into the argument, the next intertitle claims, 'The CDC fabricated the science linking Zika to microcephaly'. The accusations continue by blaming the US government for removing bans on toxic chemicals and funnelling funds to vaccine manufacturers. The rhetoric escalates to assert, 'Zika virus fear has been used as a weapon of control to terrorize the people of the Americas by violating their private property'. Zika is compared to the great 'bird flu hoax', and depicted as justification for spraying more of the chemicals that

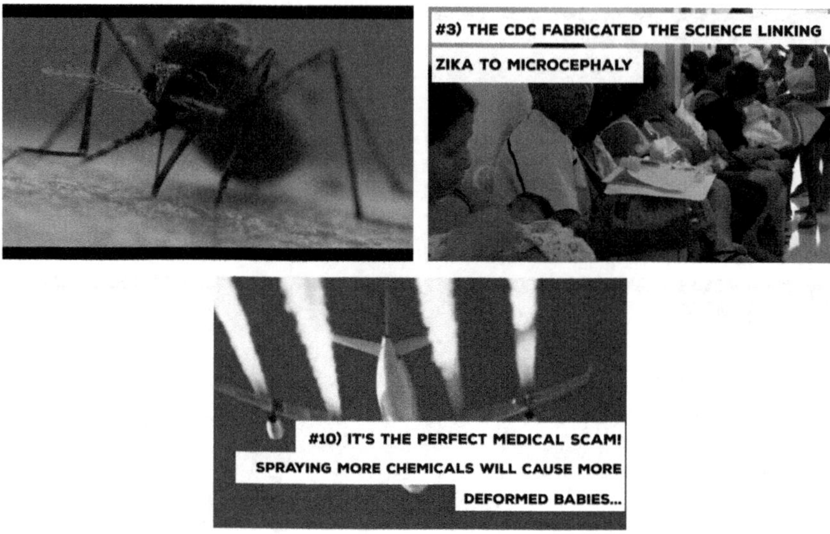

11.3. Three stills from *10 Shocking Reasons Why Zika Virus Fear Is another Fraudulent Medical Hoax and Vaccine Industry Funding Scam*, published by Brett Ryan Shaw, 6 September 2016.

the video claims caused the 'shrunken heads' in the first place. Through this rapidly paced and tightly edited montage, the film incriminates the government, the pharmaceutical industry, big agriculture, and medicine as co-conspirators who fabricate scientific evidence for monetary gain.

Comparison of the two films identified by Sharma et al.'s research revealed two contrasting sets of concerns, much as Lovero and Cardoso found in their communications with the 'Super Mães Especiais'. The core concerns of the official health communicators from the WHO were evidence-based, verifiable, and objective information from trusted, authoritative sources (such as governments and non-governmental organizations), disseminated through official channels (such as press releases, public-service announcements, and official news media). In contrast, the health conspiracy theorist was primarily concerned with presenting an emotionally charged narrative that critiqued official discourse from below, disseminated through social media. The misleading post had over ten times as many views as the relevant post. My analysis of the contrasting features of these two popular posts confirms the findings of Gyenes and Seymour, who have argued that 'distinct sub-communities form in digital public health conversations', and, among these sub-communities, public-health organizations are consistently isolated.[84] The relative unpopularity of the WHO film compared to the conspiracy

84 Gyenes and Seymour, 'Public Health Echo'.

	Epidemiology	Conspiracy theory
Sources (characters)	Mosquitoes	U.S. government/CDC/DOD; Monsanto; GMO mosquitoes; Big Pharma
Vectors (cause/effect chains)	Environmental exposure; sexual transmission	Pesticide spray; vaccine inoculation; fake blood draws
Patterns of distribution (conflicts & resolutions)	Travel to/from 'hot zones', *aedes aegypti* zones	Global capitalist cycle of exploitation & control (sell pesticide to infect, sell drug to treat)
Iconography	Close-ups of mosquitoes; health workers in space suits; aerial spraying; maps of contagion; babies with microcephaly; microscopic virus images	Close-ups of mosquitoes; health workers in space suits; aerial spraying; maps of contagion; babies with microcephaly; microscopic virus images

Table 11.1. Features of epidemiology vs. conspiracy theories of Zika virus.

film demonstrates a major challenge of health communication in the digital age: The crowded online environment surfaces sensationalistic emotional appeals more readily than carefully worded scientific statements. The widely noted 'flattening' of hierarchy online undercuts official health organizations' ability to disseminate their messages with unchallenged authority. Unlike the media environment of 1948, when the WHO presented its vision of global disease eradication in *The Eternal Fight*, the decentralized media networks of the 21st century demand more strategic forms of communication if they hope to gain viewers' attention.

Conclusion

The growing use of social networks to access news media indicates that more people are receiving information from others in their social-media networks rather than from external, official journalistic news sources.[85] While social networks can provide valuable sources of peer-to-peer healthcare, scholars have also found that information disseminated through social-media platforms can 'cultivate fear and hasten the spread of misinformation in the face of a public health threat'.[86] The concurrent rise in the popularity of social video means that the persuasive power of moving images and sound (as distinct from short- or long-form text and still images with captions alone) have the potential

85 Mitchell et al., 'How Americans'.
86 Glowacki et al., 'Identifying the Public's Concerns'.

to enact greater persuasive effects on their networks.[87] Researchers have also found that the timeliness and immediacy of social-media posts can help to curb fears during disease outbreaks, especially when the public is actively engaged and able to participate fully, not only as a receptacle for official communications.[88] In light of the need for participatory, image-based public collaboration, health organizations such as WHO and CDC must consider novel approaches to real-time, genuinely social health communications.

To demonstrate the challenge facing official health organizations, I will close with a brief discussion of a short animated public-service announcement called *Misión Zika* (2016), produced by the Cartoon Network in collaboration with the World Health Organization, the Pan American Health Organization (PAHO), and the United Nations Children's Emergency Fund (UNICEF) during the 2016 Zika outbreak. This public awareness campaign is part of the Cartoon Network's 'Movimiento Cartoon' corporate social responsibility initiative founded in 2010 to promote the well-being of children across Latin America.[89] The minute-long *Misión Zika* video was created in Portuguese to be aired in the Brazil market of the Cartoon Network Latin America, where it would reach child viewers. A rapidly edited montage of colourful cartoon superheroes from other programmes on the network such as *Powerpuff Girls* and *Ben 10*, the video is framed as a mission briefing that addresses the viewing audience as superheroes in the fight against a supervillain: the mosquito that transmits Zika virus. Purpose-designed visuals of typical mosquito breeding sites such as old tires, flower pots, garbage bins, and water bowls for pets are integrated with shots of the mission director in a high-tech animated environment. Information about how to avoid mosquito bites by wearing long-sleeved shirts and insect repellant also appears on screens in the command centre.

Much like traditional WHO health education films such as *The Eternal Fight* (1948), *Misión Zika* transmits instructions from a centralized authority, conveying the expectation that viewers will receive, assimilate, and perform the assigned behaviours. The commander's first appearance on-screen emerges through static as an interruption of regular programming, much like an emergency broadcast. To underscore the urgency of the message, the commander opens by imploring in direct address: 'Calling all superheroes, calling all superheroes! This is not a drill.' He goes on to explain, 'Our communities were invaded by extremely dangerous mosquitoes. We need all

87 McCue, 'Top 10'.

88 Glowacki et al., 'Identifying the Public's Concerns', p. 1709; see also Fu et al., 'How People React'.

89 Restrepo, 'Cartoon Movement'.

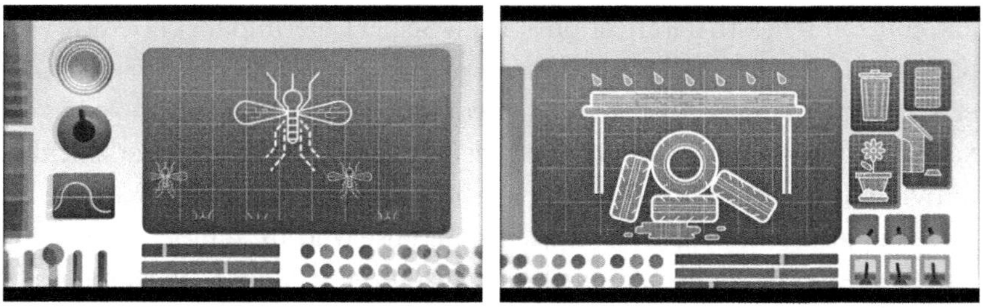

11.4. Two stills from Misi6n Zika, Cartoon Network/WHO/PAHO/UNICEF, 2016.

the help we can get'. Coupled with visualizations of the command centre as a high-tech room full of screens and control panels, this public-service announcement embraces the surveillance model of health communication. The commander watches the viewers and the mosquitoes, issuing authoritative orders from a centralized locus of information and power.

Though stylistically distinct, *The Eternal Fight* also used animation to visualize the global spread of contagion and other processes whose scale would otherwise be impossible to represent with conventional photographic film. While the cartoon format in the post-war era and today aims to address the target audience in a style and format consistent with their preferences, this approach is not open to substantive community engagement. The central authority figure issues a command, and viewers may respond through action or inaction, but, in either case, no feedback loop exists to enable direct response to the health communication. In other examples of health dataveillance discussed in this chapter, we can see that new forms of value and power emerge from data-driven practices of monitoring and control. Unlike the distributed mechanisms of dataveillance and the resistant response of citizen data-making, *Misión Zika* offers an aesthetic update to an otherwise thoroughly outdated model of asynchronous, top-down, remote transmission of expert messaging to a presumably passive viewing audience. The surface appearance has changed, but the core approach remains the same as it was when the WHO was first introduced to the world by *The Eternal Fight* in 1948.

While the emergent phenomena of datafication, dataveillance, and data-making raise new computational challenges, they do not eliminate the need for human-centred practices of interpretation and communication, particularly in the context of emerging infectious diseases and other challenges facing global health. If researchers begin to engage concepts like datafication and dataveillance as core elements of a new form of health communication, how then must we change the ways we think about the role of technologies like smartphones and apps in the context of disease communication, monitoring, and control? If health datafication is a new Social Determinant of Health, will participation in dataveillance become a predictor of health outcomes? In this emerging mediascape, distributed networks of dataveillance technologies do not necessarily equate to distributed access to power. Perhaps paradoxically, individuals and communities that are not subject to dataveillance may be more vulnerable to health disparities than those who are subject to dataveillance. In response to the manifestly uneven power relations that characterize global digital health economies, counter-narratives migrate online, fuelled by data-driven algorithms and visual iconography that foster suspicion towards official health narratives. While corporate and state techno-paternalism may succeed at data extraction, these systems fail at social engagement, leaving official health organizations to grapple with a distributed communication ecosystem (internet and mobile apps) driven by forces largely invisible to their participants. Meaningful public engagement in health communication will therefore require transparency regarding datafication and dataveillance, coupled with genuine opportunities for citizens to participate in active data-making in response to global health threats to their communities.

Works Cited

Films, Television Programmes, and Recordings

10 Shocking Reasons Why Zika Virus Fear Is another Fraudulent Medical Hoax and Vaccine Industry Funding Scam, published by Brett Ryan Shaw, 6 September 2016, https://www.youtube.com/watch?v=cHfLcEddkHI, accessed on 17 August 2018.

The Eternal Fight, photographed and directed by Victor Vicas, United Nations Film Board/Madeline Carroll Films, 1948.

Misión Zika, Cartoon Network/WHO/PAHO/UNICEF, 2016.

WHO-BROLL—14 June 2016: Press Conference after the 3rd Meeting of Emergency Committee on Zika and Observed Increase in Neurological Disorders and Neonatal Malformations, by World Health Organization, 15 June 2016, https://www.youtube.com/watch?v=USgp2fNQwR4, accessed on 17 August 2018.

Books and Articles

Ackoff, Russell L., 'From Data to Wisdom', *Journal of Applied Systems Analysis*, 16, 1 (1989), pp. 3–9.

Allen, Greg, 'Miami Steps up Mosquito Control Efforts after Suspected Zika Cases', *National Public Radio*, 22 July 2016, https://www.npr.org/sections/

health-shots/2016/07/22/487078904/miami-steps-up-mosquito-control-efforts-after-suspected-zika-cases, accessed 16 August 2018.

Baudrillard, Jean, *Simulacra and Simulation*, trans. by Sheila Faria Glaser (Ann Arbor: University of Michigan Press, 1994).

BBC Mundo, 'Cómo el virus zika se volvió tan peligroso cuando llegó a América Latina', 27 January 2016, https://www.bbc.com/mundo/noticias/2016/01/160126_zika_virus_mutacion_america_africa_asia_men, accessed on 16 August 2018.

BBC News, 'Mother Creates WhatsApp Zika Virus Support Group', 27 January 2016, https://www.bbc.com/news/world-latin-america-35414506, accessed 16 August 2018.

Belluck, Pam, 'Patch of Miami Is Ground Zero for the Zika Virus', *The New York Times*, 8 August 2016, https://www.nytimes.com/2016/08/09/health/zika-virus-florida.html, accessed 16 August 2018.

Botsman, Rachel, 'Big Data Meets Big Brother as China Moves to Rate its Citizens', *Wired*, 21 October 2017, https://www.wired.co.uk/article/chinese-government-social-credit-score-privacy-invasion, accessed 16 August 2018.

boyd, danah, and Kate Crawford, 'Critical Questions for Big Data: Provocation for a Cultural, Technological, and Scholarly Phenomen', *Information, Communication & Society*, 15, 5 (2012), pp. 662–679, doi:10.1080/1369118X.2012.678878.

Brown, Theodore M., Marcos Cueto, and Elizabeth Fee, 'The World Health Organization and the Transition from International to Global Public Health', *American Journal of Public Health*, 96, 1 (2006), pp. 62–72, doi:10.2105/AJPH.2004.050831.

Bouk, Dan, 'The History and Political Economy of Personal Data over the Last Two Centuries in Three Acts', *Osiris*, 32, 1 (2017), pp. 85–106.

Carter, Jamie, 'Why Wearables Have Become Such a Big Deal in Asia', *Wareable*, 12 May 2017, https://www.wareable.com/wearable-tech/wearables-becoming-huge-in-asia-544, accessed 15 August 2018.

Covert, Adrian, 'Facebook Buys WhatsApp for $19 Billion', *CNN Tech*, 19 February 2014, https://money.cnn.com/2014/02/19/technology/social/facebook-whatsapp/index.html, accessed 16 August 2018.

Dahlgren, Göran, and Margaret Whitehead, *Policies and Strategies to Promote Social Equity in Health: Background Document to WHO-Strategy Paper for Europe* (Stockholm: Institute for Futures Studies, 1991).

Dana, Felipe, 'Zika Virus Takes Heartbreaking Toll', *CBS News*, 28 January 2016, https://www.cbsnews.com/pictures/zika-virus-brazil-heartbreaking-toll/25/, accessed 16 August 2018.

Finley, Klint, 'Embattled Tech Companies Charge Deeper into Health Care', *Wired*, 1 March 2018, https://www.wired.com/story/embattled-tech-companies-charge-deeper-into-health-care/, accessed 16 August 2018.

Firger, Jessica, 'New Evidence Supports Zika-Microcephaly Connection', *Newsweek*, 19 February 2016, https://www.newsweek.com/

new-evidence-supports-zika-microcephaly-connection-428736, accessed 16 August 2018.

Fu, King-Wa, Hai Liang, Nitin Saroha, Zion Tsz Ho Tse, Patrick Ip, and Isaac Chun-Hai Fung, 'How People React to Zika Virus Outbreaks on Twitter? A Computational Content Analysis', *American Journal of Infection Control*, 44 (2016), 1700-1702, doi:10.1016/j.ajic.2016.04.253.

Giddens, Anthony, *The Nation-State and Violence: Volume 2 of A Contemporary Critique of Historical Materialism* (Berkeley: University of California Press, 1985).

Glowacki, Elizabeth M., Allison J. Lazard, Gary B. Wilcox, Michael Mackert, and Jay M. Bernhardt, 'Identifying the Public's Concerns and the Centers for Disease Control and Prevention's Reactions during a Health Crisis: An Analysis of a Zika Live Twitter Chat', *American Journal of Infection Control*, 44, 12 (2016), 1709–1711, doi:10.1016/j.ajic.2016.05.025.

Gyenes, Natalie, and Brittany Seymour, 'Public Health Echo Chambers in a Time of Mistrust and Misinformation: Digital Health @ Harvard, February 2017', presentation at Berkman Klein Center for Internet and Society at Harvard University, Cambridge, MA, 23 February 2017, https://cyber.harvard.edu/events/digitalhealth/2017/02/GyenesSeymour, accessed 17 August 2018.

Haselton, Todd, 'Facebook's First Response to Its Data Leak Scandal Ignores Two of Its Big Products: Instagram and WhatsApp', *CNBC*, 28 March 2018, https://www.cnbc.com/2018/03/28/facebook-new-privacy-settings-dont-address-instagram-whatsapp.html, accessed on 16 August 2018.

Holt, Lester, 'Zika Zone Triples in Miami Beach', *NBC Nightly News with Lester Holt*, 17 September 2016, https://www.nbcnews.com/nightly-news/video/zika-transmission-zones-expand-in-miami-beach-767607875611, accessed 16 August 2018.

International Data Corporation, 'Global Wearables Market Grows 7.7% in 4Q17 and 10.3% in 2017 as Apple Seizes the Leader Position, Says IDC', *IDC*, 1 March 2018, https://www.idc.com/getdoc.jsp?containerId=prUS43598218, accessed on 15 August 2018.

Kemp, Simon, 'Digital in 2018: World's Internet Users Pass the 4 Billion Mark', *We Are Social*, 30 January 2018, https://wearesocial.com/blog/2018/01/global-digital-report-2018, accessed 15 August 2018.

Kennedy, Helen, Thomas Poell, and Jose van Dijck, 'Data and Agency', *Big Data and Society* 2, 2 (2015), pp. 1–7, doi:10.1177/2053951715621569.

Kidenga Team, University of Arizona, The Mel & Enid Zuckerman College of Public Health, 'Download the Kidenga App!', 2018, https://kidenga.org/, accessed 17 August 2018.

Krumm, John, Nigel Davies, and Chandra Narayanaswami, 'User-Generated Content', *IEEE Pervasive Computing*, 7, 4 (2008), pp. 10–11, doi:10.1109/MPRV.2008.85.

LaMotte, Sandee, and Debra Goldschmidt, 'CDC Considers Travel Warning for Pregnant Women due to Zika Virus', *CNN*, 15 January 2016, https://edition.cnn.

com/2016/01/14/health/zika-pandemic-travel-warnings/index.html, accessed 16 August 2018.

Leaf, Clifton, 'The Biggest Share in the Sharing Economy', *Fortune*, 7 August 2015, https://fortune.com/2015/08/07/digital-health-data/, accessed 16 August 2018.

Lewis, Paul, 'You're Being Watched: There's One CCTV Camera for Every 32 People in UK', *The Guardian*, 2 March 2011, https://www.theguardian.com/uk/2011/mar/02/cctv-cameras-watching-surveillance, accessed on 16 August 2018.

Lomas, Natasha, 'WhatsApp to Share User Data with Facebook for Ad Targeting—Here's How to Opt Out', *TechCrunch*, 25 August 2016, https://techcrunch.com/2016/08/25/whatsapp-to-share-user-data-with-facebook-for-ad-targeting-heres-how-to-opt-out/, accessed 16 August 2018.

Lovero, Kathryn, and Claudete Araújo Cardoso, '"Super Special Moms": Grassroots, Social Media Support Group Aids the Response to Congenital Zika Syndrome', *Lancet Global Health Blog*, 14 November 2017, https://globalhealth.thelancet.com/2017/11/14/super-special-moms-grassroots-social-media-support-group-aids-response-congenital-zika, accessed 16 August 2018.

Lupton, Deborah, *The Quantified Self: A Sociology of Self-Tracking* (Cambridge: Polity, 2016).

Mason, Vanessa, 'Dear Silicon Valley, It Pays To Care about Public Health', *Fast Company,* 3 March 2017, https://www.fastcompany.com/3068726/dear-silicon-valley-it-pays-to-care-about-public-health, accessed 16 August 2018.

Mayer-Schönberger, Viktor, and Kenneth Cukier, *Big Data: A Revolution that Will Transform How We Live, Work, and Think* (London: Murray, 2013).

McCue, T. J., 'Top 10 Video Marketing Trends And Statistics Roundup 2017', *Forbes*, 22 September 2017, https://www.forbes.com/sites/tjmccue/2017/09/22/top-10-video-marketing-trends-and-statistics-roundup-2017/#76dc51897103, accessed 20 August 2018.

McNeil, Jr., Donald G., 'Houston Braces for Another Brush with the Peril of Zika', *The New York Times*, 17 July 2017, https://www.nytimes.com/2017/07/17/health/zika-virus-houston-texas.html, accessed on 16 August 2018.

McNeil, Jr., Donald G., 'How the Response to Zika Failed Millions', *The New York Times,* 16 January 2017, https://www.nytimes.com/2017/01/16/health/zika-virus-response.html?action=click&contentCollection=health&module=NextInCollection&region=Footer&pgtype=article&version=newsevent&rref=collection%2Fnews-event%2Fzika-virus, accessed 16 August 2018.

McNeil, Jr., Donald G., 'Zika Cases in Puerto Rico Are Skyrocketing', *The New York Times,* 30 July 2016, https://www.nytimes.com/2016/07/31/health/zika-virus-puerto-rico.html, accessed 16 August 2018.

McQuillan, Dan, 'Algorithmic Paranoia and the Convivial Alternative', *Big Data & Society,* 3, 2 (2016), pp. 1–12, doi:10.1177/2053951716671340.

Microsoft, 'Project Premonition Aims to Detect Pathogens before they Cause Outbreaks', *Microsoft*, 2 March 2015, https://www.microsoft.com/en-us/research/project/project-premonition/, accessed 16 August 2018.

Mitchell, Amy, Jeffrey Gottfried, Elisa Shearer, and Kristine Lu, 'How Americans Encounter, Recall and Act Upon Digital News', *Pew Research Center*, 9 February 2017, https://www.journalism.org/2017/02/09/how-americans-encounter-recall-and-act-upon-digital-news, accessed 20 August 2018.

Morozov, Evgeny, *To Save Everything, Click Here: The Folly of Technological Solutionism* (New York: Public Affairs, 2014.)

Neff, Gina, and Dawn Nafus, *Self-Tracking* (Cambridge: MIT Press, 2016).

Ostherr, Kirsten, *Cinematic Prophylaxis: Globalization and Contagion in the Discourse of World Health* (Durham, NC: Duke University Press, 2005).

Ostherr, Kirsten, 'Facebook Knows a Ton about Your Health: Now They Want to Make Money Off It', *Washington Post*, 18 April 2018, https://www.washingtonpost.com/news/posteverything/wp/2018/04/18/facebook-knows-a-ton-about-your-health-now-they-want-to-make-money-off-it/?utm_term=.254914a0b9bd, accessed on 15 August 2018.

Ostherr, Kirsten, 'Privacy, Data Mining, and Digital Profiling in Online Patient Narratives', *Catalyst: Feminism, Theory, Technoscience*, 4, 1 (2018), doi:10.28968/cftt.v4i1.288.

Ostherr, Kirsten, 'Risk Media in Medicine: The Rise of the Metaclinical Health App Ecosystem', in *The Routledge Companion to Media and Risk*, ed. by Bishnupriya Ghosh and Bhaskar Sarkar (New York: Routledge, in press).

Ostherr, Kirsten, Svetlana Borodina, Rachel Conrad Bracken, Charles Lotterman, Eliot Storer, and Brandon Williams, 'Trust and Privacy in the Context of User-Generated Health Data', *Big Data & Society*, 4, 1 (2017), pp. 1–11, doi:10.1177/2053951717704673.

Palmer, John R.B., Aitana Oltra, Francisco Collantes, Juan Antonio Delgado, Javier Lucientes, Sarah Delacour, Mikel Bengoa, Roger Eritja, and Frederic Bartumeus, 'Citizen Science Provides a Reliable and Scalable Tool to Track Disease-Carrying Mosquitoes', *Nature Communications*, 8, 916 (2017), pp. 1–13, doi:10.1038/s41467-017-00914-9.

Pariser, Eli, *The Filter Bubble: What the Internet is Hiding from You* (New York: Penguin, 2011).

Parks, Lisa, and Nicole Starosielski, eds., *Signal Traffic: Critical Studies of Media Infrastructures* (Urbana: University of Illinois Press, 2015).

Propeller Health, 'Outcomes', *Propeller Health*, no date, https://www.propellerhealth.com/outcome, accessed 16 August 2018.

Pybus, Jennifer, Mark Coté, and Tobias Blanke, 'Hacking the Social Life of Big Data', *Big Data & Society*, 2, 2 (2015), pp. 1–10, doi:10.1177/2053951715616649.

Raley, Rita, 'Dataveillance and Countervailance', in *'Raw Data' Is an Oxymoron*, ed. by Lisa Gitelman (Cambridge, MA: MIT Press, 2013), pp. 121–145.

Restrepo, Luis Felipe, 'The Cartoon Movement', Presentation at the Global Child Forum on South America, São Paolo, Brazil, 27 April 2017.

Rothman, Kenneth J., Sander Greenland, and Timothy L. Lash, *Modern Epidemiology*, 3rd ed. (Philadelphia: Lippincott Williams and Wilkins, 2008).

Ruckenstein, Minna, and Natasha Dow Schüll, 'The Datafication of Health', *Annual Review of Anthropology*, 46, 1 (2017), pp. 261–278, doi:10.1146/annurev-anthro-102116-041244.

Sharma, Megha, Kapil Yadav, Nitika Yadav, and Keith C. Ferdinand, 'Zika Virus Pandemic: Analysis of Facebook as a Social Media Health Information Platform', *American Journal of Infection Control*, 45, 3 (March 2017), pp. 301–302, doi:10.1016/j.ajic.2016.08.022.

Shtulman, Andrew, 'In Public Understanding of Science, Alternative Facts Are the Norm', *National Public Radio*, 29 May 2017, https://www.npr.org/sections/13.7/2017/05/29/527892222/in-public-understanding-of-science-alternative-facts-are-the-norm, accessed 16 August 2018.

Staletovich, Jenny, 'Air Attack against Zika Hit and Miss in Miami, CDC reports', *Miami Herald*, 16 August 2016, https://www.miamiherald.com/news/health-care/article95838697.html, accessed 16 August 2018.

Statista, 'Most Popular Social Networks Worldwide as of April 2018, Ranked by Number of Active Users (in Millions)', *Statista*, April 2018, https://www.statista.com/statistics/272014/global-social-networks-ranked-by-number-of-users, accessed on May 1, 2018.

Strasser, Bruno J., and Paul N. Edwards, 'Big Data Is the Answer ... But What Is the Question?', *Osiris*, 32, 1 (2017), pp. 328–345.

Sweeney, Latanya, 'Only You, Your Doctor, and Many Others May Know', *Technology Science*, 29 September 2015, https://techscience.org/a/2015092903, accessed 17 August 2018.

Upton, John, 'Scientists Tease out Climate Change's Role in Zika Spread', *Climate Central*, 4 August 2016, https://www.climatecentral.org/news/scientists-tease-out-climate-role-zika-spread-20582, accessed 16 August 2018.

van Dijck, José, 'Datafication, Dataism and Dataveillance: Big Data between Scientific Paradigm and Ideology', *Surveillance and Society*, 12, 2 (2014), pp. 197–208.

van Dijck, José, 'Users Like You? Theorizing Agency in User-Generated Content', *Media, Culture & Society*, 31, 1 (2009), pp. 41–58, doi:10.1177/0163443708098245.

Wallis, Lee, Paul Blessing, Mohammed Dalwai, and Sang Do Shin, 'Integrating mHealth at Point of Care in Low- and Middle-Income Settings: The System Perspective', *Global Health Action*, 10, supplement 3 (2017), doi:10.1080/16549716.2017.1327686.

Wieczner, Jen, 'Why WhatsApp Could Be a Game-Changer for American Health Care', *Fortune*, 25 August 2016, https://fortune.com/2016/08/25/whatsapp-encryption-doctors-healthcare-hipaa/, accessed 16 August 2018.

World Health Organization, *Global Diffusion of eHealth: Making Universal Health Coverage Achievable: Report of the Third Global Survey on eHealth* (Geneva: World Health Organization, 2016), https://apps.who.int/iris/bitstream/handle/10665/252529/9789241511780-eng.pdf;jsessionid=BEAC2CC3CB708BF392A2159F4C6D9300?sequence=1, accessed 15 August 2018.

World Health Organization, 'The History of Zika Virus', no date, https://www.who.int/emergencies/zika-virus/timeline/en/, accessed 16 August 2018.

World Health Organization, *Social Determinants of Health Unit?*, no date, https://www.who.int/social_determinants/SDH-Brochure-May2017.pdf?ua=1, accessed 16 August 2018.

Worth, Katie, and Catherine Osborn, 'How Brazilians Use WhatsApp to Connect on Zika', *PBS Frontline*, 23 February 2016, https://www.pbs.org/wgbh/frontline/article/how-brazilians-use-whatsapp-to-connect-on-zika/, accessed 16 August 2018.

Zang, Jinyan, Krysta Dummit, James Graves, Paul Lisker, and Latanya Sweeney, 'Who Knows What About Me? A Survey of Behind the Scenes Personal Data Sharing to Third Parties by Mobile Apps', *Technology Science*, 30 October 2015, https://techscience.org/a/2015103001, accessed 17 August 2018.

Zuboff, Shoshana, 'Big Other: Surveillance Capitalism and the Prospects of an Information Civilization', *Journal of Information Technology*, 30, 1 (2015), pp. 75–89, doi:10.1057/jit.2015.5.

About the Author

Kirsten Ostherr, PhD, MPH is the Gladys Louise Fox Professor of English at Rice University in Houston, Texas. She is the author of *Medical Visions: Producing the Patient through Film, Television and Imaging Technologies* (Oxford, 2013) and *Cinematic Prophylaxis: Globalization and Contagion in the Discourse of World Health* (Duke, 2005).

Index

General Index

Index of Persons

Index of Works

Index of Places

For Product Safety Concerns and Information please contact our EU representative GPSR@taylorandfrancis.com Taylor & Francis Verlag GmbH, Kaufingerstraße 24, 80331 München, Germany

Batch number: 10725973

Printed by Printforce, the Netherlands